EAT TO
SUCCEED

THE HAAS
MAXIMUM
PERFORMANCE
PROGRAM

Other books by Dr. Robert Haas

Eat to Win

EAT TO SUCCEED

THE HAAS MAXIMUM PERFORMANCE PROGRAM

DR. ROBERT HAAS

Recipes by Hilarie Porter, M.S.

RAWSON ASSOCIATES
New York

Library of Congress Cataloging-in-Publication Data
Haas, Robert, 1948–
    Eat to succeed.

    Bibliography: p. 313
    Includes index.
    1. Nutrition.   2. Physical fitness—Nutritional
aspects.   3. Health.   I. Porter, Hilarie.   II. Title.
RA784.H33   1986   613.2'6   85-42856
ISBN 0-89256-293-5

All rights reserved
Published simultaneously in Canada by Collier Macmillan Canada, Inc.
Packaged by Rapid Transcript, a division of March Tenth, Inc.
Composition by Folio Graphics Co., Inc.
Manufactured by Fairfield Graphics, Fairfield, Pennsylvania
Designed by Jacques Chazaud

First Edition

To my parents
and Hilarie

Contents

vii

SECTION II: THE *EAT TO SUCCEED* RECIPE BOOK

SECTION III: THE *EAT TO SUCCEED* FOOD COMPOSITION TABLES

APPENDIXES

Acknowledgments

I gratefully acknowledge the help and assistance in the creation of this book from the following people and organizations:

Hilarie Porter, M.S., for her outstanding performance in the creation, preparation, and testing of each *Eat to Succeed* recipe, and for her general assistance in all the facets of my work;

Steve Diamond, for his extraordinary computer programming, data base management, and analyses of the *Eat to Succeed* recipes;

Cher, for letting me turn her guest room into a computer center and her kitchen into a laboratory;

Kennett and Eleanor Rawson, for their excellent suggestions, editorial criticisms, and encouragement during the writing of this book;

Connie Clausen, for her professional guidance and friendship;

Steve Blechman, for supplying nutritional research data;

American, Eastern, Delta, and Pan American airlines, for supplying information on their in-flight meals;

My parents, for doing everything I didn't have time to do.

SECTION I

Eat to Succeed

ONE

Eating for Success

This book is about success—your success—in all the important areas of your life. It will work for you, just as it has for the superstar athletes, movie and television celebrities, business executives, physicians, attorneys, and others from all professions and walks of life whom I counsel. The foundation of your success, at work and at play, lies in the new maximum performance programs I've researched and created during the last several years. They will help provide you with the keys to a successful and healthy, rewarding life. And that's what eating to succeed is all about.

If you are one of over 2 million followers of *Eat to Win—The Sports Nutrition Bible*, then you've probably discovered the thrill of peak performance and better health I promised you through the *Eat to Win* program. Those benefits, however, are just the *beginning* of what you can expect to achieve if you embrace the new nutritional programs in *Eat to Succeed*.

Even though sports professionals and amateurs follow *Eat to Win* more than any other dietary program, many people may not be aware that my nutritional advice is for *nonathletic* people as well. You don't have to be a Wimbledon tennis champion or a Boston marathoner to enjoy the benefits of maximum performance. Even if you are a primarily sedentary office worker, you will benefit from *Eat to Succeed* programs.

3

Your success in life depends to a large degree on how and what you feed your body. That, after all, is where the energy for achievement comes from. I'm going to show you how to make nutrition work for you, not only in sports but also in many other important areas of your life.

Knowledge in nutrition increases dramatically every several years and *doubles* approximately every five to ten years, so you need to keep abreast of the latest information in this exciting field. *Eat to Succeed* will give you this vital new information. I've created new programs to give you the most effective means of nutritionally maximizing your performance in all aspects of your life—during business, recreation, creative thought, study, sexual activity, sleep, and musical and dramatic performances.

A NEW, SCIENTIFICALLY FORMULATED MAXIMUM PERFORMANCE WEIGHT-LOSS PROGRAM

Perhaps no other aspect of nutrition concerns as many people as does the question of weight control through dieting. Thousands eagerly grasp at fad diets that promise rapid weight loss, only to find disappointment, often subjecting themselves to nutritionally unsound, at times even dangerous regimens. At best, dieters find themselves restricted to such a narrow range of permitted foods that simple monotony soon undermines their resolve to lose weight.

Dieters who have found they lost energy as they tried to lose body fat will rejoice to discover the Haas Maximum Performance Weight-Loss Program. Here is a scientifically balanced regimen that meets your energy needs while allowing you to shed those unwanted inches. Besides providing you the full complement of nutrients essential for sustaining optimum health, it allows you to enjoy a tasty diversity of foods. You'll find more than 100 new Haas-approved gourmet recipes to move you along the road to success. And you'll learn the techniques for increasing food intake—even incorporating restaurant meals, favorite fast foods, and snacks—in such a way as to maintain weight stability once you've achieved your weight-loss goal.

EAT TO SUCCEED FOR FREQUENT FLYERS, PILOTS, AND FLIGHT ATTENDANTS

If you fly commercial or private aircraft, you should know how to protect yourself nutritionally from the little known but highly damaging effects of flying. Passengers, pilots, and flight attendants regularly use my special Frequent Flyer's Protection Program to minimize damage inflicted by radiation, lack of oxygen, dry skin, lower back strain, jet lag, and cabin pressure changes during flight. Now you can use the same type of program to help protect your body from many of the hazards of high altitude flying whenever you must travel by air.

STAYING FIT FOR THE OFFICE

Many people mistakenly believe that their office provides a relatively safe and secure environment. Unfortunately, health hazards lurk in virtually every office building, no matter how new or technologically advanced it may be. In fact, newer office buildings generally pose a greater threat/health risk than older buildings. Why? Mainly because newer office designs neglect basic human requirements for natural light and fresh air. Additionally, ordinary office equipment such as photocopiers, computers, lighting fixtures, and other electronic equipment may increase your exposure to harmful substances—toxic compounds that can cause headaches, nausea, allergic reactions, dizziness, unexplained illnesses, and may even be associated with an increased risk of cancer.

Proper nutritional protection can help minimize these hidden hazards of the office; it can also increase work performance (and therefore profits) as well as decrease workdays missed because of illness or disabling pain. The *Eat to Succeed* diet program can help protect office workers and business executives alike. This is important information that no corporation, large or small, can afford to do without.

NUTRITIONAL SUPPLEMENTS FOR MAXIMUM PERFORMANCE

I've spent years trying to find a vitamin or pharmaceutical company to devise the finest nutritional supplements in conformance with my demanding standards. I insisted that they contain pure, pharmaceutical-grade nutrients, packaged exclusively in clear hard gelatin capsules without colorings, flavorings, and other objectionable ingredients that contaminate many vitamin/nutrient formulas on the market today. Finally I found a company whose products measured up to my standards. Then I tested those products with my weekend and world class athletic clients.

When I first started my research into vitamin manufacturing, I naively believed that all companies manufactured only the purest and best products possible. I soon learned, however, that not all companies used the same quality standards, materials, testing procedures, manufacturing processes, or even the same purity of raw products to make their products. These are important differences that distinguish one brand of supplement from another as well as determine the safety and effectiveness of supplements.

For these reasons, I got in touch with Twin Laboratories, of Ronkonkoma, New York, a company that enjoyed a reputation for manufacturing only nutritional supplements of the highest quality. Scientists there were convinced that my dietary approach was scientifically sound and that it was consistent with their own research and health objectives.

After more than two years of research and development, these scientists formulated a special line of nutritional products to meet the needs of active people. They considered this revolutionary line of nutritional products so important that they created a special company, TwinSport, solely to manufacture and sell these supplements. I presently consult with them (and get paid for doing so) and I recommend their line of nutritional supplements to anyone interested in improving their health and achieving peak performance. (All my net proceeds from the sale of these products are being donated to cancer research.) See Appendix I, Nutritional Supplements: The TwinSport Formulary, for more information on these products.

FIT FOR THE ROAD

Until recently, rock and roll musicians enjoyed a less than sterling reputation for a life-style fraught with drugs, junk food, and fast living. Well, the fast living probably always will remain a staple of a rock 'n' roller's existence, but I was convinced by a friend in the music business to form a rock and roll nutritional service that would help get musicians healthy and up to their highest level of maximum performance. You see, musicians and athletes share many common attributes and nutritional needs. Musicians subject themselves to the rigors of national and international tours, often a year or longer, traveling as much or more than touring professional athletes. They live much of their professional lives on the road, eating junk food, missing vital sleep, and neglecting their bodies' needs in general. Often the only exercise they get is onstage, then later, offstage at a group party.

In May of 1984, just minutes after I appeared on the "Phil Donahue Show," a long-time friend approached me to form Fit for the Road, a nutritional service for touring rock musicians. As a former musician, I immediately saw the value and importance of this service. Music industry experts I talked to agreed that the industry sorely needed a service like Fit for the Road, so I ventured into the "unhealthy" world of rock and roll musicians to introduce them to eating for success through maximum performance foods and nutritional supplements.

The results were nothing short of astonishing. In Chapter Two you'll learn how this program helped change the health and onstage performances of some well-known music stars. If you are involved in music or other creative arts, you need this essential dietary information. Your first gold record or platinum album could be just a few healthy bites away!

SPORTS NUTRITION UPDATE

I'm going to tell you about the vital new sports nutrition information that scientists have discovered during the last two years. This information can mean the difference between mediocrity and excellence, success and failure, in virtually any sport or physical activity you enjoy. Chapters Three and Four are essential reading for anyone interested in keeping abreast of important new sports nutrition information, regardless of age, sex, or level of athletic ability.

THE SKELETON IN THE HOSPITAL CLOSET

I'm going to show you how to avoid the dangers of hospital-induced malnutrition, one of the leading causes of *completely avoidable* disability and death that you face whenever you are hospitalized. If you want to avoid nutritionally inadequate hospital meals that actually retard the healing process and if you want to protect yourself against the hazards of surgical anesthesia and other potential risks during a hospitalization, you'll want to follow my hospital nutrition guide for better healing, which includes a surgical protection plan and a get-well-soon diet program. *You can and should eat for success in the hospital because your life may depend upon it.*

NEW FOOD COMPOSITION DATA TO HELP YOU SUCCEED

Most food composition tables used by nutrition-conscious dieters lack complete, important data on food composition. Through a special arrangement with the United States Department of Agriculture and the National Technical Information Service in Washington, D.C., I have obtained up-to-date food composition data with no missing values for the six *Eat to Win/Eat to Succeed* vital nutrients. Now weight- and nutrition-conscious people can accurately and completely total their daily intakes for kilocalories, protein, fat, carbohydrate, sodium, and cholesterol. I have included a special food composition table, complete with the nutritional breakdown per serving, of all recipes in *Eat to Win* and *Eat to Succeed.* Now, for the first time, dieters will not be forced to eat in the dark.

The new Haas Maximum Performance Diet helps you control the absolute amounts of cholesterol, fats, oils, and protein you eat, and the special food composition table and nutritional information in each recipe will help you decide which foods and recipes are right for you.

COMPUTING TO WIN

As an accessory, I have created several powerful computer programs, just like those I've used to create diets for world champion athletes and celebrities who need to function at maximal performance. If you own a personal computer, you will be able to:

• Create your own *Eat to Win/Eat to Succeed* personalized diets (for your family as well)

• Graph your progress and determine how many kilocalories you've burned each day during just about any activity imaginable (including eating itself)

• Modify your favorite recipes according to *Eat to Win/Eat To Succeed* principles

• Track your weight loss, cholesterol levels, and much more

Appendix IV contains program descriptions and ordering information.

ISN'T IT TIME YOU SUCCEEDED?

People around the world continually tell me my diet has helped them succeed in areas of their life where they once failed. It's gratifying to learn about these success stories on nearly a daily basis, because, in most cases, their lives have *dramatically* changed for the better. And that's what eating to succeed is really all about—making your life the very best it can be. Isn't it time you succeeded? (To help you sustain your success, I am publishing and distributing the *Haas Health Letter*—see page 306—to provide regularly updated information on the maximum performance nutritional principles introduced in this book.)

TWO

How the Stars Eat to Succeed

World champion athletes, motion picture and television celebrities, and rock stars all share a common desire—they want to look good, feel good, and perform at their peak. Many of those who are nutritionally aware also share a common nutritional program: the Haas Peak Performance Diet.

The well-known personalities who have achieved peak performance on the diet have at the same time enjoyed resounding success in their personal and professional lives. I enjoy hearing nutritional success stories, especially when they are about those people whose artistic work adds to the pleasure and enjoyment of our daily lives. Success stories about well-known people often inspire others to emulate that success, and if the success stories in this chapter motivate you to achieve nutritional success in your life, then so much the better. You don't have to be a superstar to achieve maximum performance. I think you will find that the success stories that follow apply just as well to your own needs for maximum performance in many aspects of your personal and professional life.

CHER

Cher is a woman who has accomplished just about everything she ever set out to do. Cher has achieved success in television, legitimate theater, music, dancing, and most recently in motion pictures (having won Best Actress at the 1985 Cannes Film Festival for her performance in the film *Mask*).

One might think that Cher, who has conscientiously taken care of her body for the past twenty years, couldn't be any better physically than she already is. But that wasn't the case when she called me this year.

"I'm at the lowest point of my career, physically and mentally," she complained. "My role in *Mask* was so demanding and the pressure on me was so great to be extra thin to play my part [that of a pill-popping biker mom with a son suffering from a serious and deforming birth defect] that I starved myself. Now I've gained back all the weight I lost plus an extra eight pounds, and I'm totally burned out from dieting and stress."

As usual, Cher's timing was impeccable. We were both going to Europe at the same time. I had a European book tour for *Eat to Win*, and she had a movie and film festival tour for *Mask*. Cher invited me to stay with her in Los Angeles before we decided to go to Europe together so that we could eat and exercise together, basically the same way Martina Navratilova and I started working together.

Since I use computers to help me analyze and construct my clients' diet and supplement program, I moved my computer equipment into Cher's house. Fortunately, her daughter, Chastity, was away at school, so Chastity's room became computer central.

The next step was taking over Cher's kitchen. The first thing I did was remove the dozens of less-than-ideal supplements Cher had purchased somewhat blindly and replace them with a brand that I endorse. Next, we went shopping for peak performance foods, including those we would take to Europe with us. Then, we began an exercise program that Cher herself created using a trampoline and weights. Since Cher's personal gym surpasses most hotel gyms in quality and quantity of equipment, she had no problem maintaining her maximum performance exercise program. We even convinced some of her friends and associates in the entertainment business to adopt the program. They participated with enthusiasm. Soon there were so many trampolines that it was hard to walk through the gym.

After a month of nutrition education and training, which included discovering restaurants in Beverly Hills and greater Los Angeles (examples: Guido's for pasta and Haas-style Caesar salad; La Salsa for cholesterol-free Mexican fare), we were ready for continental cuisine. Off to Cannes we went.

Airline food posed little if any problem, because we came prepared (you'll learn the in-flight tricks to use in Chapter Five: Eating on the Wing).

We knew we'd be tempted by the easy availability of rich foods in France, but we also knew that continental cuisine includes a wide variety of maximum performance foods. In fact, we were able to enjoy maximum performance foods throughout Europe (and later Japan) while still eating in gourmet style. We never really felt we were making a sacrifice. That's the beauty of enjoying a diet based on complex carbohydrates like spaghetti, noodles, rice, bread, potatoes, vegetables, fruits, and small amounts of seafood and poultry. These foods, properly prepared, are widely available everywhere.

Our most notable meal was dinner at the elegant Eden Roc restaurant in the Hotel Du Cap, in Antibes, on the southern coast of France near Cannes. Room service at the hotel was excellent, but the food at Eden Roc was nothing less than exquisite. Did we cheat, you ask? You bet we did, but only on dessert—a one-of-a-kind chocolate soufflé made from egg whites, chocolate, and other tasty but forbidden foods that one should enjoy only on special occasions.

Cher has discovered the secrets of maximum performance and peak health. She feels that she'll be in the best shape of her life for her next motion picture and that she'll never feel burned out again, no matter how demanding the work.

DON JOHNSON

I started working with Don Johnson before *Miami Vice* became the year's biggest television success story, so I was thrilled to watch as Don's acting talents helped put *Miami Vice* at the top of the ratings chart.

Don first called me when he was bedridden with flu. I drove to his house immediately (he lives about twenty minutes away). Our first consultation led to a friendship that took us to Aspen to celebrate Christmas and ring in the new year. There's never a lack of exercise or great food at a ski resort like Aspen, and we enjoyed both to the fullest. We also enjoyed a peak performance Christmas dinner at Don's house with his girlfriend, actress Patty D'Arbanville, and friends Jimmy and Jane Buffet. Don learned how to enjoy Christmas holiday dinner the Haas Maximum Performance way: plenty of low-fat turkey, fruit stuffing, mashed potatoes and low-fat gravy, with special *Eat to Win* recipes for cranberry relish, potato casserole, pumpkin pie, plus chocolate cake (recipe in this book).

Since starting the Maximum Performance Diet, Don has consistently said that without the benefits he's derived from it, he never could have kept up the brutal pace that the success of *Miami Vice* demands. He often reports on the set at 6:00 A.M. and works late into the night. Friday nights are even more demanding; Don usually works until 6:00 A.M.

Don's success with health and fitness is more impressive than you might imagine, because he was able to overcome an extremely unhealthy life-style of drug dependence and junk food addiction. If he can do it, so can you. It's never too late, and no one is ever doomed to drug dependence if they're willing to take charge of their health. And that's the important lesson that Don Johnson wants *you* to know.

IVAN LENDL

Did things ever get so bad with your job that you wanted to quit? You're not alone. Ivan Lendl, world champion tennis player, actually contemplated quitting the game because things weren't going nearly as well as he hoped. Ivan felt that he wasn't winning nearly as many tournaments as his ability allowed, and he was losing matches to players who were less accomplished and experienced.

Ivan's agent, Jerry Solomon, asked me to help Ivan regain his fighting spirit through maximum performance nutrition.

"Can you do for Ivan what you did with Martina?" was Jerry's first question.

"Absolutely!" I answered.

I flew to the 1985 United States Open (where I first met with

Martina three years before) just before the men's finals to consult with Ivan. I told him that he would notice a measurable difference in a matter of weeks, and he did.

A blood chemistry profile revealed that Ivan's serum cholesterol was at dangerous levels, especially for a young and physically active world class athlete. Within four weeks, it had dropped into the ideal range. Ivan was able to reduce the time it took him to run 1500 meters by fifteen seconds, and he achieved a remarkable weight loss (mostly body fat) of fifteen pounds over the next two months. Ivan was ready to play again—and win.

As of this writing, Ivan has achieved the Number One world ranking in men's professional tennis by consistently beating John McEnroe (who claims he follows the "Haagen-Dasz" diet) and his old nemesis, Jimmy Connors. In 1985, on the anniversary of our first meeting, Ivan won the U.S. Open, handily trouncing McEnroe in three straight sets. (Coincidentally, Martina Navratilova, whom I have not advised since Christmas 1984—and who has reportedly changed her diet—lost some major tournaments, including the U.S. Open, to players she formerly dominated.)

The lesson you can learn from Ivan Lendl is that peak performance nutrition can help you be the best you can be. Is your job getting you down? Maybe you're not performing at your peak. Ivan learned how to eat for success and turn a sagging career around. You can, too.

REO SPEEDWAGON

Once upon a time, genuine rock 'n' rollers took pride in their ability to live as fast and as hard as their music. An evening of hard rock and hard drugs was the usual formula for a good time. That's the image most rock musicians had—until now.

Since I founded Fit for the Road, a nutritional organization that works with touring rock and pop musicians, rock 'n' rollers have begun to change their image. Some people thought I'd taken one too many vitamins when I told them I was starting a crusade to bring health and fitness to the world of rock and roll. But the skeptics have stopped their skepticism, thanks to the success of the groups REO Speedwagon and Survivor and of artists like Rosanne Cash.

Hailing from the Midwest, which has spawned dozens of well-known rock groups with reputations for no-holds-barred partying, REO Speedwagon gained a reputation for playing hard, both on- and offstage. Last year, the group; their manager, John Baruck; and road manager Tom Consolo agreed to be my first rock and roll "guinea pigs," as they referred to themselves. Since then, life hasn't been quite the same for the boys from Champaign, Illinois.

REO's *Wheels Are Turnin'* album has shot to the top of the charts, and their hit single "Can't Fight This Feeling" made it to the Number One spot on the charts. On their current tour, the group hasn't behaved like angels (I've traveled with them to monitor their progress and even performed briefly with them at several concerts—"Better stick to nutrition," jokes lead singer Kevin Cronin), but they have taken steps to protect their health and boost their onstage performance through maximum performance nutrition.

"There's definitely a certain stigma that goes with rock and roll," says Alan Gratzer, drummer for REO. "People have it in their heads that you get crazy every night on the road. But really, what your fans want is a great show, to hear you playing well. They like to read about people in bands doing drugs and stuff, but at this point it's a joke. There's definitely a new wave of health in the music business."

Rock musicians, like professional athletes, earn their living with their bodies, and very often rock musicians are just as physically active and face the same demanding travel schedules as athletes. "It doesn't matter what kind of music you call it—being on the road is being on the road," observes Rosanne Cash (Johnnie Cash's daughter). "Touring is no day at the beach, and you tend to be really hard on yourself. Let's face it, we've all abused ourselves. It takes a lot of effort to reorganize your life and take care of yourself." Frankie Sullivan, lead guitar for Survivor, another Midwest rock group with an impressive string of hit songs, agrees. Both follow the Maximum Performance Program through Fit for the Road, and both now eat for success.

REO band members are *not* people who normally like rules and restrictions. However, as lead singer Kevin Cronin noted, "It was a challenge for us, because we were real happy about our new album and wanted to do anything we could to make the tour go well. We were all positive about the tour and, really, the only thing that could've stood in our way were just the hazards of road health. So when the [Fit for the Road] program came up, it was real good timing for us."

"We haven't had to become monks or anything like that," says Kevin. "The thing is, when you do party, the better health you're in when you start, the quicker you're going to recover. And, I think, when you eat right and feel better, it just goes along that you really don't feel like trashing yourself. You can't be on a self-destructive trip if you want to give a high-energy show like we do. People don't want to pay good money to see performers who are half-conscious on stage."

REO's manager, John Baruck, observes, "The long hours catch up with a band when they've been doing it a long time. With the Fit for the Road program, we can take care of our needs and still have fun."

How's that for a new definition of the rock and roll life-style?

RUTH WYSOCKI:
HOW DIET DECKED MARY DECKER

When world class runner Tom Wysocki's doctor told him to change his diet, his wife, Ruth (a former champion runner), decided to follow Tom's new diet just to avoid having to cook two different meals each time they ate at home. Fortunately for Ruth, Tom picked the Maximum Performance Diet. Shortly after starting her new diet, and after nearly twenty years of running, Ruth Wysocki became *the* American middle-distance runner.

Just three weeks into the diet, Ruth developed the speed, strength, and power to run the fastest 800-meter race of her life. "After a couple of weeks on the diet," Tom says, "we noticed a difference in how we felt and how much better we were recovering from workouts. It was amazing how good we both felt." It was also amazing how much weight they both lost. Tom lost eight pounds and Ruth lost ten without ever trying to count calories.

Shortly afterward, Ruth experienced the ultimate victory of her career—beating the U.S. champion, Mary Decker, in the final of the 1500-meter Olympic qualifying race. With an outstanding race time of 4:00.18—the second-fastest performance ever by an American, Ruth won a place in running history. The press, true to form, emphasized that Mary Decker had lost, not that Ruth had won. However, that did not detract from Ruth Wysocki's thrill of victory. Imagine coming back from nearly five years of "retirement" to triumph at the 1984 Olympic trials over our country's leading female runner!

JEFF KEITH
EATS TO SUCCEED AGAINST CANCER

Jeff Keith may have only one leg, but he runs farther and better than most people do with two. Jeff achieved a physical feat most ordinary people only marveled at—he ran across the United States, coast to coast, stopping only to sleep, eat, and occasionally rest. In the process, Jeff helped raise money for cancer research and proved to the world that having lost a leg to cancer was no obstacle to achieving such an incredible feat.

Almost two months into his now famous coast-to-coast run, Jeff began feeling run-down, lethargic, and burned out. The daily pace and stress of running cross-country, combined with the carbon monoxide–laden automobile exhausts he breathed every step of his run, were hampering his performance. His diet of red meat, eggs, milk, and cheese proved to be more crippling to his stamina and endurance than cancer itself.

Then Jeff discovered this diet. One of his road crew introduced Jeff to the diet, and from there he learned how to eat to succeed with maximum performance foods and nutritional supplements. During the next month, Jeff lost twenty pounds and started to feel superb each day. "As each weekend passed, I began feeling lighter and better. By the end of the run, four out of five of my crew members were on the Haas diet. The supplements really helped, and I'm still on the diet. It's changed my life-style. You can't go back to your old eating habits once you are on it. And I really don't want to go back."

Jeff Keith has overcome a crippling disease with strong character, mental fortitude, hard training, and a diet designed to insure success. His achievements highlight the essentials of human success—ambition, willpower, dedication—and knowing how to eat for optimum health.

These are just a few of the success stories, and I hope they will motivate you to take charge of your health. The nutritional program that revitalized Cher, helped Don Johnson handle a demanding schedule and hectic life-style, helped put Ivan Lendl at the top of men's professional tennis, kept REO Speedwagon on tour long after most groups call it quits, and gave Ruth Wysocki and Jeff Keith the stamina and energy to achieve new heights of physical performance is the same program that can help you eat to succeed, regardless of your profession or life-style.

THREE

Nutrition Update (Part One): High-Tech Proteins

Eat-to-Winners have learned that protein robs them of maximum performance and optimal health. But for every knowledgeable Eat-to-Winner (there are now well over 2 million) who eats the correct *amount* and *type* of protein each day, there are a dozen people who still consume far too much protein for their own good. Protein is still the single most misunderstood nutrient and the source of one of the most dangerous nutritional myths in the world today.

Since the publication of *Eat to Win*, nutritional scientists have discovered some new and exciting information about the role of protein and amino acids. Unfortunately, most nonscientists will not come upon this important information for a half decade or more. This lag time is actually quite normal in the course of nutritional history. Several important nutritional discoveries have remained hidden within scientific journals for decades until someone recognized the significance of these discoveries: The proper dietary treatment for diabetes—a high-carbohydrate, low-fat diet—was actually prescribed in 1932 by a British researcher named Himsworth, writing in a well-known and respected medical journal. It took physicians and health organizations, including the American Diabetic Association, *nearly fifty years* to recognize the tremendous value and importance of an *Eat to Win*–type diet to manage and even cure diabetes. Consider how many diabetics lost their limbs to gangrene, their eyesight to diabetic retinopathy, and their hearts, kidneys, and lives to atherosclerosis because of the wrong dietary advice—advice that had been disproven for nearly half a century!

WHY PEOPLE ARE STILL CONFUSED
ABOUT PROTEIN

In 1941, the RDA (recommended daily allowance) for protein was 70 grams (about *twice* the amount humans need each day). People who followed this advice, issued by the National Academy of Science's (NAS) Food and Nutrition Board (FNB), may have suffered an accelerated onset of many of the diseases of aging, such as osteoporosis (the bone-loss disease), atherosclerosis, kidney disease, and colo-rectal cancer. Even though only five years later scientists discovered that a "reference" man weighing 154 pounds needed only 35 grams of protein per day (with a variation of plus or minus 15 percent), it was not until 1968 that the RDA for protein was reduced—and then only by a mere 5 grams!

Today, the NAS has partially corrected its poor judgment and has accordingly reduced the RDA for protein to 45 grams for women and 55 grams for men, with the recommendation that two-thirds of the protein come frrom animal sources. But the NAS still has not recognized the superiority of plant over animal protein sources for human health and fitness, and so their present recommendations are still too generous and misleading. That's why people are still confused about how much and what kind of protein they should consume.

It's time we learned a lesson from history in order to avoid repeating the mistakes of the past. Let us now settle the protein controversy once and for all. Here, then, is the official *Eat to Succeed* position on protein:

THE MAJORITY OF YOUR PROTEIN CALORIES SHOULD COME FROM GRAINS, CEREALS, LEGUMES (SUCH AS BEANS, PEAS, LENTILS), AND A VARIETY OF VEGETABLES, *NOT* FROM ANIMAL SOURCES.

The amino acid patterns of plant proteins, including starches, provide the optimal pattern for superb health, vitality, fitness, and degenerative disease prevention. Scientists have demonstrated this fact in the laboratory and in free-living populations throughout the world. Why, then, do hospital dietitians and health organizations still want us to stuff eggs, beef, cheese, dairy products, and other animal protein sources down the gullets of our children? The non-scientific reasons are beyond the scope of this book. However, the scientific rationale for these recommendations is *nonexistent* and therefore unjustifiable and immoral.

The problem, as I learned firsthand, starts with the formal education of nutrition and medical students who go on to become dietitians and serve on nutritional advisory boards like the one that establishes the RDA's.

Since medical students still receive little or no nutrition education (and what little nutritional education they do receive is generally incomplete and outdated), let's examine what nutrition students learn about protein in U.S. colleges and universities. These are the students who eventually go on to become hospital (registered) dietitians. I can write from my own personal experience because I received my Master of Science degree in Nutrition and Food Science from Florida State University—a university with nutrition coursework and programs recognized and approved by the American Dietetic Association.

My training in organic chemistry, medical biochemistry, human physiology, histology (microscopic anatomy), biology, embryology, oncology (the study of cancer cells), and medical pharmacology was excellent and provided me with a more extensive scientific background to study and understand nutrition than many registered hospital dietitians possess. My nutrition courses, however, left much to be desired.

By the time I began my formal study of nutrition, I had already learned more *correct* information about diet and degenerative disease than some of my professors apparently had, since some appeared overweight or had a diet-related disease (peptic ulcer disease, hypertension, hypercholesterolemia, etc.). A few of them even smoked cigarettes.

Perhaps the most inappropriate example of dietary behavior I saw at the time was a picture of an officer of the American Dietetic Association (the ADA is a private organization that certifies nutrition students as registered dietitians once they have passed a minimum coursework load, a written test, and an internship). I was somewhat shocked to see what appeared to be a patently *obese* person smiling at me from a page in their journal. This was the nutrition organization that I intended to join, an organization that influenced many national nutritional policies concerning very serious health issues!

So if you still follow the advice of many dietitians to eat steak and eggs, plenty of dairy products, or peanut butter to get your daily protein, read this chapter very carefully. My protein recommendations could do more than boost your daily energy level and help slow down your body's rapid rate of aging. *They could save your life.*

EAT TO SUCCEED PROTEIN PRINCIPLES

Let's begin by recognizing three important protein principles:

1. Vegetable protein is *complete* protein; vegetable protein possesses an amino acid pattern that is actually *superior* to animal proteins for promoting health and vitality. (This doesn't mean, however, that you must become a vegetarian.)

2. Most of your daily protein requirement should be met by complex carbohydrate foods such as potatoes, rice, vegetables, legumes, and pasta, *not* chicken, fish, pork, or beef.

3. Excessive protein consumption—in general, greater than 14 percent of your daily total calories—can prematurely age your body, cause loss of vitamins and minerals, drain your energy, dehydrate you, and promote degenerative diseases such as cancer, heart attack, stroke, kidney failure, high blood pressure, health problems during pregnancy (and perhaps damage to the fetus as well), diverticulosis, hemorrhoids, and constipation.

And now, based on the most recent protein research, there's a fourth protein principle that you should know about to help you be the best you can be, at work and at play:

4. The *branched chain* amino acids (BCAA's) *leucine, isoleucine,* and *valine,* when added to your diet, can help build muscle, improve recovery time from surgery, and help improve the quality of your daily protein intake needs.

This is vital new information for all Eat-to-Winners. The three BCAA's, available in a special supplement formula you'll learn about later in this chapter, can help increase *the quality* of your protein intake while helping to keep *the quantity* of protein to *safe and effective* levels.

VEGETABLE PROTEINS ARE COMPLETE PROTEINS

Ironically, the myth of complete (animal) versus incomplete (plant) proteins has been perpetuated through the years by the very groups who are charged with preserving our health—dietitians and physicians. In fact, the most scientifically inaccurate and dangerous diets based on high-protein consumption have been promoted during the last thirty years in best-selling diet books written by physicians!

Let me now and forever dispel the false notion that animal foods provide complete proteins and that plant foods provide incomplete (and by inference, inferior) proteins. The truth is that plant proteins are complete proteins, with amino acid patterns that produce *superior* rather than inferior results in humans when compared to animal protein amino acid patterns. Understanding this protein principle is essential to your achieving the best of health and vitality for the rest of your life—with the added benefit of slowing down and even *reversing* the ravages of aging.

Humans need to get *at least* eight and *perhaps ten* amino acids from food. When scientists began to examine human protein needs in the early 1920s, they experimented with rats, although rats have markedly different protein requirements, life-span, and metabolism than those of humans. Scientists came to the false conclusion that the ideal amino acid pattern for human food choices was the same pattern on which rats thrived. *That single misconception did more to set back twentieth-century nutrition than any other error in the history of nutritional science.* My nutrition professors believed it, taught it, and based their own diets around it.

Essentially, scientists then (and some even now) mistakenly believed that because rats grew best on animal protein amino acid patterns commonly found in eggs, milk, beef, cheese, and poultry, then humans, too, should thrive best on these very foods. *Nothing could be farther from the truth.*

PLANT PROTEIN SOURCES PROVIDE THE BEST NUTRITION FOR HUMANS

I don't believe that humans were meant to be strict vegetarians, but I do know that plant sources of protein should provide the bulk of our daily protein needs, supplemented with small amounts of animal protein.

A diet based largely but not exclusively on foods such as potatoes and pasta and brown rice can provide more than the RDA of highly usable, cholesterol-free low-fat protein. That's why 60 to 80 percent of the daily calories of the *Eat to Succeed* diet comes from cereals, grains, and vegetables, including potatoes, and beans, peas, or lentils. *The less cereals, grains, and vegetables you eat, the more protein your body requires.*

Scientific studies have shown that:

• The human requirement for protein is lower than the current RDA.

• The "ideal" protein foods—eggs, milk, beef—possess an amino acid pattern that is inconsistent with optimal health and protein metabolism in humans. (However, such foods in large amounts are great for rats.)

• The currently estimated levels of protein intake of most Americans promote osteoporosis, cardiovascular disease, cancer, dehydration, diabetes, kidney and liver damage, premature aging, high blood pressure, diverticular disease, vitamin and mineral deficiencies, and more.

Many science educators, including myself, have long wondered how this deplorable and inexcusable condition can persist year after year. The answer, I suspect, is a combination of intentional igno-rance (many health care professionals live on and enjoy diets high in animal protein sources), and/or an incomplete understanding of diet and its relation to disease.

If you wait for the rest of the world to acknowledge the truth about protein—remember that nutritional truths generally have taken decades to gain acceptance by the scientific community at large—then you will pay a high price.

EAT TO SUCCEED WITH HIGH-TECH PROTEINS

Discovery of the role of the branched chain amino acids (BCAA's) leucine, isoleucine, and valine represents an important advance in modern protein research. The BCAA's, unlike any other amino acids, act as a direct source of energy for muscles. In fact, after a meal, the BCAA's account for most of the amino acids that enter muscle tissue. BCAA's also can reduce your protein needs and supply energy during exercise, stress, and illness, including bacte-rial infection and weight loss.

A large number of studies have shown that BCAA's, particularly leucine, promote muscle growth and general protein synthesis. Bodybuilders who eat properly can now rely on these naturally occurring amino acids instead of dangerous steroids to achieve maximal muscle growth. (See the formula given below.)

Some nutritionists have recommended that active people eat more protein than sedentary people because exercise increases protein needs. This is both a half truth and a potentially dangerous recommendation. Your protein needs can be better met not by increasing the quantity of protein in your diet (and most likely, the fat and cholesterol content as well), but by supplementing your diet with a balanced formula containing the BCAA's, the amino acids arginine and ornithine, and related vitamins (such as below).

Eating for success means rejecting the advice of those coaches, trainers, dietitians, and other people who still insist that you should increase your protein intake if you enjoy regular physical activity.

HOW TO USE HIGH-TECH PROTEINS

Even though the BCAA's occur in ordinary foods such as chicken and fish, you may want to supplement your diet with these three amino acids plus arginine and ornithine (and the vitamins involved in their metabolism) to help you eat for success. Here is the optimal high-tech amino acid muscle-building (anabolic) and fat-burning formula I recommend to my clients:

L-arginine	225 mg.
L-ornithine	225 mg.
BCAA mix	225 mg.
L-carnitine	25 mg.
Vitamin B-6	5 mg.
Pantothenic acid	10 mg.

DIRECTIONS: Take three capsules *in between* meals during the day and three capsules in the evening *on an empty stomach*, just before retiring, if possible.

This high-tech formula, made by TwinSport and sold throughout the country in health food stores, provides a state-of-the-art nutrient mix to help you eat for success. This is a valuable formula not only for those people who want to build more muscle, but also for dieting people who need to help insure that their reduced-calorie diet contains adequate protein and L-carnitine to help burn unwanted fat (see Chapter Four).

High-tech proteins, when used properly, can help you eat to succeed. You should, however, consult with a physician before taking any dietary supplements, especially if you have a medical condition that requires medication, surgery, or special testing, monitoring, or attention. If your physician is unfamiliar with the metabolic role of the BCAA's, refer him/her to the reference section at the end of this book. It contains medical journal citations that explain the mode of action of the BCAA's and describe how they can be used to improve your protein status under a variety of conditions.

FOUR

Nutrition Update (Part Two): The New Fat Fighters and Energy Boosters

L-CARNITINE: FAT BURNER?

There is a substance that is absolutely essential in your body if you are to burn fat. Just as important, your body requires this substance for protein metabolism, muscle contraction, athletic endurance, and maintaining a healthy heart. It's called L-carnitine.

Scientists have learned that L-carnitine is made in small quantities by the body and that we also obtain it from many of the foods we eat. While we still don't know how much L-carnitine is essential for optimal health, growth, and energy production, we do know that several groups of people may need more L-carnitine than their bodies can make or absorb from food. These groups at risk of L-carnitine deficiency include prematurely born babies, people with heart disease, diabetics, the chronically ill, physically active people, dialysis patients, people on intravenous liquid diets, people with low blood sugar, cancer patients, and the elderly.

A report prepared for the Food and Drug Administration (FDA) by the Life Sciences Research Office of the Federation of American Societies for Experimental Biology in 1982 concluded that "orally administered L-carnitine as a therapeutic agent may have beneficial effects in patients with carnitine deficiency states, renal disorders requiring hemodialysis, certain cardiovascular conditions, certain types of hypoglycemia, and type IV hyperlipidemia [elevated blood fats]."

HOW L-CARNITINE WORKS

L-carnitine is an amino acid–like substance that transports fats within cells so they can be burned for energy instead of being stored as fat. L-carnitine thus plays a unique role in fat metabolism, because without it the body cannot burn fat. L-carnitine actually carries fat into special sites (called mitochondria) within each cell that burn fat and carbohydrates for energy. L-carnitine mistakenly has been called a vitamin when actually it is not, because the body can synthesize it from amino acids, with the help of vitamin C, the B vitamins, and iron. The body can also absorb L-carnitine from food and L-carnitine dietary supplements.

L-carnitine is so essential for fat metabolism that people on carnitine-deficient diets experience high levels of blood fats (triglycerides) until their diets are supplemented with it. Several researchers have suggested that some overweight people may not fully utilize the L-carnitine that their body manufactures (perhaps due to genetics and/or the metabolic derangements caused by obesity itself) and consequently must rely on supplemental L-carnitine to successfully reduce body fat.

L-CARNITINE AND THE HEART

The FDA report just cited and the research I have listed in the reference section at the end of this book suggest that people with heart disease, including atherosclerosis, may benefit from supplemental L-carnitine. In 1979, a team of scientists tested the effects of L-carnitine (500 milligrams or more per day) on fourteen heart patients and discovered that they showed improved heart function when engaging in physical activity. Other scientists, working with laboratory animals, have concluded that L-carnitine protects a weak or diseased heart from ventricular arrhythmias (disturbances in the electrical system of the heart that controls its beating) and helps prevent the buildup of fats in the heart muscle. Additional studies have shown that heart patients taking nitroglycerin for angina pectoris (pain in the chest, neck, or arms due to atherosclerosis) reported fewer angina attacks and needed less of the drug when their diet was supplemented with L-carnitine. Studies have also demonstrated that L-carnitine lowers serum cholesterol and blood fats in normal and cardiac patients.

SOURCES OF L-CARNITINE

Source	TOTAL CARNITINE CONTENT* (MILLIGRAMS PER 3½ OUNCES)
L-carnitine supplements (average per capsule dosage)	250
Chicken muscle	7.5
Yeast	2.4
Cow's milk	2.0
Wheat germ	1.0
Chicken liver	0.6
Bread	0.2
Cauliflower	0.1
Peanuts	0.1

*The U.S. RDA for L-carnitine has not yet been established.

Adapted from Leibovitz, *Carnitine: The Vitamin Bt Phenomenon* (New York: Dell, 1984).

L-CARNITINE AND FAT

L-carnitine is absolutely essential for the transport of long-chain fatty acids across the inner membranes of the mitochondria. What this means is that without L-carnitine cells cannot burn fat efficiently for energy. L-carnitine is present in a number of ordinary foods such as wheat germ, cauliflower, chicken, beef, cow's milk, and lamb. The body synthesizes L-carnitine from two simple amino acids, lysine and methionine, and this synthesizing process, which takes place in the liver and kidneys, requires vitamins C, B-3, B-6, and iron.

Once synthesized in the liver and kidneys, L-carnitine is transported in the blood to skeletal and heart muscles, where it accumulates in muscle cells. There L-carnitine becomes involved in a large number of metabolic processes, which include:

• Controlling the amount of sugar the body makes from protein
• Protein metabolism (breakdown of specific amino acids)
• Sperm maturation and motility
• Transporting signals between cells in the brain
• Lowering serum cholesterol and triglycerides
• Reversing some of the harmful effects on the immune system that result from intravenous hospital liquid diets
• Boosting endurance
• Lowering recovery pulse rate after exercise
• Burning body fat more efficiently

L-CARNITINE AND THE NEWBORN

The ability of newborn and premature infants to synthesize L-carnitine is limited. Investigations have shown that neonates and premature infants who receive intravenous nutritional formulas not containing L-carnitine suffer from impaired fatty acid oxidation (fat-burning). Since neonates rely on fatty acid oxidation for most of their energy, a carnitine deficiency can seriously jeopardize their health. A recently published review of the scientific literature on the newborn's requirement for dietary L-carnitine concluded that:

• Neonates have a critical need for L-carnitine because they depend heavily on fat-burning for energy.
• Plasma and tissue concentrations of L-carnitine in the neonate are low in comparison to those found in older children and adults, indicating an increased need for L-carnitine to insure proper fat metabolism.
• At birth, the ability to synthesize L-carnitine is not fully developed.
• The lack of an outside supply of L-carnitine in the infant diet results in significant reduction in plasma concentrations of L-carnitine, thereby compromising energy production.

While an absolute L-carnitine deficiency in children and adults is rare, those under stress or involved in sports and victims of heart disease, low blood sugar, diabetes, and obesity may suffer from a decreased supply. Low L-carnitine levels may interfere with efficient energy production, heartbeat regulation, and protein synthesis. Present evidence suggests that supplementary L-carnitine may one day become an essential nutritional supplement for those groups of people at risk of carnitine depletion.

L-CARNITINE AND ATHLETIC PERFORMANCE

Athletes use L-carnitine as an ergogenic (energy-enhancing) substance. The first human clinical study measuring the physiological effects of L-carnitine supplementation in well-trained endurance athletes, conducted at the University of Wyoming in 1985, demonstrated that L-carnitine supplements can boost endurance, lower recovery pulse rate, and burn body fat.

Scientists in the Department of Health Sciences at the University of Wyoming recently conducted a pilot study to determine the effectiveness of L-carnitine when used by collegiate cross-country runners and wrestlers. The results of the study showed that L-carnitine was related to lowering body weight and body fat and improving (lowering) pulse recovery time after physical activity. Runners lost 14.3 percent of their body fat, and wrestlers lost 33.6 percent of their body fat during the thirty-day test period. While there may have been additional reasons for this impressive weight loss (such as increased physical activity or decreased caloric intake), the scientists who conducted the study concluded that L-carnitine (at a dosage of 500 milligrams per day) can be of benefit for improving heart muscle function, lowering body weight and body fat, and increasing aerobic power.

Don't be misled by these and other findings as they are reported in the months and years to come. L-carnitine is not really a miracle fat-burning substance, but rather a vital and necessary substance that you may require in supplemental form in order to burn fat *most efficiently*, keep blood fats and cholesterol at safe levels, and reach your highest level of maximum performance.

L-CARNITINE HELPS CORRECT
HOSPITAL-INDUCED DIETARY PROBLEMS

Hospital dietitians have long overlooked the importance of L-carnitine to their patients on liquid or intravenous diets. Diabetic, cardiac, and dialysis patients very often require special diets while hospitalized, and these diets and the special liquid diet formulas hospital dietitians use may be carnitine-deficient.

Since hospital dietetic staffs have not fully recognized the vital role of L-carnitine and other important nutrients in keeping their patients in optimal health, I always insist that my clients *do not* eat hospital food but rather have a friend or mate make and bring them *Eat to Win/Eat to Succeed* recipes and the nutritional supplements I recommend (see Appendix I for a complete list) that contain all the nutrients needed to protect against hospital-induced malnutrition. Hospital-induced malnutrition is a problem that you will probably face sooner or later and is so important that I have devoted a separate chapter to the problem to help you avoid an L-carnitine deficiency and other potentially dangerous but *completely avoidable* hospital-induced dietary problems.

COENZYME Q_{10}

Coenzyme Q_{10} plays a vital role in the maintenance of normal heart function and energy metabolism in general. The body needs coenzyme Q_{10} to utilize fully the energy it derives from proteins, fats, carbohydrates, and alcohol.

Body stores of coenzyme Q_{10} can become depleted with physical activity, illness, drug use, and aging. Coenzyme Q_{10} has also been shown to offer protection from free radical damage. (Free radicals are harmful substances that form in the air, in foods, and in the body itself and can accelerate aging, promote heart disease, cancer, and other health problems.)

Coenzyme Q_{10} supplementation represents a safe and nontoxic way to boost physical performance (especially in people with heart disease) and protect against free radical damage and associated health problems. Recent research has convincingly demonstrated that people with angina pectoris (pain in the neck, chest, jaw, or arms from coronary artery blockage) can exercise harder and longer without chest pain and reliance on drugs such as nitroglycerin with the aid of coenzyme Q_{10}. I predict that coenzyme Q_{10} will become a nutritional supplement commonly used by all people who want to boost endurance, and I believe that physicians will soon begin to prescribe it routinely to help their cardiac patients improve the quality of their active life. (See Appendix I for nutritional supplements that contain coenzyme Q_{10}.)

HIGH-TECH WATER—
THE WAVE OF THE FUTURE?

For nearly one million years, the best drink for active people, from cavemen to this year's Wimbledon champions, has been pure water. With such an unrivaled historical precedent and impressive record of success, one might assume that water would continue to enjoy the Number One spot as the drink of champions for at least another million years. Scientific progress, however, pays little attention to precedent; plain old water may soon become a nutritional dinosaur, at least for active people who want to achieve maximum physical performance.

During the last two years, food technologists and sports nutritionists have formulated a new breed of beverage that I call high-tech water. Some versions of it are now available to the public, and several more will be marketed shortly. Scientists have succeeded in transforming ordinary distilled water into a nutritionally enhanced beverage that can rapidly and effectively supply the body with several important energy nutrients that research has shown to be effective in increasing endurance and stamina.

High-tech water is much more than warmed-over Gatorade. It is, in fact, a truly scientific blend of salts, polymers, mineral–amino acid compounds, and fat and amino acid–carrier molecules that the body needs to burn the metabolic fuels that fire muscular activity. Formulas differ, according to manufacturer, and some will most likely prove more effective than others in extending the limits of human endurance. There is, however, one common attribute shared by all high-tech waters—glucose polymers. These are long-chain branched molecules of an ordinary sugar, constructed much like beads strung together in a necklace, and they account for much of the success of high-tech water. Other substances, such as magnesium aspartates and sodium phosphate, may play an important role in boosting the energy potential of water. In order to help you choose the high-tech water that's right for you, I've created a high-tech water primer, which follows.

GLUCOSE POLYMERS

Recent research has demonstrated that three primary factors affect physical performance, duration of activity, and recovery from activity during prolonged exercise:

- Dehydration (loss of body water)
- Carbohydrate depletion (running out of glycogen)
- Hyperthermia (elevated body temperature)

In the past, water has been the most effective nutrient in retarding the performance-robbing effects of dehydration and hyperthermia, while high–complex carbohydrate diets have helped slow glycogen depletion. Due to their high osmolarity (concentration of salts and sugars) and the high osmotic pressure they exert, activity drinks like Gatorade don't leave the stomach soon enough to safeguard peak performance. Water may actually be drawn into the stomach *away* from working muscles to help reduce the sudden high concentration of salt and sugar in the stomach, thus sapping muscle performance. Most activity drinks contain enough glucose (sugar) to delay stomach emptying.

Glucose polymers, however, exert less osmotic pressure and are rapidly absorbed into the bloodstream from the stomach and small intestine and carried to active muscles to be used as energy. Since the delivery of water and sugars to the body depends on the stomach emptying, use of the polymerized form of glucose will shorten the time and increase the amount of water and carbohydrate (fuel) delivered to the muscles, thereby providing rapidly available energy and replacement of lost water. Glucose polymer solutions can prolong exercise times.

Maltodextrin is the glucose polymer generally used in the new high-tech water formulas. It is made in the laboratory by breaking down ordinary cornstarch into smaller carbohydrate units. Maltodextrin plays an essential role in the efficacy of high-tech water; however, there are several other ingredients that also provide high-tech water with energy-giving power. Your favorite high-tech water should contain them to insure maximum performance.

POTASSIUM AND MAGNESIUM ASPARTATES

Magnesium plays a vital role in converting carbohydrates to energy, controlling heartbeat, activating enzyme systems, and muscular contraction. Dr. Kenneth Cooper, of the Aerobics Institute in Dallas, Texas, has shown that runners experience a decrease in blood levels of magnesium during long-distance running. Dr. Roy J. Shepard, of the University of Toronto, has discovered that distance runners lose significant amounts of magnesium in their sweat.

Potassium is essential for stimulating nerve impulses, maintaining the delicate acid-base balance in the body, and in the conversion of glucose to glycogen (stored carbohydrate that makes up the body's priority fuel reserve). Potassium also helps to widen blood vessels during exercise, increasing blood flow to help carry heat away from exercising muscles.

Several research studies have reported that taking potassium and magnesium aspartates (salts of aspartic acid) can increase stamina and oxygen uptake and aid recovery from exercise. They believe that these aspartates help reduce blood levels of ammonia (an ordinary but toxic by-product of protein metabolism and muscle tissue breakdown) that become elevated during exercise. Some scientists believe that potassium and magnesium bound to aspartic acid in salt form reach their intended destination within the cells much quicker than when taken in other forms.

SODIUM PHOSPHATE

Sodium phosphate is the sodium salt of phosphoric acid, a common substance found in ordinary cola-type beverages. Sodium phosphate, unlike sodium chloride and other sodium compounds, does not appear to raise blood pressure in sodium-sensitive animals.

Phosphates participate in the energy-producing systems in the body and help regulate the body's acid-base balance. The fatigue-fighting effects of phosphates were recognized as early as World War I, when German soldiers were given phosphate-supplemented diets to combat battle fatigue.

Recently researchers at the University of Florida demonstrated that sodium phosphate could significantly elevate the ability of muscles to remove and use oxygen from the blood and decrease buildup of lactic acid, a substance that causes muscle fatigue. Sodium phosphate appears to increase levels of 2,3-DPG (2,3-diphosphoglycerate), a substance normally made during carbohydrate metabolism. 2,3-DPG ordinarily increases muscle tissue's oxygen uptake and reduces lactic acid accumulation that can painfully retard and even prevent muscular contraction, thus impeding movement. Dr. George Sheehan, noted cardiologist, author, and runner, recently stated, "A dose of sodium phosphate may lift the runner to new levels of performance." (Runner's World, October 1984)

While water will still remain the primary and most effective ingredient in the new high-tech waters, current research suggests that the addition of glucose polymers, potassium and magnesium aspartates, and sodium phosphate, can additionally boost energy and endurance while helping to fight fatigue. Two companies, Ross Laboratories and Twin Laboratories, have already developed high-tech liquids (sold in health food stores and supermarkets) that contain some or all of these energy-giving substances in addition to vitamins and minerals. (Ensure, made by Ross Laboratories, can be used as a beverage and/or a meal replacer; QuickFix, made by TwinSport, is an energy-enhancing activity beverage and thirst quencher.) The Coca Cola company is expected to place its version of high-tech water, called Max, into national distribution sometime soon.

Performance-conscious athletes who now eschew alcoholic beverages in favor of sparkling water may soon pass that up in favor of these new souped-up waters. In fact, the day may not be too far off when restaurant waiters routinely inquire, "How would you like your water, regular or high-tech?"

FIVE

The Haas Maximum Performance Diet

Exciting nutritional discoveries since the publication of *Eat to Win* now make it possible for you to reach new heights of performance and success, at work and at play, with the new Maximum Performance Diet and Weight Loss Program and the scientific use of nutritional supplements.

The Maximum Performance Diet has a newly defined range of protein, fat and oil, and simple and complex carbohydrates. *Recent research has shown that we can enjoy certain types of oils and carbohydrates more than others and not jeopardize our health or performance.*

MAXIMUM PERFORMANCE HAAS-APPROVED RANGE
(upper and lower limits)

Complex carbohydrates (starches)..... 60–85% of daily calories
Simple carbohydrates (sweets)........ 5–10% of daily calories
Protein (animal and vegetable)....... 10–20% of daily calories
Fats (animal and vegetable) .... 5–25% of daily calories

Adjust your daily intake so that your nutrient consumption falls within the recommended ranges indicated. These new ranges and values permit a greater variety of food choices, including more oils from the monounsaturated group (the main source is olive oil) and more marine oils, such as EPA (eicosapentanoic acid), DHA (docosahexanoic acid), and related oils from seafood. Since oils tend to enhance the palatability of foods and recipes, these new modifications in the Maximum Performance Diet add flavor and help move your serum cholesterol, triglycerides, and blood clotting times into the maximum performance range.

Your range of complex carbohydrate intake can also be modified, according to the changes you make in your oil and protein intake. For example, if you increase your use of olive and marine oils, your daily carbohydrate consumption would vary accordingly. Thus, you now may enjoy a more varied diet and still consume enough complex carbohydrate to give you power to spare.

With the newer knowledge of the positive role played by the BCAA's, you actually can eat less high-protein foods (and less fat and cholesterol) when you supplement your diet with BCAA's. Protein research has shown that people can eat a diet with as little as 4 percent of daily calories from protein (mostly vegetable sources) and still remain healthy. A 4-percent protein diet would contain 30 grams of protein per 3000 calories (about the same amount of protein as is provided by 4.5 ounces of water-packed tuna or 5 cups of cooked spaghetti).

I'm not advocating a 4-percent protein diet. However, people who have eaten high-protein diets for many years and sustained kidney damage (as many Americans have done for decades) or those with renal diseases that require very low protein intakes can actually improve their health and kidney function on a low-protein (approximately 40 grams per day), BCAA-supplemented maximum performance diet. It's also comforting to know that on any given day, should your protein intake fall as low as 5 percent of your daily calories or reach as high as 20 percent, you will not jeopardize your health, as long as you return to a more moderate range (10 to 15 percent) the majority of the time. Due to the wide range of biologic variability, some people thrive on very-low-protein diets, and some extremely active people seem to do well on protein intakes that range between 15 and 20 percent of their daily calorie consumption. For the vast majority of us, however, I recommend that we stay within the 10 to 15 percent range as much as possible.

My new Maximum Performance Guidelines focus on a more liberal range of protein, fat, and cholesterol intake on each of the three levels of the program. In light of recent nutritional evidence concerning marine fats and oils, I have revised my dietary recommendations for these nutrients and have listed them later in this chapter.

LATEST NUTRITION RESEARCH SUPPORTS MAXIMUM PERFORMANCE DIET RECOMMENDATIONS

When *Eat to Win* became a Number One best-selling hardcover book for 1984, nutritional scientists took careful note of the reasons for its unprecedented success. When first published, several critics incorrectly reported that my dietary recommendations were low in calcium. (One persistent critic had written a sports nutrition book that sold less well.) They obviously did not read *Eat to Win* carefully, because, in addition to the calcium from the recommended list of foods (which includes milk, yogurt, cottage cheese, dark green leafy vegetables, and legumes—all rich sources of calcium), I stated that I always recommended calcium supplements, especially for active women, in a dosage from 500 to 1000 milligrams. (The U.S. RDA for calcium is 800 milligrams.) Another critic claimed that I recommended megadoses of fat-soluble vitamins A, D, E, and K. Again, it's obvious that this critic did not read my book carefully, because I never recommended megadoses (or any doses, for that matter) for these vitamins.

Nearly every critic agreed that my dietary recommendations were sound and healthy. (I was pleased to read that a member of the American Dietetic Association's Sports and Cardiovascular Nutrition Committee stated that *the Haas diet was the same type of diet now recommended by most registered dietitians*). A few critics who thought that it was healthy to eat several eggs each week, along with other high-fat, high-cholesterol foods, wound up with egg on their faces: Since *Eat to Win* was published, a ten-year government-sponsored study clearly and conclusively demonstrated that "normal" serum cholesterol levels—200 to 300 milligrams per 3½ ounces of blood—dramatically increase the risk of cardiovascular disease. In *Eat to Win,* I recommended that everyone achieve a blood cholesterol level of only 160 milligrams or below. Recently the American Medical Association (AMA) radically changed its position on the ideal range of blood chemistry values for cholesterol. The newer AMA recommendations are now much closer to my recommendations for levels One, Two, and Three of the Haas Maximum Performance Program. There is still room for improvement in the latest AMA recommendations, but that too will come with time. Still, the AMA has performed an important service to the American public by revising for the better its long-standing notions about ideal blood chemistry values.

Finally, when I cautioned active people that the U.S. RDA's for certain vitamins and minerals were too low in some cases, critics who still believed in the four-food-group concept ("You can get all the vitamins and minerals you need by selecting your foods from the four food groups") complained. Now the latest nutritional research has shown that active people do indeed need more of certain vitamins and minerals than the RDA's suggest. Most people cannot practically obtain all the nutrients they require for maximum performance and optimal health from food alone, no matter how well constructed their diet is.

HOW TO USE THE FRIENDLY FATS

In *Eat to Win,* I recommended that people use fish and fish oil supplements to help control their blood levels of cholesterol and triglycerides. All published research since that time has established that my recommendations were sound and effective. Certain oils derived from seafood have a beneficial effect in lowering the blood values of substances that increase our risk of heart attack, stroke, high blood pressure, and certain diet-related cancers. I call them the "friendly fats," and indeed they are. There is also evidence that monounsaturated oils—olive oil is the most common—may also exert a beneficial effect on serum cholesterol or, at the least, do not adversely affect it. That is why I recommend that you choose olive oil if you must use oil in any recipe or cooking technique. To reduce your intake of fat, I also recommend the use of PAM, a vegetable spray that provides only one gram of fat per application. PAM provides a very-low-fat alternative to cooking oil and makes it easy to enjoy sautéed or fried vegetables or other stove-top foods while still staying within the Haas-recommended guidelines. While some purists may take issue with the fact that PAM uses partially hydrogenated vegetable oil, I believe that it is a much healthier alternative than using larger amounts of most cooking oils to fry and sauté foods.

NUTRITIONAL SUPPLEMENTS AND THE HAAS DIET

A recent survey of registered dietitians has shown that despite the official nutritional dogma of the American Dietetic Association, which states that people can get all the nutrients they need from a "balanced" diet chosen from the four food groups (a concept that should have disappeared with the dinosaurs), *48 percent of registered dietitians surveyed now recommend nutritional supplements for their clients.*

Recent sports nutrition research has shown that *Eat to Win* was correct in stating that physical activity increases one's needs for vitamins and minerals (despite the protestations of critics). It can no longer be argued that active people don't require nutritional supplementation. The published facts have proved the opposite. Chapters Three and Four contain vital new information in this regard to help you be the best you can be, as does Appendix I.

More and more nutritionally aware physicians have begun to recommend nutritional supplements. Virtually every major medical/nutritional journal today contains research and communications from physicians and researchers who have determined that people can and should use nutritional supplements to prevent, manage, and even cure health problems. I predict that in the not too distant future, physicians will increasingly recommend over-the-counter nutritional formulas and supplements in place of the many less-than-healthful medications so commonly prescribed today. Several pharmaceutical companies, already aware of this trend, have begun aggressive marketing of vitamin/mineral supplements. Others are lobbying for legislation to make ordinary vitamin/mineral formulas available only by prescription. Such legislation could create enormous profits for the drug companies, increase the cost of nutritional supplements, place the prescribing of supplements in the hands of nutritionally untrained professionals, and deny you the right to manage your own health.

THE ASPARTAME CONTROVERSY AND THE HAAS DIET

When aspartame (Equal and NutraSweet) was introduced to American consumers shortly after receiving FDA approval, I recommended its use as a sugar substitute (while still permitting people to use real sugar, but in small quantities). Is aspartame really safe?

According to a recent and thorough investigation of all available evidence on the sweetener by the American Medical Association, aspartame has been judged to be safe. A recent AMA report, published in the *Journal of the American Medical Association* (July 19, 1985), supports the FDA's contention that the maximum projected intake of aspartame by most children and adults is far below any level even suspected of being toxic. When scientifically conservative organizations such as the American Medical Association and the Food and Drug Administration report that after careful study they judge aspartame to be safe for human consumption, that at least inspires confidence that aspartame and aspartame-containing products (Equal for direct consumer use and NutraSweet for use by food manufacturers in their products) pose no appreciable health threat. *And yet, neither the AMA nor the FDA has ever stated that sugar, at the present level of American consumption, is safe!*

It is estimated that as a nation we consume 125 pounds of sugar per capita per year. Unlike aspartame, sugar has been shown to raise serum cholesterol, blood fats, and uric acid, to compromise the effectiveness of the immune system, and to promote hypoglycemia and dental caries (cavities). If a public scare over table-top sweeteners is appropriate, it should be over sugar, not aspartame. Could sugar withstand more than ten years of careful scientific scrutiny, as aspartame has, and pass the AMA's and FDA's tests today? I think not. That's why Equal is *still* the table-top sweetener of choice on the Maximum Performance Diet.

HAVE A BLOOD CHEMISTRY PROFILE TODAY!

The Maximum Performance Diet contains four levels, and one of them is right for you. This is the most scientific approach to deciding which foods and recipes best suit your unique biological needs. But you first must have a simple blood chemistry profile made to determine whether you should begin at Level One, Two, or Three. This relatively quick and inexpensive test has already helped save millions of lives by alerting physicians to potential health hazards in time to prevent them in many cases.

If you don't discover your five vital values—total cholesterol, HDL cholesterol, triglycerides, sugar, and uric acid—then you are eating in the dark. This is valuable information you must know in order to help prevent serious health problems and achieve a high-quality, maximum performance life-style. Do yourself a favor. Visit a local health-testing center or see your physician and get a simple blood chemistry profile that measures these five vital values. It could well be the best money you ever spent.

THE OPTIMAL RANGES FOR YOUR FIVE VITAL VALUES

As you move from Level One, Two, or Three to *the new Maximum Performance Level Four,* you will find that the absolute amounts and total percentage of simple carbohydrates (sweets), protein, and fats will generally increase. However, complex carbohydrates (starches) will always provide the *greatest proportion* of your daily kilocalories. On the Haas Maximum Performance Program, starches always remain your *primary foods.*

LEVEL ONE BLOOD CHEMISTRY VALUES

If any one of your five vital values falls within the ranges listed below, begin with Level One:

Total cholesterol.	200 or more
HDL cholesterol	30 or less
Triglycerides	150 or more
Glucose	100 or more
Uric acid, women	6 or more
men	7 or more

Eat within these guidelines:

Total dietary cholesterol: no more than 75 milligrams per day
Total fats and oils: no more than 10 grams of fat per day
Total protein: no more than 50 grams per day
Liquid meal replacement (your favorite brand, any flavor—see Appendix II): up to two meals per day

Add your favorite brand of sports nutrition supplements (see Appendix I for recommended formulations).

LEVEL TWO BLOOD CHEMISTRY VALUES

Once you have achieved the following blood chemistry profile, move on to Level Two:

Total cholesterol.	160
HDL cholesterol	45 or more
Triglycerides	125–150
Glucose	85–95
Uric acid, women	5 or less
men	6 or less

Eat within these guidelines:

Total dietary cholesterol: no more than 100 milligrams per day
Total fats and oils: no more than 15 grams of fat per day
Total protein: no more than 60 grams per day
Liquid meal replacement (your favorite brand, any flavor—see Appendix II): up to two meals per day

Add your favorite brand of sports nutrition supplements (see Appendix I for recommended formulations).

LEVEL THREE BLOOD CHEMISTRY VALUES

Once you have achieved the following blood chemistry profile, move on to Level Three:

Total cholesterol. 130
HDL cholesterol . . . . 65 or more
Triglycerides . . . . 75 or less
Glucose . . . . 85 or less
Uric acid, women . . . . 4 or less
　　　　　 men . . . . 5 or less

Eat within these guidelines:

Total dietary cholesterol: no more than 150 milligrams per day
Total fats and oils: no more than 20 grams of fat per day
Total protein: no more than 65 grams per day
Liquid meal replacement (your favorite brand, any flavor—see Appendix II): up to two meals per day

Add your favorite brand of sports nutrition supplements (see Appendix I for recommended formulations).

LEVEL FOUR BLOOD CHEMISTRY VALUES

Once you have achieved the following blood chemistry profile, move on to Level Four:

Total cholesterol . . . . 120 or below
HDL cholesterol . . . . 70 or more
Triglycerides . . . . 70 or less
Glucose . . . . 70 or less
Uric acid, women . . . . 3.5 or less
　　　　　 men . . . . 4.0 or less

Eat within these guidelines:

Total dietary cholesterol: no more than 150 milligrams per day
Total fats and oils: no more than 25 grams of fat per day
Total protein: no more than 70 grams per day

Liquid meal replacement (your favorite brand, any flavor—see Appendix II): up to two meals per day

Add your favorite brand of sports nutrition supplements (see Appendix I for recommended formulations).

THE HAAS MAXIMUM PERFORMANCE 28-DAY EAT-AT-HOME DIET

The Maximum Performance Diet is well known for its delicious low-calorie/low-fat/low-cholesterol recipes. In keeping with that tradition and your expectations, Hilarie Porter, M.S., has once again outdone herself and created over 100 new peak performance recipes.

If you enjoy easy-to-make gourmet food that promotes better health, energy, and vitality, you'll enjoy these daily menus I've put together for eating at home. These menus are ideal for entertaining at home because your guests will never know they are eating "healthy" foods—foods that help lower their risk of diet-related maladies such as heart disease, cancer, high blood pressure, diabetes, and obesity.

Each daily menu is based on Haas-approved *Eat to Succeed* recipes, which are marked with an asterisk and are contained in the recipe section in this book. Each recipe includes a nutritional breakdown per serving for six nutrient values: calories, protein, fat, carbohydrate, cholesterol, and sodium. This means that you can enjoy these recipes on the Haas Maximum Performance Diet and/or the Haas Maximum Weight-Loss Program because you know whether a dish's caloric and nutritional values fall within the recommended guidelines for each level—One to Four—of the diet. If you are following a physician-prescribed low-sodium or low-cholesterol diet, for example, simply add up those values and determine which recipes meet your dietary needs.

You may enjoy the daily menus as often as you wish. Mix and match them if you choose, *but always take note of their nutritional content*. By doing this, you will not over-consume protein, fat, cholesterol, calories, or sodium.

Since many of these delicious and filling recipes probably provide less calories than you're accustomed to eating, you may begin to lose weight just by substituting them for your usual meals, depending upon your unique metabolism. If you wish to maintain or gain weight, simply adjust the portion size of each recipe you eat (while paying attention to its nutritional values) to achieve the body weight at which you feel best. *Use the nutritional values given with each recipe and those listed in tables in the food composition section of this book to help you select the proper amounts of your favorite recipes and foods.*

You will find helpful cooking and shopping tips to make eating to succeed at home easily manageable at the beginning of Section II of this book. Note in particular the recommendations to:

• Use PAM vegetable cooking spray instead of vegetable oil, margarine, or butter whenever possible for nonstick, tasty cooking.
• Use Equal brand low-calorie sweetener as a sugar substitute.

THE HAAS MAXIMUM PERFORMANCE RECOMMENDED FOOD LIST

Recommended Complex Carbohydrate Foods

Use these foods in amounts consistent with your level of the Haas Maximum Performance Diet. Complex carbohydrates should always supply the majority of your daily kilocalories. If you are trying to lose weight, follow the Haas Maximum Weight-Loss Diet in Chapter Six.

Oatmeal	Whole-grain bread	Whole wheat flour
Rice flour	(made without egg yolk)	White potatoes
Shredded wheat	Sourdough bread	Brown rice
Millet	Puffed brown rice	Sweet potatoes
Cornmeal	Whole-grain pasta	Cornstarch
Whole-grain noodles	Corn	Arrowroot

Recommended Complex Carbohydrate Vegetables

In general, enjoy vegetables as you desire. Limit your intake of beans, peas, or lentils to two cups each day, so as not to exceed your protein limit.

Broccoli	Green peas	Mustard, turnip,
Zucchini	Artichoke	and/or collard greens
Cucumber	Tomato	Chickpeas
Cabbage	Cauliflower	Navy beans
Pinto beans	Lettuce (all types)	Kidney beans
Lima beans	Peppers	Pinto beans
Lentils	Carrots	

Recommended Dairy Foods

Up to two cups per day may be used (if desired).

Skim milk	Cottage cheese (up to 1% fat)
Nonfat dry milk	Plain yogurt (up to 2% fat)
Buttermilk (up to 1% fat)	

Recommended Oils

Use these oils to enhance the flavor of foods or to reduce blood fats, but do not exceed the limits set by your level of the Haas Maximum Performance Diet.

Marine oils such as eicosapentanoic acid (EPA) and docosahexanoic acid (DHA) (from salmon, mackerel, lobster, vegetables)

Olive oil (extra virgin type)

Recommended Condiments, Sauces, Toppings

These can be eaten as desired within reason. Limit soy sauce, steak sauce, barbecue sauce, ketchup, and Worcestershire sauce to *one tablespoon per day.*

Vinegar (any type)	Tabasco sauce
Lemon juice	Taco sauce
Lime juice	Tamari soy sauce
Wines (sherry, sauternes,	(dilute 50:50 with water)
vermouth, red, white)	Tomato paste or sauce
Mustard (including Dijon)	Salsa (made without avocado)
Uncreamed horseradish	Ketchup
Vanilla or lemon extract	Vegit
Worcestershire sauce	Mrs. Dash
Steak sauce (e.g., A-1 brand)	All herbs and spices
Barbecue sauce	Any no-oil dressing

LEVEL ONE
DAY 1

BREAKFAST
*Apples and Brown Cereal
Beverage

LUNCH
*Pasta e Fagioli (1 cup)
Salad with approved dressing (unlimited)
Beverage

DINNER
*½ Turkey-Stuffed Potato
Steamed vegetables (unlimited)
Salad with approved dressing (unlimited)
*½" slice Banana Nut Loaf Cake
Beverage

DAY 2

BREAKFAST
Approved whole grain cereal with ½ cup skim milk
½ sliced banana or ¼ cup raisins
Beverage

LUNCH
*Spinach Salad
½ whole wheat bagel or 1 slice whole wheat bread
Beverage

DINNER
8 ounces freshly cooked pasta† with
*Eggplant Sauce
Salad with approved dressing (unlimited)
*½" slice Banana Nut Loaf Cake
Beverage

*Recipe appears in Section II.
†Use 4 ounces dry pasta—it will double in weight when cooked.

DAY 3

BREAKFAST
Oatmeal with ½ sliced banana or ¼ cup raisins
Beverage

LUNCH
*Lentil Barley Soup (1 cup)
Salad with approved dressing (unlimited)
Beverage

DINNER
*Chicken and Broccoli Stir Fry
Salad with approved dressing (unlimited)
1 fruit

DAY 4

BREAKFAST
2 slices whole wheat bread or 1 whole wheat bagel
*Applesauce (½ cup)
Beverage

LUNCH
*1 Chicken Curry Muffin
Salad with approved dressing (unlimited)
Beverage

DINNER
*Broiled Shrimp
Steamed vegetables and brown rice
Salad with approved dressing (unlimited)
1 fruit

*Recipe appears in Section II.

DAY 5

BREAKFAST
*Need-No-Syrup Banana Pancakes (2)
Beverage

LUNCH
*Chickpea and Pasta Salad (1 cup)
Whole wheat bagel or 2 slices whole wheat bread
1 fruit
Beverage

DINNER
*½ Turkey-Stuffed Potato
Steamed vegetables
Salad with approved dressing (unlimited)
*1" square Apple Cake

DAY 6

BREAKFAST
*Mushroom Onion Scramble
1 slice whole wheat toast or ½ whole wheat bagel with
*1 tablespoon Fruit Spread
Beverage

LUNCH
*Chicken Fried Rice
Salad with approved dressing (unlimited)
1 fruit
Beverage

DINNER
*½ Neptune's Potato
Salad with approved dressing (unlimited)
*1 Sweet Potato Muffin
Beverage

*Recipe appears in Section II.

DAY 7

BREAKFAST
*Cinnamon French Toast (2 slices)
*Applesauce (½ cup)
Beverage

LUNCH
*Chunky Chicken Noodle Soup (1 cup)
Salad with approved dressing (unlimited)
Beverage

DINNER
*Baked Cannellini
Salad with approved dressing (unlimited)
1 fruit
Beverage

DAY 8

BREAKFAST
*1 Sweet Potato Muffin
1 fruit
Beverage

LUNCH
*Potato Pancakes (3)
Salad with approved dressing (unlimited)
Beverage

DINNER
*Chicken Brown Rice Pie
Steamed vegetable platter
Salad with approved dressing (unlimited)
*½" slice Pumpkin Apple Bread
Beverage

*Recipe appears in Section II.

DAY 9

BREAKFAST
2 slices whole wheat toast or 1 whole wheat bagel with
*1 tablespoon Fruit Spread
Beverage

LUNCH
*Black Bean Soup (1 cup)
Salad with approved dressing (unlimited)
1 fruit
Beverage

DINNER
*Rolled Stuffed Eggplant (2–3 rolls)
Salad with approved dressing (unlimited)
*1 Banana Date Muffin
Beverage

DAY 10

BREAKFAST
*½" slice Bran Date Bread
1 fruit
Beverage

LUNCH
*Carrot Salad Waldorf (1 cup)
1 slice whole wheat bread or ½ whole wheat bagel
Beverage

DINNER
*Quick Tomato Sauce over 8 ounces freshly cooked pasta†
Salad with approved dressing (unlimited)
1 fruit
Beverage

*Recipe appears in Section II.
†Use 4 ounces dry pasta—it will double in weight when cooked.

DAY 11

BREAKFAST
*Corn Cakes (2)
*Applesauce (½ cup)
Beverage

LUNCH
*Hearty Vegetable Soup (1 cup)
Salad with approved dressing (unlimited)
Beverage

DINNER
*Ziti Casserole
Salad with approved dressing (unlimited)
*½" slice Fruitcake
Beverage

DAY 12

BREAKFAST
*½" slice Pumpkin Apple Bread
1 fruit
Beverage

LUNCH
*Tuna Bean Salad
1 fruit
Beverage

DINNER
*Corn and Brown Rice Stir Fry
Salad with approved dressing (unlimited)
*½" slice Pumpkin Apple Bread
Beverage

*Recipe appears in Section II.

DAY 13

BREAKFAST
*Hot Brown Rice Cereal
Beverage

LUNCH
Baked potato
Salad with approved dressing (unlimited)
1 fruit
Beverage

DINNER
*Vegetable Rice Casserole
Salad with approved dressing (unlimited)
*Pumpkin Brown Rice Cereal (½ cup)

DAY 14

BREAKFAST
*Cheddar Scramble
1 slice whole wheat toast
Beverage

LUNCH
*Vegetable Potato Salad (1 cup)
1 fruit
Beverage

DINNER
*Black Bean and Rice Casserole
*Squash Amandine
1 fruit
Beverage

*Recipe appears in Section II.

DAY 15

Repeat breakfast menu given for the first fourteen days for days 15 through 28.

LUNCH
*Tabbouleh
1 fruit
Beverage

DINNER
*Baked Barley
Salad with approved dressing (unlimited)
*½" slice Banana Nut Loaf Cake
Beverage

DAY 16

LUNCH
*Split Pea Soup (1 cup)
Salad with approved dressing (unlimited)
1 fruit
Beverage

DINNER
*Mexican Rice (1 cup)
*Apple Raisin Salad (½ cup)
Steamed vegetable platter
Beverage

*Recipe appears in Section II.

DAY 17

LUNCH
*Chickpea and Pasta Salad (1 cup)
1 slice whole wheat bread or ½ whole wheat bagel
1 fruit
Beverage

DINNER
*Poached Salmon
*Carrot Casserole (½ cup)
Salad with approved dressing (unlimited)
1 fruit
Beverage

DAY 18

LUNCH
*Corn Chowder (1 cup)
Salad with approved dressing (unlimited)
Beverage

DINNER
Baked potato topped with
*Garden Dip
Steamed vegetables (unlimited)
*Pumpkin Brown Rice Pudding (½ cup)
Beverage

*Recipe appears in Section II.

DAY 19

LUNCH
*Squash Amandine (1 cup)
*Hash Brown Potatoes
1 fruit
Beverage

DINNER
*Noodles Romanoff
Salad with approved dressing (unlimited)
*1 Cherry Almond Muffin
Beverage

DAY 20

LUNCH
*Cauliflower Broccoli Salad (1 cup)
*Mashed Potatoes (½ cup)
1 fruit
Beverage

DINNER
*Indian Rice Casserole (1 cup)
Salad with approved dressing (unlimited)
1 fruit
Beverage

*Recipe appears in Section II.

DAY 21

LUNCH
*Grape and Chicken Salad
1 slice whole wheat bread or ½ whole wheat bagel
1 fruit
Beverage

DINNER
*Broccoli Macaroni Bake (1 cup)
Salad with approved dressing (unlimited)
*1 Cherry Almond Muffin
Beverage

DAY 22

LUNCH
*Baked Lentils (1 cup)
Salad with approved dressing (unlimited)
1 fruit
Beverage

DINNER
*Onion Potato Pie
Steamed vegetable platter
Salad with approved dressing (unlimited)
1 fruit

*Recipe appears in Section II.

DAY 23

LUNCH
*Cucumber and Onion Dip with assorted raw vegetables (¼ cup)
*Shrimp Cocktail
1 fruit
Beverage

DINNER
*Zucchini and Cauliflower Italian, served over 8 ounces brown rice
    or freshly cooked pasta†
Salad with approved dressing (unlimited)
1 fruit
Beverage

DAY 24

LUNCH
*Oriental Salad
1 fruit
Beverage

DINNER
*Tomato Broccoli Pie
Baked potato
Salad with approved dressing (unlimited)
1 fruit
Beverage

---

*Recipe appears in Section II.
†Use 4 ounces dry rice or pasta—it will double in weight when cooked.

DAY 25

LUNCH
*Carrot Salad Waldorf
1 slice whole wheat bread or ½ whole wheat bagel
Beverage

DINNER
*Sweet Potato Discipio (1 potato)
Salad with approved dressing (unlimited)
*½" slice Fruitcake
Beverage

DAY 26

LUNCH
*Chicken Salad Supreme
1 fruit
Beverage

DINNER
*Navy Bean Soup (1 cup)
Salad with approved dressing (unlimited)
1 fruit
Beverage

*Recipe appears in Section II.

DAY 27

LUNCH
*Potatoes Parmesan
Salad with approved dressing (unlimited)
1 fruit
Beverage

DINNER
*Zucchini Corn Casserole
Salad with approved dressing (unlimited)
*½" slice Pumpkin Apple Bread
Beverage

DAY 28

LUNCH
*Corn Salad (1 cup)
1 slice whole wheat bread or ½ whole wheat bagel
1 fruit
Beverage

DINNER
*Potato Cheese Bake (1 slice)
Salad with approved dressing (unlimited)
1 fruit
Beverage

*Recipe appears in Section II.

LEVEL TWO:
ADDITIONAL RECIPES*

Your blood chemistry profile determines the level at which you should be eating. Refer back to the tables on pages 42–44 for the eating guidelines to follow at your level.

When changing levels, your food intake can be increased *up to the limits* indicated in the guidelines for the next level. The additional recipes indicated here and for levels Three and Four are suggested substitutions for dishes in the same food category given in the Level One menu plan. However, *do not make wholesale substitutions* down the line. Refer to the Nutritional Information Per Serving indicated in Section II for the recipes provided (or refer to the *Eat to Succeed* Food Composition Tables in Section III) to ensure that nutrient intake remains within the guidelines established for your level.

In addition to substituting recipes listed here or below for levels Three and Four, you may choose to increase the serving size of dishes recommended for Level One. Just be sure that you *take the added nutrient content into account* in each case. Whether substituting recipes or increasing the size of servings, your total nutrient intake must stay within the guidelines given for your level. Section III of this book has been specially provided so that you can also incorporate other foods into your diet *judiciously* and observe the nutrient guidelines for your level.

BREAKFAST
Corn Cakes

APPETIZERS
Crabmeat Dip

SALADS AND
SALAD DRESSINGS
Lobster Salad
Shrimp Salad

SIDE DISHES
Creamed Corn

ENTRÉES
Cornish Hens
Rice-Stuffed Green Peppers
Stuffed Shells

SAUCES AND SPREADS
Apple Cranberry Sauce
Pesto

*All recipes given in Section II.

BREADS AND MUFFINS
Pecan Cranberry Bread

DESSERTS
Fruitcake

LEVEL THREE AND LEVEL FOUR: ADDITIONAL RECIPES*

BREAKFAST
Hawaiian Pancakes
Nova Scramble

APPETIZERS
Onion Dip
Salmon Spread

ENTRÉES
Chicken Tetrazzini
Chili
Creamy Lasagna
Veal Lasagna
Veal-Stuffed Eggplant

BREADS AND MUFFINS
Sesame Sweet Bread

DESSERTS
All-in-One Apple Pie
Brownie Cakes
Carob Nut Loaf
Fudgies
Merv's Favorite Chocolate-Covered
   Cherry Cake
Pineapple Upside-Down Cake
Pumpkin Brown Rice Pudding
Raspberry Preserve Bars

*All recipes given in Section II.

SIX

The Haas Maximum
Weight-Loss Program

Here, at last, is a weight-loss plan you can succeed on because it works while you work—and play. I've designed it for people like myself, who normally have such sluggish metabolisms that we can't seem to lose weight unless we eat less than 800 kilocalories a day (that's *less* than the amount of kilocalories *in the average American dinner*) and exercise.

The Haas Maximum Weight-Loss Program provides about 800 delicious kilocalories each day so that you'll lose body fat regardless of your age, sex, or body type. This means that you can enjoy dining in or out on pasta, potatoes, corn, salads, Haas-style milkshakes and other desserts, and still be able to lower your body fat—permanently.

It is now possible to enjoy eating more delicious and nutritious foods than traditional weight-loss diets allow and still stay slender for life if you use the plan I'm going to reveal in this chapter. Over a half-century of research on weight-loss schemes and products has convincingly demonstrated that very few people ever successfully lose the weight they want *and* keep it off. I believe that once you understand why these methods fail, you will understand why and how you can successfully and permanently lose that "tire" tummy or those "thunder" thighs that increase your chances of suffering from heart disease, cancer, arthritis, stroke, and diabetes.

HOW THE PROGRAM WORKS

The weight-loss program introduced here works because it uses three primary elements that insure prompt weight loss and maximum energy.

• A specially formulated liquid meal replacer that contains a scientific blend of fiber, protein, carbohydrate, energy vitamins, and minerals

• Complex carbohydrate foods, the kind that world class athletes uses to fuel the fires of strength, energy, and stamina while staying slim

• fat-burning, high-energy nutrients such as L-carnitine, Co-enzyme Q_{10}, and the branched chain amino acids to help speed up weight loss while maintaining muscle if you are inactive or while building muscle if you enjoy sports and exercise.

LIQUID MEAL REPLACERS: PAST AND PRESENT

The modern era of American weight loss began in 1959, when Mead Johnson introduced Metrecal, a meal replacement powder that, when mixed with water, tasted pretty much like powder mixed with water. Each glass full of this mixture contained 300 kilocalories, and the recommended weight-loss plan called for three servings per day for a total of 900 kilocalories. Unfortunately, even though Metrecal's sales grew, so did the bodies of a weight-conscious American public. We remained a nation of fatties.

By 1977, a new generation of still-overweight Americans tried other liquid and powdered weight loss meals and snacks: Sego (made by PET) and Carnation's Instant Breakfast (later rechristened as a lower-calorie product, Slender); that was the *good news* for frustrated fatties. But still we remained a nation of unsuccessful, overweight dieters, and the bad news came two years later. Its name was liquid protein.

THE HIGH-PROTEIN, LOW-CALORIE NUTRITIONAL NIGHTMARE

Americans, clearly losing their battle for girth control, eagerly embraced a new weight-loss product that would eventually become known as the Black Friday of the weight-loss industry. The dieter's doomsday was set in motion with the publication of a best-selling diet book that promoted the use of a protein drink derived from the breakdown of animal connective tissue (collagen hydrolysate).

According to the Center for Disease Control, at least sixty dieters died mysteriously while following the 300- to 400-kilocalorie liquid protein regimen. In seventeen cases of fatality involving people who had used liquid protein as the sole source of nutrition for two months or longer, investigators determined there was no sign of any disease that would otherwise account for their untimely deaths. Subsequent investigations revealed evidence that ventricular arrhythmias (electrical disruptions in the heart that cause it to beat asynchronously and eventually fail) were the immediate cause of death, probably due to the exclusive ingestion of liquid protein.

Prominent coverage by the news media of the liquid protein–associated fatalities that occurred in 1977–78, coupled with warnings issued by the Food and Drug Administration, led to the almost overnight cessation of the liquid protein craze. Although subsequent investigations into the deaths associated with liquid protein use have never fully determined the precise cause of death, many scientists believe that liquid protein diets as well as very-low-calorie diets consisting solely of protein should be discouraged. The questionable safety of high-protein/low-calorie diets should concern dieters who use some of the newer over-the-counter (OTC) very-low-calorie weight-loss plans that are popular today.

THE VALUE OF LIQUID MEAL REPLACERS IN WEIGHT LOSS

Liquid meal replacers, used in conjunction with solid foods and meals, remain a feature of some of the most popular weight-loss plans today. Liquid meal replacers are currently marketed as powders to be reconstituted as beverages, soups, or desserts. In contrast to the now generally abandoned liquid protein products (which, surprisingly, are still available as OTC diet products), these new diet powders contain high-quality protein, vitamins, complex and simple carbohydrates, trace minerals, and even fiber, none of which were used in the original liquid protein products. The popularity of liquid meal replacers is reflected by their sales—well over 5 million Americans gulped down one brand (The Cambridge Diet) within the first two years it was introduced to the United States. *This represents a rate of use at least twenty-five times higher than the rate reported with the original liquid protein products.*

Many manufacturers of the newer weight-loss meal replacers have learned a lesson from the liquid protein tragedy. Their new formulations can help dieters avoid the potential health problems associated with the nutritionally incomplete original formulas. Here are the essentials you should look for before you choose a low-calorie meal replacer (and I'll help you do that in the next section):

• *Protein.* A high-quality protein source—from nonfat dry milk or egg white—is an essential for any meal replacement formula. Each serving should contain neither too much nor too little protein. Powdered meal replacer products should provide between 15 and 20 grams of high-quality protein per serving. This amount of protein, in conjunction with essential carbohydrates (the second most important constituent of a top-quality meal replacer), will help keep your body from digesting its own vital protein (from organs and muscles) during weight loss.

• *Carbohydrate.* The primary complex carbohydrate you should look for is called *maltodextrin.* (Several popular meal replacers use this as the primary source of carbohydrate.) Complex carbohydrates from maltodextrin, as well as from the starches, such as pasta and potatoes, that you will enjoy on the Haas Maximum Performance Weight-Loss Program, actually help *reduce* your daily protein requirements, because carbohydrates spare the body's limited store of protein for essential uses instead of burning protein for energy.

Meal replacers may also contain simple carbohydrates for sweetness, and the best natural sweetener tested to date is fructose. Fructose has special properties that render it preferable to sucrose (common table sugar). Various sugars have differing effects on how well muscles store glycogen—stored energy in the form of a carbohydrate produced within the body. Stored glycogen is like money in the bank to anyone who wants a reserve of energy. Fructose-containing meal replacers are much better than glucose-containing products, because the former promote glycogen storage and result in a much lower rate of muscle glycogen depletion, without requiring insulin to enter the muscle cells. Since insulin can promote glycogen depletion and lead to fatigue from low blood sugar, select meal replacers that use either fructose or aspartame (NutraSweet) as a sweetener.

• *Minerals and trace minerals.* The meal replacement product you choose must contain vital minerals such as calcium, magnesium, iron, and zinc for strong bones, proper muscular function, healthy blood, a strong immune system, and general good health. But you also need trace minerals such as manganese, chromium, selenium, and molybdenum to protect against heart disease, diabetes, and diet-related or environmentally induced cancers. While the body requires trace minerals in much smaller amounts than minerals like calcium or magnesium, they are just as vital as any other class of nutrients.

• *Fiber.* Fiber is essential for maintaining optimal intestinal and cardiovascular health. The meal replacement product you select should contain the *right* type of fiber, one that helps to lower serum cholesterol and blood fats as well as improve bowel function. Water-soluble fibers such as oat bran, soy bran, and guar gum help you excrete cholesterol and its related metabolic products as well as carcinogenic waste products manufactured by bacteria that ordinarily live in your intestine. The type of fiber that stimulates proper bowel function and elimination, psyllium seed husks, for example, should be present in any first-rate meal replacer.

Should you use a liquid meal replacer to help you lose weight and keep it off permanently? Today's nutritionally balanced meal replacers permit safe and effective weight loss without the risk of nutritional deficiency *as long as you do not use them as your sole source of nutrition and as long as you consume at least 800 kilocalo-*

ries each day from meal replacers and solid, well-balanced foods. Here's why.

Liquid protein and other very-low-calorie regimens share a common danger. Research has documented that the death rate in people on liquid protein weight-loss plans may not be significantly different from that in people who, *under a physician's supervision,* follow a very-low-calorie, high-quality protein regimen supplemented with vitamins and minerals. This suggests that the *total amount of daily kilocalories is just as important* as the protein quality, vitamins, and minerals in any weight-loss regimen. That is why the Haas Maximum Weight-Loss Program is *not* a very-low-calorie plan (500 or less kilocalories per day), but rather a nutritionally complete plan that relies on the scientific and prudent combination of a nutritious meal replacer and solid foods and meals eaten at home or in restaurants. The Haas Maximum Weight-Loss Program provides maximum weight loss at a safe and effective rate. The use of nutritionally fortified meal replacers and nutritional supplements insures maximum performance.

PICKING THE PROPER MEAL REPLACER

There are a number of liquid meal replacers now on the market that may be used in conjunction with a daily solid meal or meals. Among those I found available in supermarkets, groceries, health food outlets, and some pharmacies are:

TwinSport Endurance Meal
    Replacement & Weight
    Control Formula
Your Life Natural Weight Loss
    Plan
Slim Fast
Dietene
Ensure

Carnation Do-It-Yourself Diet
    Plan
Pillsbury Instant Breakfast
Carnation Instant Breakfast
Slender Diet Meal for Weight
    Control
Meritene

You will find a detailed breakdown of the formulation, calorie count, and nutrient content of each of these products in Appendix II.

THE HAAS MAXIMUM WEIGHT-LOSS PLAN
FOR EATING IN AND OUT

My clients have achieved successful weight loss by following this simple plan, at home or out, whenever they want to shed unwanted body fat quickly and safely. Use your favorite liquid meal replacer for one or two meals each day, *but always eat at least one solid meal*.

BREAKFAST

1 serving of your favorite brand of meal replacer (see list above and Appendix II)

or

1 Haas breakfast recipe (see cookbook section) *and* 1 glass Endurance brand QuickFix drink (or make your own by using a low-calorie fruit-type dry beverage mix made with NutraSweet—e.g., Crystal Light, Wyler's lemonade, or Country Time lemonade—and adding the contents of your favorite multivitamin/mineral capsule to the mix before adding water)

LUNCH

1 serving of your favorite brand of meal replacer

or

1 Haas entrée recipe

or

1 approved restaurant entrée (see eating-out guidelines later in this chapter)

or

1 baked potato with Haas-approved topping, plus a large mixed salad with no-oil dressing

DINNER

1 serving of your favorite brand of meal replacer

or

1 Haas entrée recipe

or

1 approved restaurant entrée (see eating-out guidelines later in this chapter)

plus the following:

1 glass Endurance brand QuickFix or your own low-calorie substitute formula
A large garden salad with no oil dressing
Any green, orange, or yellow vegetable (approximately ½ to 1 cup serving)
1 fresh fruit (e.g., banana, papaya, apple, a half grapefruit, or orange). However, avoid avocado.

SUPPLEMENTS

TwinSport Endurance brand Anabolic Formula on an empty stomach (see package label to determine dosage)

or

You may formulate your own anabolic formula, as long as you avoid supplements that contain objectionable contaminants such as artificial colors and flavors. Here is a suggested formula, per capsule:

L-arginine	225 mg.
L-ornithine	225 mg.
Branched chain amino acids (isoleucine, leucine, and valine)	225 mg.
Vitamin B-6	5 mg.
Pantothenic acid	10 mg.

plus

TwinSport Endurance brand Diet Aid capsules with each meal. These contain additional fiber to reduce blood levels of cholesterol and fat and to promote intestinal health and optimal bowel function. They are not the appetite-suppressant-type of capsules that contain the potentially dangerous drug phenylpropanolamine. See package label to determine dosage. A suitable self-formulated substitute is virtually impossible to prepare in this case.

plus

1 TwinSport Endurance Fitness Pak or other brand multivitamin/ mineral pack taken at breakfast or lunch (not both).

SNACKS

One snack each day is permitted, as long as it is on the following list:

2 cups of popcorn (hot-air popped is preferred)
1 cup unsweetened applesauce
2 puffed brown rice cakes with unsweetened apple butter
1 serving of any Haas recipe snack (see Section II)
4-ounce serving of low-fat frozen yogurt
1 serving of any of the following cereals with ½ cup skim or nonfat
    dry milk (use Equal sugar substitute if you desire additional
    sweetener):

Shredded wheat	Quaker 100% Whole Wheat
Grape Nuts	Nutri-Grain
Oatmeal	Health Valley cereals
Wheatena	Erewhon cereals

An average day on the Haas Maximum Weight-Loss Program provides the following nutrition:

Calories	900	Fat	5 grams
Protein	45 grams	Cholesterol	20 milligrams
Carbohydrates	170 grams		

Caloric breakdown: 75% carbohydrate, 20% protein, 5% fat, and over 100 percent of the U.S. RDA for vitamins and minerals

Please note that on reduced-calorie weight-loss plans, a more generous protein intake of 15 to 20 percent of daily kilocalories is permitted. Once weight maintenance is begun, protein intake normally returns within the range of 10 to 15 percent of daily kilocalories.

ESSENTIAL GUIDELINES
FOR SUCCESSFUL WEIGHT LOSS

There are five *iron-clad* Haas Maximum Weight-Loss Program guidelines to follow that will help you eat to succeed:

1. Always eat *at least* 800 kilocalories each day, from liquid meal replacers and conventional foods. The bulk of scientific evidence indicates that consuming any less than 800 kilocalories may pose health risks similar to those experienced by liquid protein users. Research has shown that medically supervised, very-low-calorie diets, even those supplemented with vitamins, minerals, and fiber, do not provide the body with enough kilocalories to sustain optimal health. The mortality rate associated with these diets does not differ appreciably from that associated with the infamous liquid protein diet. The message is clear. You must consume *800 or more* kilocalories each day of highly nutritious meals (solid and liquid) that contain high-quality protein, trace minerals, fiber, and supplementary vitamins and minerals.

2. Never use liquid meal replacers as the *sole source* of nutrition. The human body was designed to function best on a *combination* of solids and liquids. Achieving and maintaining peak health during the relatively stressful period of weight loss depends on supplying the body with nutrition-dense foods and supplemental nutrients.

3. Maintain a regular exercise regimen, such as brisk walking, climbing stairs, cycling, swimming, jogging, racquet sports, martial arts, rowing, skiing, or other aerobic activity that elevates your heart rate to 120 beats per minute or more and generally causes you to break a sweat. Physical activity or sports should last a minimum of thirty continuous minutes, with at least an additional five-minute warm-up and cool-down period.

Regular aerobic exercise provides important benefits to the cardiovascular system, skeletal system, muscular system, and brain. Combined with the Haas Maximum Performance Program, it can help prevent and reverse the symptoms of common degenerative diseases, as well as keep you younger and fitter. Research studies have clearly established that diet and exercise can positively prevent many of the degenerative effects of aging that scientists formerly believed were inevitable.

During periods of reduced caloric intake, you should not increase your normal level of regular aerobic activity, but rather try to maintain it as you reduce your intake of calories. The double benefits of exercise and reduced calorie intake for weight reduction may seem obvious, but there is also a hidden benefit. Exercise seems to establish a new level of metabolism, one that permits you to continue to lose weight, if you desire, and keep it off *after* you've gradually increased your caloric intake back to normal levels.

4. Use liquid meal replacers occasionally as snacks or desserts after you have reached your desired weight. In the cookbook section, I have provided dessert-type drinks made from liquid meal replacers that provide a nutritious alternative to conventional high-fat, high-calorie treats. Even though you may have succeeded in reaching your desired weight, you may still use liquid meal replacers as tasty treats to enhance the nutritional value of the Haas Maximum Performance Diet.

5. Always consult with your physician before you begin any weight loss or dietary regimen. Even though most physicians receive little or no nutritional training, many of them have begun to study nutrition and incorporate nutritional treatments into their medical practices. My own physician, for example, now regularly studies the nutritional literature and often uses diet instead of drugs to treat diet-related health problems. Even if your own personal physician does not practice clinical nutrition, he or she will still be able to advise you whether or not you should undertake a weight-loss or special dietary program based on your medical history and present state of health.

My advice on this matter: Do yourself a favor. If you don't have a nutritionally aware physician, shop around until you find one.

GENERAL EATING-OUT GUIDELINES

Use liquid meal replacers for breakfast and one other meal. Eat a solid-food lunch or dinner consisting of any appropriate Haas menu or entrée suggestion from the following eating-out list:

• *Chicken or turkey* (baked, broiled, or barbecued): 3½ ounces. *Always* remove the fatty skin before eating poultry.

• *Lobster tail* (steamed, broiled, or boiled without butter): 4 ounces after removing shell. Serve with lemon juice and/or red cocktail sauce.

• *Fish* (baked, broiled, boiled, or grilled): 4 ounces any type. Choose salmon or mackerel because they are rich in EPA (eicosapentanoic acid) and other marine oils that help lower serum cholesterol and blood fats.

• *Pasta* (spaghetti, linguini, macaroni, mostacelli, etc; choose whole-grain varieties whenever possible): up to 1½ cups of cooked pasta with marinara, tomato, or red clam sauce with up to 1 tablespoon grated Parmesan or Romano cheese.

• *Bean burrito* (made with vegetable oil, not lard): one only, *without* sour cream, guacamole, or cheese.

• *Baked potato* with butter substitute topping (such as Butter Buds), or use low-fat cottage cheese, plain low-fat yogurt, or low-sodium condiments such as Vegit or Mrs. Dash as toppings.

• *Turkey or chicken:* 4 ounces on a sandwich made with rye or whole-grain bread (sourdough is permitted) with unlimited lettuce, tomato, onions, peppers, mushrooms, sprouts

• *Bean, pea, or lentil soup:* 8- to 12-ounce bowl

Additional Suggestions

• Use Equal sweetener as a table-top sweetener instead of sugar or saccharin-containing sugar substitutes.

• Use Vegit or Mrs. Dash as a condiment in place of table salt.

• Use mustard as a condiment for sandwiches instead of high-fat spreads like mayonnaise, vegetable oil, butter, or margarine.

• Use QuickFix or another fruit-type beverage made with Nutra-Sweet if you desire a sweet-tasting beverage.

• Use low-sodium bottled mineral water, such as Perrier, whenever you desire water.

• Use alcohol, including light beer, wine, and hard liquor, no more than twice a week in the following quantities:

Light beer: 24 ounces per week
Wine (red or white): two 3½-ounce glasses per week
Hard liquor (e.g., vodka): 3 ounces per week

One type of alcoholic beverage and the corresponding permitted amount may be substituted for another type of alcoholic beverage— e.g., one light beer (12 ounces) = one 3½-ounce glass of wine = 1½ ounces hard liquor.

• Use fresh garden salads with a variety of vegetables with a no-oil dressing (commercial brand or Haas recipe) at least once each day whenever possible.

• If you require additional calories on any given day (e.g., if your level of physical activity increases), select additional foods from the complex carbohydrate group. These foods include all whole grains, cereals, vegetables, fruits (but avoid avocado and olives whenever possible), pasta, potatoes, and whole-grain breads.

APPETITE SUPPRESSANTS

Appetite suppressants are drugs, and in my opinion their use constitutes abuse. I'm not especially concerned about prescription medications used to curb appetite, since most physicians refuse to prescribe them because they are potentially dangerous and because dieters usually develop a tolerance to them after one or two weeks. Nonprescription appetite suppressants pose the greatest threat to dieters, because they have a much larger abuse potential. Anyone can buy them in just about every supermarket and drugstore in this country.

The active ingredient in these appetite suppressants is called *phenylpropanolamine*. To the untrained eye, the chemical structure of phenylpropanolamine is barely distinguishable from that of amphetamine (speed) and for good reason. There is only one atom of oxygen that distinguishes amphetamine from phenylpropanolamine.

In the body, phenylpropanolamine acts like weak amphetamine. It can speed up the heart rate, increase blood pressure, and precipitate anxiety attacks, chest pain, nausea, dizziness, and heart palpitations. Dieters usually become immune to its appetite-suppressing effect in a matter of days to weeks after they begin using it.

No scientific study ever has proven that appetite suppressants containing phenylpropanolamine work in the long run. However, there are many published reports in the medical literature that have documented the potentially harmful effects of this drug in humans. Phenylpropanolamine is on my "don't take" list of diet aids, and I hope it's on yours as well.

A SAMPLE 14-DAY
MAXIMUM WEIGHT-LOSS MENU PLAN

For additional variety and convenience, here is a two-week weight-loss plan based exclusively on Haas recipes and your favorite brand of meal replacer. Choose your favorite meal replacer for breakfast and one other meal, either lunch or dinner. For the remaining meal and any snacks, follow the diet plan given here.

For variety, you can vary any day's menu by substituting recipes from Section II or by selecting any single eating-out entrée from the list. For additional variety, you may also choose one entrée from the Haas Maximum Performance 28-Day Eat-at-Home Meal Plan, as long as you use liquid meal replacers for one or two meals per day.

You can repeat the menu plans that you enjoy as often as you wish and eliminate those that you enjoy less.

DAY 1
Chicken Salad Supreme
Snacks: Apple
         2 cups hot-air-popped popcorn

DAY 2
Turkey-Stuffed Potato
Snacks: Apple

DAY 3
Chickpea and Pasta Salad
Snacks: Banana
       Baked potato with approved topping

DAY 4
Baked Cannellini
Snacks: Salad with approved dressing
       Apple

DAY 5
Shrimp Salad
Snacks: Banana
       2 cups hot-air-popped popcorn

DAY 6
Ziti Casserole
Snacks: Salad with approved dressing

DAY 7
Broiled Shrimp
Snacks: Salad with approved dressing
       Apple

DAY 8
Chicken Tetrazzini
Snacks: Salad with approved dressing
       Banana

DAY 9
Oriental Salad
Snacks: Baked potato with approved topping
       Apple

DAY 10
Mexican Rice
Snacks: Salad with approved dressing
        Banana

DAY 11
Poached Salmon
Snacks: Baked potato with approved topping
        Apple

DAY 12
Rice-Stuffed Green Pepper
Snacks: Salad with approved dressing
        Banana

DAY 13
Tomato Broccoli Pie
Snacks: Salad with approved dressing
        Banana
        2 cups hot-air-popped popcorn

DAY 14
Chili
Snacks: Salad with approved dressing

SEVEN

Eating on the Wing

E very commercial airline flight you take exposes you to a host of hazards that can cause a variety of health problems from fatigue to accelerated aging to cancer. Even though frequent flyers, including passengers, flight attendants, and flight crews (pilots, copilots, and navigators) suffer more damage than the occasional passenger, *everyone* can help protect him- or herself against the hazards of high altitude flight.

Here is the nutritional protection plan I use to protect my own body from hazards of high flight. It's the same plan used by many pilots and flight attendants. These professionals use my nutritional advice because it protects against radiation damage, air pollution, and low oxygen levels in aircraft cabins and helps fight the fatigue associated with flight across time zones. Just as important, it provides them with the maximum performance nutrition they need to succeed in their jobs. Now *you* can benefit from the protection program by following the nutritional advice in this chapter.

HOW I DISCOVERED THIS PLAN

Last year, I logged nearly 200,000 air miles, many at very high altitudes on the Concorde, a supersonic transport (SST) that flies 60,000 feet high at twice the speed of sound (MACH II). I knew from past research that the higher one flies, the more radiation one is exposed to. Since an SST flies roughly two times higher than most commercial airlines, I exposed myself to a relatively high dosage of damaging radiation.

Exposure to radiation is cumulative, and so the damage adds up, flight after flight, year after year. Combined with other commonly occurring toxic hazards of flying, such as decreased cabin oxygen levels, exposure to cigarette smoke (including cigar and pipe tobacco smoke on Concorde flights from continental Europe and the United Kingdom to New York), and the stress of a fast-paced travel schedule, airline delays, and time zone changes, I decided to investigate what I could do to protect myself against the unavoidable exposure to these hazards.

After two years of investigation and research, during which I obtained research reports from the National Aeronautics and Space Administration (NASA), the Federal Aviation Administration (FAA), and the Airline Pilot's Association (ALPA) and interviewed flight attendants and pilots, I developed my own Frequent Flyer's Protection Plan. It works for pilots and flight attendants, and it will work for you.

THE HAZARDS OF FLYING

Usually, the first hazard of flying that comes to mind is the spectacular airline accident sensationalized by the press. But there are also other, less spectacular but potentially harmful hazards of flying that perhaps you never knew existed.

I'm most concerned with damage from the four hazards I consider to be harmful but preventable—radiation, ozone, tobacco smoke, and jet lag. Here's how to protect yourself against these hazards as you fly at speeds between 500 miles per hour to twice the speed of sound.

RADIATION

Cosmic rays, pi mesons, alpha particles, gamma rays—is this dialogue from *Star Wars?* No, these are terms used to describe galactic cosmic radiation, the invisible particles of energy that can accelerate aging, damage all organs of the body, and even cause cancer. Our entire atmosphere, from the ground up, constitutes a radiation shield that does a good job of protecting us from overexposure. At regular commercial airline and supersonic transport altitudes, our exposure to these potentially harmful rays and particles of energy can increase dramatically.

As if that weren't enough, we also have to be concerned with *solar* cosmic radiation. This consists of cosmic radiation emitted by our sun. Following a solar flare, during which the sun gives off tremendous energy, there are dramatic increases in ultraviolet radiation, X rays, and other damaging types of cosmic energy. In the case of a giant solar flare that occurred on February 23, 1956, high-energy radiation continued to bombard the earth for two days after the flare. Again, on August 4, 1972, another solar flare bombarded the earth with high-intensity and long-lasting radiation. These are just two of the more spectacular solar flare-ups; there are many smaller ones each year.

From the standpoint of possible radiation hazard to airline passengers, especially at SST altitudes, it has been estimated that a single flight during the time of a major solar flare could expose passengers to more than 500 millirems (abbreviated to "mrem"—a unit used to measure radiation levels), the upper limit of "safe" exposure for *an entire year* for people on the ground. Twenty-five percent of the adult population flies commercially at least once each year and many people fly twenty-five times or more each year (I'm one of them). Infrequent flyers are, of course, exposed to less in-flight radiation, but nevertheless they run the risk of overexposure, depending upon the eleven-year solar cycle (which determines how much radiation from the sun we're exposed to) and the altitude and latitude of their flight (which determines how much cosmic radiation gets to you through the atmosphere). Flight crews are exposed to approximately 160 mrem each year under normal conditions; frequent travelers generally sustain a 63-mrem exposure per year.

On the basis of a dose-effect relationship, the National Academy of Sciences (NAS) has determined that the incidence of disease from radiation exposure during air travel can be estimated. The NAS believes that genetic damage to DNA might result after several generations (remember, radiation damage is cumulative), resulting in up to seventy-five serious disabilities in the entire U.S. population. Additionally, the NAS has estimated that airline flying results in up to forty-three cancer deaths per year in the flying population of the United States. These estimates, according to the FAA Advisory Committee on Radiation Biology Aspects of Supersonic Transport, may be "substantially in error"—*on the low side.*

FAA scientists believe that biological damage from "fast" neutrons (part of the cosmic ray package) may actually be more lethal than previously assumed, and they have convincing research to support their concern. They have also pointed out that the data on the incidence of leukemia in nuclear blast survivors of Hiroshima and Nagasaki indicate that neutron-induced leukemias were caused by only *one-fourth* the neutron dose previously assumed. (The Japanese experience has been used as a primary source of data for estimating cancer risks from radiation.) Neutron levels in the atmosphere are currently being reinvestigated because initial measurements show that airline passenger exposure is higher than previously thought.

That's the bad news from the FAA. The half-good news is that there is some evidence that the latency period for radiation-induced cancer may be longer in some cases of low-dosage radiation exposure than the human life-span. But that also means that while you may not die from radiation-induced cancer, *your child-to-be or their children might.*

Pilots, copilots, navigators, and flight attendants receive annual radiation doses that are higher, on the average, than those suffered in almost any other industry. SST crews probably receive more than the 500-mrem per year maximum permitted individual members of the general public. Such considerations, according to the FAA, might warrant designating SST crews as high-risk, occupationally exposed persons. If this is done, then every SST flight crew member must be informed of his/her exposure and must agree to accept the risk such designation carries as a condition of employment. Every Concorde SST carries a radiation monitor, which consists of three miniature Geiger counters, and pilots are instructed to monitor radiation levels on each flight. If radiation reaches critical levels, pilots have been instructed to descend to lower altitudes. There are at least two recorded instances in which the crew and passengers of an SST on a routine flight very likely received a single radiation dose in excess of the 500 mrem annual safety limit. Under normal conditions, the highest average dose on a single SST flight has been calculated to be 6 and 7 mrem per hour of flying time. On more than 99 percent of the flights measured in 1976–77, the average radiation level was less than 4 mrem/hour. (The Concorde flight from London to New York takes about three hours and eighteen minutes.)

The highest radiation levels recorded (15.2 mrem/hour) on routine Concorde flights occur on the North Atlantic route between Paris and the United States. At this value, the 500 mrem maximum dose per year for the general public would be reached in thirty-three flying hours, or roughly five round-trips between Paris and New York. Flight crews on conventional aircraft are at a somewhat reduced risk of radiation damage. However, their frequent flying schedules can still boost their risk to unacceptable levels. On conventional commercial airline carriers, the dose may be half that sustained at SST altitudes, but since radiation damage is cumulative, today's safety limit may be tomorrow's danger zone.

OZONE

Recently, ozone, a colorless gas that forms in the atmosphere between 35,000 and 150,000 feet (and a gas that is created by automobiles and electrical equipment such as photocopiers), has been singled out as a potentially toxic substance that may jeopardize the health of flight crews and passengers. Scientists have recently measured high ozone levels in aircraft cabins flying at 18,000 feet and have discovered alarmingly high concentrations on commercial aircraft.

Flight crews began reporting what appeared to be symptoms of ozone poisoning (eye, nose, throat, and chest irritation) in increasing numbers just after the oil crisis of 1973, when higher prices for jet fuel sent airliners to higher altitudes where thinner air meant more miles per gallon. In 1976, Pan American began nonstop service between New York and Tokyo with the new Boeing 747SP (a higher-flying, longer-range aircraft). These flights flew through northern latitudes known to contain very high concentrations of ozone.

In 1978, the Federal Aviation Administration (FAA) proposed to limit ozone concentrations in airplanes to 0.1 part per million (ppm) on the average, with a maximum allowable concentration of 0.3 ppm. The Airline Pilots Association (ALPA) claimed that exposure under the FAA proposal allowing exposures of up to two hours at 0.3 ppm could seriously damage health. Airline industry spokespersons, on the other hand, claim that exposures should be allowed to go even higher than those proposed by the FAA. Data from the National Air and Space Administration's (NASA) Global Air Sampling Program (GASP) show that ozone in commercial aircraft cabins sometimes reaches 1.2 ppm—four times the peak level set by the FAA.

Donald Tierny, past president of the American Thoracic Society, claims that passengers with heart and lung problems may be at risk of increased dangers. He cautions that while exposures of 0.2 ppm may not immediately affect an asthmatic, for example, they could trigger a delayed reaction because ozone could make asthmatics "very sensitive to agents that produce asthma, and this effect could last for several days. I would be doubly concerned with an asthmatic with a common cold," he warns.

When I contacted the FAA and ALPA and researched the published scientific literature on ozone toxicity, I discovered that the most vocal complainers were not airline passengers, but flight attendants. I suspect that there are two reasons for this: (1) Most passengers are not aware of the problems associated with ozone exposure and don't report their symptoms to the airlines; (2) flight attendants probably have more problems with ozone exposure because they work during flights, often pushing metal carts that weigh several hundred pounds and often at an incline—L1011 wide-body aircraft, for example, fly at an exaggerated angle, making cart-pushing much more strenuous than it would be on other types of aircraft). A passenger at rest breathes about 5 liters of air per minute while a flight attendant pushing a heavy cart up and down an aisle breathes 20 liters per minute and thus inhales many times more ozone.

I'm therefore especially worried about flight attendants' exposure to ozone, because ozone is a mutagen (a mutation-causing substance) and is known to cause biochemical changes in the blood of exposed persons. It is still unknown if the high rates of miscarriages and children with birth defects among flight attendants are a result of chronic or acute ozone exposure. That's why I recommend my program to every flight attendant and flight crew member I talk to. I urge all airlines to adopt this program for the safety of their employees, and I urge you to follow this program whenever you fly.

SELECTED SAMPLE OZONE CONCENTRATIONS

Location of Source of Ozone	Concentration (ppm)
Electric typewriter	<0.002 to 0.014
Clean air	0.020 to 0.050
Average airline cabin limit (FAA)	<3-hour average of 0.100
Airliner cabin (average)	<0.002 to 0.200
Office photocopy machines	0.003 to 0.204
Inside—office building	up to 0.220
Inside—private residences	up to 0.230
Hospital, intensive care units	0.230 to 0.260
Maximum ozone limit—airline cabin (FAA)	0.300
Smog alert (first stage), Los Angeles County	0.500 or above
Outside in smog conditions	up to 0.900

TOBACCO SMOKE

Tobacco smoking should be prohibited on all public transportation, especially commercial airline carriers. Tobacco smoke poses as much a health threat to nonsmokers as it does to smokers. In fact, research indicates that passive or sidestream smoke may eventually be more harmful than direct smoke inhaled by smokers.

The extremely high temperatures of a lighted cigarette produce hundreds of toxic substances that jeopardize human health; tobacco is also a prime source of radioactive material. Filter cigarettes of the very-low-tar variety produce higher amounts of carbon monoxide than nonfiltered cigarettes. It's the carbon monoxide, along with dozens of other chemicals—not the tar—that scars the cardiovascular system and leads to heart attack, stroke, and other life-threatening health problems. Tobacco smoking is also directly responsible for the epidemic of lung cancer that now affects more women than men for the first time in history. (This is due to the head start men had in taking up smoking during the first half of the twentieth century.)

Nonsmoking passengers have every right to expect airlines to prohibit tobacco smoking on board aircraft, yet the most any airline will do is to establish smoking and nonsmoking sections. This is foolish. Based on air-flow patterns in the aircraft cabin, passengers are exposed to smoke from the smoking section no matter how far away they sit in the nonsmoking section. Pity the poor nonsmoking flight attendants who are forced to work in the smoking section for hours, days, months, and years on end.

No one knows just how much damage the combination of tobacco smoke (with its radioactive particles), cosmic radiation, low cabin oxygen levels, and pressure changes really causes. Moreover, the possibility of an in-flight fire, second in seriousness only to an actual airline crash, increases dramatically when passengers are permitted to smoke. Even though airline carriers prohibit smoking in aisles and lavatories and on takeoff and landing, many passengers still continue to disobey these safety rules, causing serious life-threatening incidents.

JET LAG

Jet lag poses a major inconvenience and exerts stress on passengers who fly across several time zones and disorient the synchronicity of their internal biological clocks. Such a disruption generally occurs when people cross three or more time zones. The daily (diurnal) cycles within our bodies—such as the wake-sleep cycle, the work-rest cycle, the hunger-satiety cycle, and certain hormonal cycles—are all more or less interdependent. Jet lag can throw them all out of balance.

In 1959, scientists first used the term *circadian* to denote a time period that approximates twenty-four hours; thus, *circadian* means the same thing as *diurnal* (daily). The circadian body cycles or periodicities have been recognized for centuries, but their significance to human performance and behavior are just now being realized. In our own Declaration of Independence, one of the colonists' grievances against King George III complained of the fatiguing nature of long-distance travel: "He has called together legislative bodies at places unusual, uncomfortable, and distant . . . for the sole purpose of fatiguing them. . . ." Another eighteenth-century American published the suggestion that valuable time could be gained by instituting what would later be called "daylight saving time." This suggestion was published in 1784 in the *Journal of Paris*; the author was Benjamin Franklin. No one took Franklin's suggestion seriously until the twentieth century, testimony to the tenacity with which we cling to our sleep-wake cycles.

Circadian rhythm research has shown that our internal biological clockwork consists of many subsystems that oscillate in tune with each other. As a result of jet travel across time zones, we can disrupt these subsystems and throw the time clocks for a loop, causing the normal twenty-four-hour cycle to become a twenty- or twenty-eight-hour cycle.

Despite what you may have heard or read, travel across time zones by itself does not cause the time clock disturbances that result in jet lag. The most influential disorienting factor is the *environment* in which you land. How many hours of daylight or night remain relative to your point of origin? Are you eating breakfast when your body thinks it's midday? Have you lost sleep as a result of air travel? These are the real causes of jet lag. They disrupt your internal rhythms, although the extent of disruption varies from person to person. Internal control systems react differently and uniquely; they provide a biological fingerprint of one's own internal clock system, and no two people respond in quite the same way.

There is a popular jet lag diet that claims to prevent jet lag through nutrition, based on the misconception that food—specifically the ratio of protein to carbohydrate and the timing of food intake—will speed up or slow down the multitude of internal biological clocks. As a nutritionist, I would enjoy being able to control my own biological time clock with food. The theory looks okay on paper, but it just doesn't work. *Exposure to light and synchronizing your eating, sleeping, and activity schedule to your new surroundings does work*. When I recently accompanied Cher to the Cannes Film Festival, then to Paris, back to Cannes, then to London, New York, Los Angeles, Tokyo, Los Angeles (then proceeding on my own to New York, Miami, Chicago, New York, and back to Miami), I never once experienced jet lag. Cher, however, suffered from jet lag in every city because she maintained her normal Los Angeles sleep-wake patterns.

When Wiley Post, the record-setting global flier of the 1930s, set out on his eight-day trans-global flight of 1931, and later, during his seven-day solo trans-global flight of 1933, he observed the effects of altered sleep-wake cycles and meal schedule on his flying proficiency. He attributed his successful missions to preventing the fatigue of jet lag.

The FAA has conducted experiments on the effect of time zone shifts on body temperature, heart rate, respiratory rate, loss of water from the palms of the hands, reaction time, decision time, urinary output, subjective fatigue, and changes in intellectual ability. Other research groups have investigated changes in excretion of steroids and other hormones, sodium, and potassium. Scientists have discovered that recovery (readaptation to one's normal environment) occurs more slowly after west-to-east travel than after east-to-west travel.

There are many variables that account for the symptoms of jet lag. The important ones are:

• Time of departure
• Sunlight
• Change in sleep patterns
• Direction of flight
• Age

• Physical condition
• Travel experience
• Stress
• Temperature changes
• New social environment
• Intake of food and beverage during the flight

Since research shows that it can take up to nine days or more to recover from jet lag, it is important, especially for pilots and air crews, flight attendants, and travelers charged with important responsibilities at home and abroad, to minimize or completely prevent jet lag. Nor are vacations a pleasure when you are too tired to enjoy yourself and the company of others.

There are things you can do to prevent jet lag in yourself and in employees who need to operate at peak levels. Just as importantly, you can minimize the hazards of in-flight radiation, ozone, and tobacco smoke damage.

Adjusting sleep patterns to conform to new surroundings can be difficult if not impossible without taking sleep medications. Most physicians I've questioned recommend diazepam (trade name: Dalmane) because it has little effect on the rapid-eye movement (REM) phase of sleep, which is known to be essential to maintaining optimal moods, clarity of thought, and efficiency. Pilot lore abounds with alternative methods for inducing drug-free sleep. Hot baths, long walks, and the amino acid tryptophan have all been used with some measure of success. The best non-drug formula I've used as a sleep aid is called Lights Out, which is sold in health food stores. This nonprescription formulation contains vitamins and nutrients that bind to the same brain receptors as prescription sleep aids.

EAT TO SUCCEED AGAINST RADIATION AND AIR POLLUTION: FOR PILOTS, FLIGHT ATTENDANTS, AND PASSENGERS

Antioxidants and nutritious low-fat meals and beverages offer effective and readily available protection against the hazards of in-flight radiation, ozone, and cigarette smoke. Nutritional supplements described in Appendix I help protect flight crews on major U.S. airlines, and they can do the same for you. Three products that are used routinely by flight attendants and passengers I counsel are QuickFix beverage, Twinsport Endurance Meal Replacer, and antioxidant supplements. Here's how to use them during your next flight:

• Use QuickFix as a fluid and electrolyte replacer. Dry cabin atmosphere can deplete your skin of vital moisture, and cabin pollution, including radiation and cigarette smoke, can damage your lungs, eyes, skin, and internal organs. QuickFix contains low-calorie protection against these hazards in the form of antioxidants to help prevent free-radical damage. It also replaces essential water losses and supplies energy nutrients to combat fatigue.

• Use an approved meal replacer (see Appendix II) instead of airline meals or snacks to enjoy a nutrient-dense, low-calorie drink. Since you can easily bring this powder on board and mix it with milk, you can enjoy this radiation/pollution protection in liquid meal form on every flight anywhere in the world.

• Use an antioxidant formula (e.g., Endurance Multivitamin Fitness Paks—see Appendix I) to supply added protection against free-radical damage caused by cigarette smoke, radiation, and ozone.

If you enjoy airline food (despite the almost universal complaint that it is bland and overcooked), you should know what to eat and what to avoid to help make your flight less hazardous. Most airlines offer a wide variety of foods for people with special dietary needs. Commercial airlines want to cater to your dietary needs because they want you as a customer. Despite the jokes about airline food, some airlines actually serve nutritious and delicious meals that conform to just about everyone's tastes and nutritional needs. The trick lies in knowing what the airline offers and *ordering your special meal well in advance of the day of departure.* Here, courtesy of American Airlines, is the variety of special meals you can enjoy while flying to your next destination:

Bland-soft	Kosher
Diabetic	Strict-vegetarian

Lacto-ovo vegetarian   Low-cholesterol
Low-sodium   Low-carbohydrate
Low-calorie

Dietetic snacks are also available upon request on snack flights.

American Airlines claims that all these special meals have been medically reviewed and approved. American Airlines' Traveler Menu has been designed with the approval of the American Heart Association, in accordance with AHA guidelines.

The typical American Airlines' coach meal consists of a package of honey-roast peanuts (½ ounce), a salad of iceberg lettuce and mandarin orange slices topped with a vinaigrette dressing; an entrée of boneless, skinless leg of chicken (dark meat) with tomato, pepper and mushroom sauce, noodles, and green beans; two slices of malt bread, one pat of butter on the side; and apple-walnut cake for dessert.

With a few minor adjustments you can turn this meal into an *Eat to Succeed*–approved maximum performance menu:

• Avoid the honey-roast peanuts and apple-walnut cake.

• Enjoy the salad with your own oil-free dressing that you bring with you, or ask for fresh lemon wedges and squeeze lemon juice over the salad.

• Make a chicken sandwich with tomato and the two pieces of malt bread topped with mustard; scrape off the pepper mushroom sauce and enjoy the noodles and green beans.

• Drink plain water or salt-free carbonated water (hard to come by on airlines) or QuickFix.

Transcontinental and international flights generally serve incredibly good food in first class. I had the best airline meal of my life on a Pan American Airlines flight from Los Angeles to Miami (flight #441). I won't tell you what I ate (I used up my cheating ration for one week), but it was delicious. If there are times when you feel like deviating from your healthy diet, save them until you are a captive customer on the Concorde, Regent Air, or other first-class flights that serve gourmet low-fat meals. Eastern Airlines, for example, has just instituted truly gourmet foods and beverages (worth the cheat)

on flights to Great Britain. Once on the ground, however, it's back
to the straight and narrow.

SPECIAL AIRLINE MEAL CHOICES

American Airlines thoughtfully offers the following menu selections
as alternatives to regular in-flight meals:

California quiche. Made with low-fat cheese, egg substitute,
onion, and diced green chili peppers in a light pie crust and
garnished with seasonal fresh fruit.

Comment: A clever recipe that avoids the traditional high fat/high
cholesterol of traditional quiche.

Fresh fruit salad. Chilled fresh seasonal fruits, cottage cheese
topped with walnuts, and a special fruit dressing.

Comment: Not as low-calorie as it sounds, but nutritious nevertheless.

Fresh vegetable plate. Greek-style pasta salad served in a green
pepper surrounded by a variety of crudites and served with an
herbed yogurt dip.

Comment: An excellent choice but avoid the traditional olives.

The great American hamburger. Broiled chopped choice steak,
served on grilled seeded bun with lettuce, sliced tomatoes, Spanish
onion, dill pickle, and potato chips.

Comment: Skip this one unless you want to use up your cheating
ration for the whole week.

American seafood platter. Crab meat in fresh tomato half with
chilled shrimp, artichoke heart, and vegetable garnish; served with
lemon and red cocktail sauce.

Comment: This one's cholesterol city, so avoid it if you're trying to
lower your cholesterol. If your serum cholesterol is excellent, this is
a nutritious, very low-fat meal.

Seafood Cassolette. Lobster chunks, scallops, and baby shrimp in
a creamy white wine sauce with shallots; served with rice pilaf.

Comment: Same as above, except that this dish has a higher fat content due to the creamy white wine sauce. I'd prefer the American seafood platter if I were choosing between the two.

American deli plate. Sliced turkey, ham, and roast beef accompanied by an artichoke salad, asparagus spears, and tomato wedge; served with Dijon mustard.
Comment: Eat the turkey on a roll or bread topped with tomato and Dijon mustard; give the ham and roast beef to a passenger on the Atkins diet.

For Pilots and Flight Attendants

Do you know what the best safety feature is on commercial aircraft? Radar? Seat belts? No, it's the flight attendants.

On November 22, 1964, a TWA Boeing 707 crashed on takeoff at Rome's Fiumicino Airport. In addition to the regular crew of five flight attendants, this flight carried another six TWA flight attendants, five of whom were flying as "deadheads" (off-duty) and one who was traveling with her parents on vacation.

After the aircraft skidded to a stop, it was engulfed in flames. Seconds later, a fuel tank exploded and twenty seconds after that a second, larger explosion rocked the aircraft, killing all passengers and crew members still aboard and many others already outside the aircraft in the immediate vicinity. Two of the on-duty flight attendants were killed and the three survivors were seriously injured. All six of the off-duty flight attendants died. The bodies of five of the off-duty flight attendants were found aboard the aircraft, and from survivor accounts and body placements, it was apparent that most of these flight attendants died while assisting other passengers to escape.

The primary duty of a flight attendant is not to serve drinks, meals, or supply pillows, blankets, or playing cards. *The primary duty of the flight attendant is to save lives.*

It is in takeoff and landing, when a disproportionate number of fatal air crashes occur, that a flight attendant's training and dedication to duty are critical. In an air crash, flight crews in the cockpit experience the fullest impact forces and are often killed or seriously injured. Even if they are uninjured, their full attention must be devoted to emergency shutdown procedures to minimize post-crash fire hazards. Only the second officer is assigned to assist in an evacuation.

The success or failure of emergency evacuation—measured in human lives—depends upon the performance of the flight attendants. Very often, flight attendants are women who, alone and unassisted, must manually open doors weighing hundreds of pounds, manhandle window exits weighing half as much as they do, deploy escape slides, and assist passengers, which includes lifting disabled or elderly people and small children. To perform these duties, female flight attendants must be in the best of mental and physical condition and, above all, uninjured in the crash.

In order to keep mentally and physically at their peak, flight attendants use my nutritional advice and recommended food and supplements. Since commercial airlines provide no nutrition education or maximum performance foods and supplements to their employees, I was gratified to learn that during the last two years, scores of airline employees had embraced the Haas Peak Performance Diet. I feel much more secure when, upon learning that I'm on board, the pilot and flight crew come out to report their excellent results on my diet. That's when I know the plane is in the hands of a peak performance pilot and crew.

A Special Note for Pilots

The National Transportation Safety Board (NTSB) has determined that pilots are the cause of accidents in approximately 83 percent of all nonfatal accidents and 87 percent of fatal accidents. Pilot incapacitation can result from heart attack, stroke, seizure, hypoglycemia (low blood sugar), or other medical emergencies. Some pilots may knowingly ingest chemicals and drugs that alter their mood and impair their professional performance. In this respect, alcohol is the drug of greatest abuse. Statistical analyses of pilots killed in civil aviation accidents indicate that about 10 percent of the pilots had blood alcohol concentrations of 0.05 percent, a level that definitely affects a pilot's ability to fly an aircraft safely. About 20 percent of all pilots killed in aircraft accidents have some alcohol in their blood. Maximum performance nutrition and nutritional supplements can help protect against some of the toxic effects of alcohol ingestion, but it can *never* prevent the effects of alcohol that impair pilot performance. If you are a pilot, *don't drink and fly (or drive)!*

A SPECIAL NOTE TO FLYERS WITH HEALTH PROBLEMS

Passengers with lung disease, heart disease, or asthma may need to take precautions in addition to the nutritional protection discussed previously. At sea level, we are exposed to 14.7 pounds of pressure per square inch of our body surface. At this pressure, our lungs can fill with the necessary amount of oxygen our bodies require. As we ascend to higher altitudes (commercial aircraft fly between 28,000 and 43,000 feet; the Concorde flies at about 58,000 feet), we experience a significant decrease in pressure and a decrease of oxygen delivery to the lungs. Even though aircraft cabins are pressurized, they can only partially offset the pressure change associated with high-altitude flight; cabin pressures only reach about 12 pounds of pressure per square inch.

Healthy people usually experience no problems with this decrease in oxygen to the body. However, people who suffer from a medical problem that already limits the supply of oxygen to their body may experience problems such as pain in the chest and difficulty with breathing. If you have a medical condition such as asthma, emphysema, or cardiovascular disease, you should call the airline at least forty-eight hours before your flight and discuss your problem with the airline's flight surgeon. The flight surgeon can determine if you might need supplementary oxygen during the flight, depending upon your condition, the altitude, and the duration of the flight.

AN IN-FLIGHT EXERCISE PROGRAM
FOR AIRLINE PASSENGERS

American Airlines has provided these in-flight exercise tips to help make long airline flights more comfortable by stimulating circulation and relaxing muscles:

1. Lean head forward as far as possible. Feel a stretch down the back of your neck. Lean head to the side (keep face front) and feel the stretch down the side of the neck. Lean to other side.

2. Let head drop back (jaw relaxed), and look up at the overhead compartment of the row behind yours. Arch upper back as you look up. Feel stretch under your chin.

3. Hug yourself (right hand on left shoulder, left hand on right shoulder). Lean head forward, cave in upper chest, and pull your shoulders forward. Feel stretch down the back of the neck and between your shoulder blades.

4. Push shoulders forward and cave in upper chest and stomach. Push shoulders back and arch lower back. Keep head straight. This exercise moves the rib cage to front and loosens muscles in the center of the back.

5. Relax your shoulders and arms and make a circle with one shoulder at a time by moving it forward, raising it up, pushing it back and down. Then reverse the exercise; begin with moving the shoulder back.

6. Press elbows down onto armrests and press shoulders down as hard as you can. Feel stretch across top of shoulders.

7. Grasp the right armrest with your left hand and turn your upper body around to the right to look behind you. Turn to the left, grasping the left armrest with your right hand. Feel stretch down each side of your back.

8. Reach up toward light or air vent without rising from your seat. Breathe in as you reach up, and exhale as you lower your arm. Stretch as you reach, using one hand and then the other.

9. Loosen seat belt slightly, and lean over to the floor as if to pick up something you've dropped or to adjust packages under the seat in front of you. Reach down as far as possible, and then sit up slowly. This stretches lower back and back of thighs.

10. Sit up straight and pick one foot up off the floor by raising your whole leg about an inch off the seat. While maintaining this position, make circles in the air with the raised foot by rotating your ankle. Circle your foot to the right eight times and to the left eight times. Place the foot back on the floor and repeat with other foot. This exercise not only stretches the ankle but all sides of the lower leg as well. (An added benefit is that while you are holding your leg up, you are pulling in and tightening the stomach muscles.)

"In doing all exercises, move the part of your body as instructed as far as possible to feel the greatest stretch. Push your head forward as far as it will go, raise your shoulders or push them back as far as they will go, et cetera. Even circle your foot as far as it will circle to stretch your toes and arches."

EIGHT

The Skeleton in the Hospital Closet and the *Eat to Succeed* Hospital Food Survival Kit

There is a skeleton in the hospital closet. You don't often read or hear about it, yet it's a serious, even life-threatening problem that many physicians and hospital dietitians don't care to discuss. It is a problem you should know about before you are hospitalized for any reason. The skeleton in the hospital closet is the nutritional nightmare of misinformation and sub-optimal nourishment given to unwary patients by hospital dietitians.

People often ask me to recommend a nutritionist or diet-care organization that can help them with a diet-related problem. Nutritional counseling, like tennis or golf lessons, can be excellent or poor, depending on the ability of the professional who helps you. You may have heard or read that you should consult a registered dietitian (sometimes called an "R.D.") for nutritional advice. While there are many competent R.D.'s in public and private practice, you should know something about R.D.'s and other types of nutritionists before you select a diet-care professional.

WHAT IS A REGISTERED DIETITIAN?

In general, a registered dietitian is a person who has earned a bachelor's degree in nutrition, including food science, from a regionally accredited college or university, and who has applied for membership and met the minimum requirements established by the American Dietetic Association (ADA). Not all ADA members are registered dietitians. The ADA is a private nongovernment organization that confers the designation R.D. on applicants who meet the minimum membership standards it has established. ADA membership is voluntary. In fact, many highly qualified and competent nutritionists employed by federal, state, and local governmental agencies have chosen not to become members of the ADA and not to become registered dietitians.

The ADA lobbies in Washington on various diet and health issues that affect public policy and dietary recommendations subsequently made to the public. The ADA also has a public relations department that deals with the public media. The ADA trains its spokespersons to communicate its official positions on nutrition issues to the American public through television, radio, magazines, newspapers, journals, etc. The ADA also has an active publications department to disseminate information on a wide variety of health-related issues to physicians, dietitians, and consumers. We'll review some of this information shortly.

The basic difference between a registered dietitian (most of whom hold only a bachelor's degree) and a nutritionist with a master's or doctoral degree in nutrition is that the non-R.D. nutritionist often is better educated in biological, biochemical, and nutritional sciences than the registered dietitian. In my opinion, minimal training often fails to provide the practitioner with enough nutritional and scientific background to prescribe diets and nutritional supplements for people with acute nutritional problems.

That's why I believe that the real skeleton in the hospital closet is the nutritional care offered in many institutions. To understand why a group of well-meaning health-care professionals would recommend sub-optimal foods and diets, one must understand the nature of the training many dietitians-to-be receive before they earn their degrees.

NUTRITIONAL KNOWLEDGE WE'RE TAUGHT IN COLLEGE

I hold two advanced nutritional degrees—a master of science degree from a fully accredited U.S. university and a doctoral degree from an international university recognized by the British and Canadian governments. Additionally, I have taken college coursework in advanced biological, nutritional, and biochemical sciences, far beyond the science requirements established by the ADA for membership. Sadly, with the exception of my vigorous training in premedical and medical studies, much of my formal nutrition coursework was fraught with error. Only my own determination to learn the real nutritional truths gave me the proper grounding as a nutritionist and health educator.

Our present educational system, especially at the graduate level, stifles individual thinking, creativity, and the pursuit of ideas that go against departmental policy, philosophy, and accepted thinking. Students who refuse to subscribe to the current nutritional line followed by conventional nutritional organizations may jeopardize their degrees because the granting of a graduate degree is based on subjective considerations (i.e., the personal feelings, beliefs, and judgments of the student's professorial committee) as well as on "objective" criteria such as test performance and grades (and very often, grades in graduate school are arbitrary and inaccurate indications of a student's knowledge and abilities).

In graduate school, my classmates and I, some of whom went on to become registered dietitians, were taught that:

• Cholesterol had nothing to do with atherosclerosis.

• High-fiber diets (considered high solely because they provided more fiber than the fiber-depleted American diet) were dangerous and caused vitamin/mineral deficiencies.

• Animal protein was healthier than vegetable protein.

• Animal protein was complete; vegetable protein was incomplete.

• Diabetics must limit their intake of carbohydrate to less than 40 percent of their daily kilocalories.

• Sodium was the primary cause of high blood pressure.

• Gastrectomy (surgical removal of part of the stomach and intestines) was an acceptable method of managing stubborn obesity.
• Special diets played no role in boosting physical performance.
• Low-fat diets caused vitamin/mineral deficiencies.
• If you selected foods from the four food groups, you wouldn't need to take vitamin supplements.

My own research told me that all of this dogma was incorrect and, fortunately, a few of my classmates came to the same conclusion. We quietly began a systematic search of the medical/nutritional literature and began to discover the real nutritional truths that our professors neglected to teach us. Just as fortunately, nutritionists such as Nathan Pritikin were beginning to challenge such beliefs.

Pritikin, whom I later came to know, had no college degrees or formal nutritional training, yet he knew more about human nutritional needs than any registered dietitian I've met. The ADA and American Medical Association, however, severely criticized his diet. All of the criticism to date has been scientifically unsubstantiated. In fact, the principles of a low-fat, low-cholesterol, and high-fiber diet have been vindicated by hundreds of current studies, including those conducted and sponsored by the U.S. government.

NUTRITIONAL FALLACIES STILL BEING ADVANCED

Among the nutritional fallacies still being foisted on the public by the nutrition establishment are these:

• *The Zen macrobiotic diet, rather than being healthier than usual eating patterns, is dangerously deficient.*
This represents an inaccurate and unfair condemnation of a very healthy diet and way of life—a nutritional eating plan that has been credited with prolonging the life of people seriously ill with cancer, heart disease, and other degenerative health problems. In fact, one physician, Dr. Anthony Sattilaro, has medically documented his own success in eliminating his cancer with the macrobiotic diet.

The ADA claims that the macrobiotic diet is "very dangerous when followed strictly." Actually, the opposite is true. Had the ADA consulted with the Macrobiotic Foundation in Boston, they would have discovered that their condemnation is based on an older version of the macrobiotic diet as published by George Ohsawa. One of Ohsawa's versions of the macrobiotic diet (Diet 7) *is* nutritionally unbalanced and could lead to nutritional deficiencies if followed for an extended period of time. But that version of the macrobiotic diet has long since been discredited and abandoned.

The macrobiotic diet as practiced *today* is a very well balanced and health-supporting diet. While it includes many foods that we in the United States are unaccustomed to eating (and contains foods not generally sold in supermarkets or offered in most restaurants), there is nothing dangerous or unbalanced about it. In fact, the new macrobiotic diet is much healthier (lower in fat, cholesterol, and overprocessed foods and higher in fiber) than the diet recommended by the ADA.

• *Fats are "essential for absorption of fat-soluble vitamins," as they "both carry the vitamins and improve the ability of the body to absorb them."* (See page 16 of the ADA booklet *Food Facts Talk Back.*)

Meticulous absorption studies in laboratory animals and in humans (as well as epidemiologic studies of whole populations that eat an extremely low-fat diet) have consistently demonstrated that dietary fat is *not* essential for the absorption of fat-soluble vitamins (you will find supporting references in the bibliography at the end of this book).

This is yet another example of the ADA's scientifically inaccurate statements based on an outdated and disproven nutritional mythology still being touted as gospel to students today. Of the fat-soluble vitamins (A, D, E, and K), two can be toxic and lethal (A and D), one can lead to life-threatening food-drug interactions and jeopardize blood clotting (vitamin K). Moreover, vitamin D is not a vitamin but a hormone manufactured in the skin in response to sunlight and activated in the liver and kidneys. Sunlight, not dietary fat, is the critical factor in assuring adequate vitamin D. Finally, the more fat (oil) you consume, the *more* vitamin E your body will require.

• *The milk group of foods "is especially important for calcium and phosphorus; it also provides protein, riboflavin, and other nutrients."* (See page 18 of *Food Facts Talk Back.*) The following are the ADA's prescribed "servings needed daily" to maintain optimum health in the individuals indicated:

Adults .... 2 or more cups
Children 10 and under .... 2 to 3 cups
Preteens and teens........................ 4 or more cups
Pregnant and nursing women............... 4 or more cups
Pregnant teens............................. 5 to 6 cups

This ADA recommendation is unjustifiable and potentially dangerous. Why? Milk at that proposed level of intake can actually promote calcium loss rather than prevent it. An unsuspecting pregnant teen, if she were to follow the ADA's advice, would bombard her poor body with 50 grams each of fat and protein and more than 200 milligrams of cholesterol—from milk alone! She could run the risk of a vitamin D overdose (400 IU are added to each quart). Such large amounts of vitamin D, fat, and cholesterol are clearly inappropriate for her health and well-being.

Many nutritional scientists would disagree with the claim that the milk group is "especially important for calcium and phosphorous." The vegetable kingdom is richly endowed with calcium, and you can easily get all the calcium you need from vegetables. Besides, the human requirement for calcium did not evolve on milk; dairy cows have been used for only the last 10,000 years, and not in all cultures even then. Moreover, a large segment of the world's population loses the ability to digest milk upon reaching adulthood. Milk is a leading cause of food allergy and intestinal distress for vast numbers of people.

Milk and milk products can be part of a healthy diet (as long as the reliance is on skim or very-low-fat milk), but not at the levels recommended by the ADA. The American diet is already dangerously high in phosphorous, so there is no need to drink milk to get more. Ironically, in recommending alternatives to milk for getting calcium, the ADA points to spinach, which is in reality a poor source of biologically available calcium because it contains oxalic acid, which binds calcium and inhibits its absorption in the body.

As long as fallacies like these continue to be disseminated by the nutritional establishment, the nutritional knowledge applied in institutions, including schools *and* hospitals, will continue to be deficient.

THE NEW NUTRITION

Today, a nutritional revolution is changing the attitudes, beliefs, and practices of R.D.'s and nutritionists across the country. More and more diet-care professionals are departing from party-line nutritional dogma and embracing a new type of nutrition founded on scientific fact and evidence rather than outdated and biased information. The new nutrition, which includes the above mentioned principles plus reduced-protein foods and nutritional supplements and emphasizes the need for regular aerobic exercise, has forced old-guard nutritionists to rethink their outmoded positions and dietary recommendations. Just as *Eat to Win* started a sports nutrition revolution, I believe that *Eat to Succeed* will help usher in a new, more healthful approach to nutrition in general. Unlike many dietary recommendations of the past, my diet does make a positive difference in health, stamina, endurance, and energy.

Health care organizations like the Pritikin Longevity Centers (which also employ enlightened R.D.'s and M.D.'s), Bio-Nutronics (which employs a staff of nutritionists, enlightened registered dietitians, and physicians), the Kushi Institute, and the Cooper Institute respond to the needs of a nutrition-conscious public with sound dietary advice. These are just a few of the diet-care organizations that can provide you with sound nutritional care (their addresses and telephone numbers are listed in Appendix III).

Hospitals are just beginning to recognize that they need to modify the nutritional care they deliver to their patients. Doctor's Hospital in Hollywood, Florida (also listed in Appendix III), now offers a special VIP program in nutritional care based on the Haas diet and the nutritional principles of *Eat to Win/Eat to Succeed*. More and more physicians in private practice now recommend these diets to their own families and patients for a variety of reasons—from achieving better health to gaining a new zest for life.

In the balance of this chapter, I'll tell how to eat to succeed in the event that you must be hospitalized or undergo surgery. I will show you how to protect against the harmful effects of general anesthesia and how to heal faster and stronger from surgery. Staying healthy and fit in the hospital is a matter of knowing how to eat to succeed— and how to avoid the skeleton in the hospital closet.

Not all hospitals jeopardize their patients' health from hospital-induced malnutrition, mind you, just the vast majority. But you *can* and should eat to succeed in the hospital. In fact, the difference between surviving the trauma of surgery and the poisons used for anesthesia, avoiding life-threatening infections, and preventing hospital-induced malnutrition often depends on your nutritional status. Many people don't discover the critical role that nutrition plays before, during, and after hospitalization until they have suffered from hospital-induced problems. Sadly, some people never get a second chance. According to Charles B. Inlander, Executive Director of the People's Medical Society, hospital malnutrition causes an estimated 50,000 *preventable* U.S. hospital deaths each year. For patients who don't have the benefit of a complete, scientifically based nutrition program such as that at Doctor's Hospital in Hollywood, Florida, I present the following *Eat to Succeed* Hospital Food Survival Tips—to help you avoid hospital-induced malnutrition and to help protect against the hazards of anesthesia, surgery, and infection. These tips will also help improve your chances of healing faster and stronger during recovery in the hospital and, later, at home.

EAT TO SUCCEED HOSPITAL FOOD SURVIVAL TIPS

SURVIVAL TIP #1

• *Take your own vitamin/mineral supplements with you.*
Hospital dietitians set themselves and *you* up for failure because they operate under the false principle that "you can get all the nutrients you need from a balanced diet." Dietitians actually create hours of unnecessary calculations for themselves by attempting to

construct unrealistic diets to provide 100 percent of the Recommended Daily Allowance (RDA) for vitamins, minerals, kilocalories, and protein. This type of busywork is nonproductive for at least three reasons:

1. The RDA's are *arbitrary* values that do not apply to a hospitalized individual's needs for nutrients—disease, injury, medications, and surgery all alter your need for vitamins and minerals. RDA's, in many cases, may not be sufficient to compensate for increased nutritional demands during a hospitalization.

2. Two ordinary breakfast cereals (Kellogg's Product 19 and General Mills' Total) supply 100 percent of the RDA for nutrients that a hospital dietitian will spend hours trying to work into a menu of bland, overcooked, overprocessed, and nutritionally incomplete hospital foods—and for much less kilocalories, fat, and cholesterol.* *Nutritionally enriched cereals and/or vitamin/mineral supplements, which most hospitalized patients should be given routinely, eliminate any need for the dietitian's drudgery of time-consuming calculations.*

3. The RDA's do not address the *full* spectrum of nutrients required for health. Surgery, anesthesia, bed rest, liquid diets, nausea, fatigue, medications, and stress all may drastically increase your need for nutrients (especially trace minerals and fiber) already in short supply in an overprocessed hospital diet. Simply meeting the RDA for a *few* nutrients does not insure that your nutritional needs will be met. In fact, it *insures that they will not be met.*

There are many excellent nutrient formulas you can use to help protect against hospital-induced malnutrition. I recommend the following to help you recover faster and stronger. (See Appendix I for a complete breakdown of nutrients provided.)

QuickFix

We have discussed how this delicious orange-flavored fluid, an electrolyte replacement beverage that supplies potassium and mag-

---

*The 100 percent of RDA provided by Total or Product 19 is in a serving with milk and for selected nutrients only. Neither cereal provides 100 percent of RDA for all nutrients required by the body.

nesium aspartates, can help nourish people under physical stress, including hospitalization. It contains complex carbohydrates, B-complex vitamins, vitamin C, and other nutritional factors required for optimal health. It is a low-calorie beverage that contains no artificial colors, flavors, or preservatives.

Endurance Weight Gain Powder

Many hospitalized patients require extra kilocalories to help prevent malnutrition, and this beverage mix (just add skim milk) provides extra protein, vitamins, minerals, trace elements, and essential fiber. You can easily mix it right in your hospital room—a meal in a minute.

Endurance MultiVitamin Fitness Paks

A multivitamin/mineral insurance formula to help prevent nutritional deficiency due to reduced calorie intake or stress and trauma such as are associated with hospitalization. This formula contains no coatings, binders, or colors that might cause adverse reactions in people with allergies or on special diets, and it is free of corn, wheat, yeast, milk, and egg products.

Endurance Anabolic Formula

This formula contains the branched chain amino acids (BCAA's), L-carnitine and the urea cycle intermediates arginine and ornithine, as well as the vitamins necessary for their metabolism. This anabolic formula promotes positive protein balance and promotes muscle-building, thereby reducing the risk of hospital-induced protein malnutrition.

SURVIVAL TIP #2

• *Try to find a hospital that serves natural, unprocessed foods and low-fat, low-cholesterol menus.*
This may seem like a tall order, but a few calls to local hospitals should help you determine ahead of time which of them offer the most up-to-date nutritional care. Hospitals may even send you sample menus.

SURVIVAL TIP #3

• *Bring your own food to the hospital or have friends or relatives prepare* Eat to Succeed *recipes and bring them to you.*

Of course, you should let your physician and the hospital dietetic staff know exactly what you are doing (and that applies to the vitamin/mineral formulas you are taking at the time), in the event that they may be inappropriate for your specific condition. However, in most cases, you will be doing yourself a favor by taking charge of your own health and avoiding hospital-prepared foods.

Don't let the hospital intimidate you. You have the right to a healthful diet, and you are entitled to the best food possible. After all, it's *your* health at stake, not the doctor's or the dietitian's. *Ask their advice as to what foods to eat.* If it seems sound, then it probably is, but politely request an explanation for any advice that doesn't seem to make sense. This is particularly important when you are taking medications. Many foods are contra-indicated because they may adversely affect the beneficial actions of prescribed drugs.

SURVIVAL TIP #4

• *Avoid foods such as uncooked vegetables and fruits that may contain bacterial contamination, if you are undergoing chemotherapy or radiation therapy or taking immunosuppressant drugs.*

Research has shown that nearly 50 percent of the infections contracted by cancer patients (the people who are most likely to have a depressed immune system) were acquired in hospitals. Always request that your foods be properly and thoroughly cooked and avoid raw or suspect foods that have been left open or unheated for any length of time.

SURVIVAL TIP #5

• *Avoid meat and other foods that have a tendency to obstruct the esophagus or trachea if you are taking sedatives or if you cannot sit upright to eat.*

Choking to death, even while hospitalized, is not that uncommon. If you are taking sedatives, hypnotics, or other medications that make you tired or drowsy, or if you are elderly and/or you don't have a full set of teeth (or if you have poor-fitting dentures), you should observe this rule. If possible, always chew your food until it is liquefied in your saliva.

SURVIVAL TIP #6

• *Always check with the nurse or physician to be sure that they have the right dietary prescription for you.*
Health-care professionals are human and therefore do make mistakes. The wrong diet has been given to the wrong patient more than once, sometimes with disastrous results. Better safe than sorry.

Finally, you should know that as a hospital patient you have certain rights clearly spelled out by the American Hospital Association's *A Patient's Bill of Rights*. Contact your local hospital to request a copy of this document. Eating for success in the hospital means taking charge of your health and exercising your right to enjoy maximum nutritional protection against hospital hazards.

EATING TO SURVIVE SURGERY

The nutritional state of your body—*your* nutritional status—often determines your ability to recover from poisonous anesthesia and the trauma of surgery itself, and how fast and well your body will heal. Proper nutrition can also help reduce the risk of post-surgical depression and other complications.

Many dietitians have learned from practical experience that surgical patients often require many times the RDA's in order to thrive. The trouble is that many liquid formulas and hospital meals are deficient in one or more of the vital nutrients. The burden is thus placed upon the unsuspecting patient to prevent nutritional deficiencies before and after surgery. Since sub-optimal nutrition for surgical patients can and does seriously jeopardize health and recovery, here is a suggested method for protecting against some of the damage and health complications caused by anesthesia toxicity and nutritionally incomplete hospital feeding formulas and menus.

WHAT ANESTHETICS DO

Anesthesia is a wonderful and welcome medical procedure that permits surgeons to accomplish medical miracles. Before the development of anesthesia (during the 1840s), surgeons were limited to performing amputations and minor procedures such as treating superficial wounds. Surgery within the abdomen, chest, or skull was considered impossible. Anesthesia, however, is the scientific use of deadly poisons in precisely the right amounts to eliminate pain and, in some cases, consciousness as well. Surgical candidates should understand the anesthetizing procedure as well as how to protect themselves from the potential damage that these poisons can cause.

As a surgical candidate (perhaps for abdominal surgery), you may be given a sedative or hypnotic drug the night before surgery to help you sleep. The next morning, you may be given an injection of another drug to help you relax. Prior to surgery, however, an anesthesiologist (a physician who specializes in delivering and controlling the correct amount of anesthetics during surgery) may administer pure oxygen through a face mask. This allows the patient to survive *without* breathing for about two minutes while he or she is given the anesthetic.

To induce anesthesia for most operations in the chest and abdominal area, the anesthesiologist uses muscle relaxers/paralyzers and barbiturates. The former may include dangerous poisons such as curare and must be carefully administered so that the toxic effect does not overwhelm the system and prove fatal. The latter must be similarly administered to keep their effect as depressants under rigorous control. Usual practice is to administer these drugs in gradual increments, monitoring vital body functions all the while.

But these are just the first foreign substances introduced into your body. Now the anesthesiologist brings out the heavy stuff. First, a mixture of nitrous oxide (the same laughing gas your dentist uses) mixed with oxygen. Since nitrous oxide alone is insufficient to induce the profound anesthesia required for most surgical procedures, the anesthesiologist supplements this gas mixture with halogenated gases such as enflurane, isoflurane, and halothane. These anesthetics affect the heart and cardiovascular system and must be delivered with precision. An error of less than 1 percent could be lethal. Next the anesthesiologist administers more curare to relax abdominal muscles completely, and at this time he must connect the patient to a respirator that takes over the patient's breathing.

Once the surgery is completed, guess what . . . That's right—more drugs. Now that surgery is over, it's time to give the patient the antidote. Once accomplished, and the patient is again breathing, the anesthesiologist and attending physician check the patient's blood volume and composition and determine that all body functions are normal. Finally, the patient is awakened just enough to respond to the ministrations of a recovery room nurse.

The anesthesiologist's job is analogous to the job performed by air traffic controllers. Constant monitoring of vital measurements and readjustments that literally determine the difference between life and death are routine procedures. Is it any wonder that malpractice insurance for anesthesiologists is astronomically high? Most surgical procedures that require anesthesia today are so safe that survival rates are the highest in history. Surviving surgery, however, marks the beginning of your recovery—a compromised recovery that can lead to serious health problems or total recovery of the best of health. Which do you prefer?

As mentioned above, nutrition can help minimize the bodily damage caused by the multitude of poisons administered during anesthesia, and it can help insure a safe and speedy recovery and help reduce healing time. Eating to succeed in the hospital means much more than preventing hospital-induced malnutrition. It means protecting yourself from the damaging effects of anesthesia and providing your body with the right nutrients to help you heal faster and stronger. It is with that end in mind that I have formulated the *Eat to Succeed* Surgical Protection Plan.

THE *EAT TO SUCCEED* SURGICAL PROTECTION PLAN

Caution: Always check with your physician, surgeon, and anesthesiologist to determine if they know of any medical reason why you should not eat specific foods or take certain vitamin or mineral supplements prior to surgery. (Some surgeons, for example, don't want patients to take massive doses of vitamin E because vitamin E may affect blood clotting times.)

1. Surgery and the poisons used to anesthetize you throw your body and its metabolic machinery into shock. You should, therefore, *begin eating to succeed at least two weeks before surgery.* This means faithfully following the Haas Maximum Performance Diet and fortifying your body with nutritional supplements. Some surgical procedures require that you subsist on a liquid diet during recovery. Endurance meal replacers and Endurance brand nutritional supplements (listed in Appendix I) provide high-intensity nutrition and *fiber,* often missing in hospital liquid formulas. Quick-Fix also can provide liquid nutrition if you must limit your intake of or avoid solid foods. The liquid supplements that I recommend for my clients provide nutritional insurance both before and after surgery.

2. If your post-surgery meal prescription consists of light foods with a low nutrient density (such as gelatin desserts, cola beverages, broth), you should insist on light or liquid meals that supply adequate protein, fiber, vitamins, minerals, and trace elements along with other important nutrients, unless medically contraindicated. Here is a list of light foods you can choose from (with your physician's permission) to help prevent nutritional deficiency:

- Any *Eat to Succeed* beverage recipe made with Endurance brand drink mixes
- Any *Eat to Succeed* soup recipe
- Vegetable broth made from broccoli and/or other green vegetables
- Puree (e.g., baby food) of bananas or carrots
- Instant mashed potatoes made with water or skim milk
- Vegetable juice cocktail

- Bean, pea, or lentil soups
- Sweet potatoes or yams
- Corn puree (made simply by placing cooked corn kernels in a blender or food processor)
- Unsweetened applesauce
- Oatmeal with Equal sugar replacer, cinnamon, and raisins

3. If your physician permits you to eat solid foods, request that all meals be prepared without oil, margarine, butter, or fatty toppings, including conventional salad dressings, because fats and oils can retard the healing process by increasing inflammation and by reducing the oxygen-carrying capacity of blood. My "don't eat" list includes meat, egg yolks, cheese, avocado, mayonnaise, peanut butter, and ice cream.

4. Use vitamin/mineral supplements, *with your physician's permission,* each day to insure proper nutrition. Include a formula that contains the branched chain amino acids, urea cycle amino acids, and accessory nutrients involved in their metabolism to promote positive nitrogen (protein) balance.

5. If medically permissible, consume enough kilocalories to prevent weight loss during hospitalization. Use a nutrient-dense weight-control formula such as the Endurance brand listed in Appendix I or other meal replacers listed in Chapter Six.

6. If medically permissible, go for a walk after you eat, even if it's only up and down the hospital hall. Physical activity, even walking, can help prevent important mineral losses due to bed rest, and walking after a meal will help lower blood fats (triglycerides).

7. If medically permissible, drink plenty of fluids such as water, fruit juice, high-tech waters (such as are described in Chapter Four), and nutrient-rich vegetable broths.

Eating to succeed can make a dramatic difference in your recovery from surgery and help you heal quickly and correctly. It all begins with proper nutrition. Start by putting the right nutrients in your body and eliminating the harmful ones. Let Mother Nature do the rest.

NINE

Feed a Cold, Fight a Fever

Even though the *Eat to Succeed* Maximum Performance Diet provides all the nutrients you need to enjoy optimal health and protection against powerful health problems such as diabetes, diet-related cancers, and cardiovascular disease, you may on rare occasions still catch the common cold. Do you know *what* and *how* to eat in order to fight the fever, aches, and pains that accompany the common cold? Eating to succeed, in this case, involves more than sipping a bowl of chicken soup. You *can* succeed in fighting a cold through nutrition, and this is how you do it.

THE DOCTOR WAS RIGHT—ALMOST

"Drink plenty of liquids, eat something light, take aspirin, stay warm, and get lots of rest" was the advice my physician gave me whenever I asked what I should do for my common cold. This is a time-tested, common-sense prescription that just about everyone has heard and followed while fighting the common cold. It's good advice, as far as it goes. Fighting a cold, *Eat to Succeed* style, however, requires that you choose specific foods and beverages to help reduce uncomfortable symptoms such as sore throat and runny nose and stimulate your immune system to fight off the infection.

WHAT IS A COLD?

Many people mistakenly believe that colds and flu (influenza) are the same thing. In reality, these are distinctly different disorders caused by different types of viruses. Both share common symptoms—scratchy or sore throat, nasal and sinus congestion, and fever. Flu, however, causes more severe and generalized symptoms such as an ache-all-over feeling, higher fever, and tiredness that may persist for weeks after an infection.

More than one hundred rhinoviruses can cause the common cold. Not everyone who is exposed to these cold viruses will catch a cold, usually characterized by tearing eyes and upper respiratory symptoms of sneezing, runny nose, and scratchy throat. In some cases, the infection may spread to the lower respiratory system (lungs) and cause bronchitis, which is characterized by a deep cough, wheezing, and difficulty in breathing.

A cold is a viral infection, and antibiotics, so commonly prescribed for people suffering from ordinary cold viruses, cannot kill the microorganism responsible for the cold, as they would in ordinary bacterial infection. *Antibiotics such as tetracycline and penicillin have no effect against the viruses that cause the common cold—or any other viruses, for that matter.* If your physician prescribes antibiotics for you during your next cold, it may be because he or she believes that you may be suffering from a secondary *bacterial* infection such as strep throat, which can be prevented and cured by antibiotics. Antibiotics may also help prevent secondary infections in people who suffer from chronic bronchitis, emphysema, or other pulmonary disorders.

There are three classes of influenza viruses—types A, B, and C . Type A flu is the most common, and there is an oral medication called amantadine, which can be used to prevent and help cure this type of flu. Worldwide epidemics of Type A influenza occur every three years or so. Outbreaks of Type B flu occur roughly every five years, while Type C flu viruses seem to affect local regions and cause only sporadic outbreaks of mild illness.

The bad news is that the virus that causes the commonest type of flu, Type A, is constantly undergoing change, with an *entirely new strain appearing every decade.* These new strains are the ones responsible for millions of deaths, such as in the Great Flu Pandemic of 1917–18 and the infamous Hong Kong and Asiatic flu epidemics of recent years. When new strains of flu viruses appear, epidemics follow because people's immune systems are not equipped to fight the new strain.

The good news is that we probably don't have to worry about "killer" strains of flu viruses because researchers constantly monitor flu viruses; when a new strain appears, they quickly develop an effective vaccine. Researchers occasionally goof, however, such as in the case of the recently predicted swine flu epidemic that never materialized. Public health officials now recommend annual flu vaccinations for people at high risk of developing serious medical problems as a result of influenza—those with heart disease, emphysema, diabetes, kidney problems, severe anemia, or depressed immune systems, and anyone over the age of sixty-five.

Most physicians usually do not recommend specific diets or foods to help the immune system fight the common cold. However, the medical profession has recently discovered that mother, God bless her, was right. Chicken soup actually can help reduce the severity of symptoms of the common cold!

CHICKEN SOUP—A COMMON CURE FOR THE COMMON COLD?

Many of us smile whenever we hear about the seemingly magical powers that chicken soup exerts over the common cold. Could something as ordinary as chicken soup help cure the common cold?

Well, yes and no. Chicken soup, it seems, actually does help the body rid itself of the cold virus, because the hot vapor that we breathe in as we sip chicken soup helps wash the virus down the nasal passages and throat, an environment favored by cold viruses. While there is nothing inherently magical in the nutritional composition of chicken soup (any hot broth will provide the same beneficial effect), there is nothing wrong with enjoying chicken soup or any other light soup (see accompanying list) during your next bout with a cold. Soup is indeed good food!

HAAS-APPROVED SOUPS
FOR THE COMMON COLD

Chicken

Tomato*

Pasta e fagioli (Italian bean and
   pasta, recipe included in this
   book)

Minestrone

Vegetable

Onion (without cheese)

Barley*

Kidney bean

Lentil*

* Made without cream, oil, butter, or margarine

FEVER AND FLUIDS, FLUIDS, AND MORE FLUIDS

A cold-causing virus may predispose you to dehydration (loss of body fluids) through sweating from fever or diarrhea. A significant loss of body fluids (about 5 percent of your total body weight) can disrupt the body's ability to control fever and fight infection.

The body uses the relatively high temperature of a fever to create an unfavorable environment for microorganisms and to keep you from overexerting yourself while you are fighting a cold; chills that often accompany fever are the body's way of generating additional heat. Human bodies, like car engines, will overheat and malfunction if they run out of coolant—too high a fever over too long a time, especially in children, can damage the brain and lead to a coma, so it is critical to provide the body with enough liquids to prevent overheating. Fortunately, brain damage from fever is rare, but you should always take the proper precautions to prevent fever-induced health problems.

The normal body temperature of young children, unlike that of adults (which is 98.6 on the average), ranges between 97.1 to 100 degrees Fahrenheit, depending on the time of day, the child's level of physical activity, and the site at which the temperature is measured. A good rule of thumb is that rectal temperature is 1 degree Fahrenheit higher and axillary (armpit) temperature is 1 degree lower than oral temperature.

Once a child's temperature rises above 100 to 101 degrees Fahrenheit, the child has a fever and a doctor should always be consulted, even if only by telephone. The degree of fever does not always indicate the seriousness of the illness—some children may run a low body temperature with very serious illness while others run higher temperatures (103 to 104 degrees Fahrenheit) and have a minor illness.

Fever in children and adults is not a disease, but a symptom of illness, of a viral infection, for example. Measles, chicken pox, and other viral and bacterial infections are all common causes of fever in children. Since fever is part of the body's natural defense system for overcoming infection, it is usually unnecessary to worry about lowering it unless body temperature exceeds 103 degrees Fahrenheit, or unless the high fever lasts longer than seventy-two hours or is accompanied by other symptoms such as nausea or vomiting.

In order to keep fever at safe levels and prevent possible dehydration, it is important to provide the body with enough fluid to balance losses due to fever, vomiting, and diarrhea. Fluid loss due to fever shares a common attribute with exercise-induced fluid loss—neither immediately alerts the body's thirst center to the increased need for fluids. How much and what type of fluids should you drink during your next cold?

USE THIS TWO-STEP RULE FOR MAXIMUM HYDRATION

• *Rule One: Select fluids that contain no fat and very little sugar.* (I prefer drinks sweetened with NutraSweet or Equal instead of table sugar.) The body cannot absorb more than one to two pints of fluid per hour from the stomach and intestines. Therefore, at the first sign of a cold or fever, select one or more fluids from the Haas-approved fluid list and drink 1 to 2 pints during the first hour to insure maximum hydration and at least one cup of fluid (see Rule Two for fluid choices) every two hours thereafter, unless advised otherwise by a physician.

• *Rule Two: Drink water as your primary fluid, but consume at least 8 fluid ounces of one or more of the following choices twice each day:*

QuickFix
Orange juice (unsweetened)
Grapefruit juice (unsweetened)
Apple juice (unsweetened)
Any fruit-type beverage sweetened with NutraSweet, such as Crystal Light (any flavor), Country Time lemonade, Wyler's lemonade, Kool-Aid (any flavor), Linden Flowers Tea (use Equal sweetener and lemon or lime juice, if desired)
Hot water with lemon juice and/or Equal sweetener

SHOULD YOU TAKE VITAMIN C FOR THE COMMON COLD?

Maybe. There is now clear evidence that supplemental doses of vitamin C can decrease the severity of symptoms associated with the common cold and can decrease the number of days you will miss at work or school. Studies have not shown, however, that megadoses of supplemental vitamin C (greater than 500 milligrams per day) will *prevent* colds.

Taking large doses of vitamin C can cause the formation of free radicals (reactive substances that can injure and destroy healthy tissue) unless other antioxidants (such as vitamin E) are present in your diet as well, so I recommend taking a multivitamin in addition to supplemental vitamin C. The Haas Maximum Performance Diet provides between 150 and 1000 milligrams of vitamin C, depending upon the food and beverage choices you make, so take this into account when calculating your daily vitamin C intake.

Nutritionists still remain divided on precisely what the optimal dose of vitamin C per day is. Some say the RDA of 60 milligrams per day is satisfactory; others claim that the body may need as much as 2 or more grams—2000+ milligrams—per day during a cold. This question may not be resolved for many years, and taking extremely large doses of vitamin C without also taking other nutrients that work with vitamin C may produce undesirable health effects.

The commonest effect of taking too much vitamin C is diarrhea and dehydration, precisely what you are trying to avoid during a cold and fever. In general, vitamin C consumed in amounts up to 2 grams per day, especially while infected with a cold virus, does not appear to cause diarrhea or any other inappropriate effect in the majority of people who have been studied under clinical conditions.

People with sensitive stomachs or medical conditions affected by acid (vitamin C is a weak acid) should use *calcium ascorbate,* the calcium salt of vitamin C. This form of vitamin C is just as potent as regular vitamin C, generally does not cause acid stomach, and provides additional calcium as well. Synthetic vitamin C is just as effective as vitamin C derived from natural sources and usually much cheaper. However, purists who don't mind paying extra may use "natural" vitamin C.

FOODS THAT FIGHT COLDS

Unfortunately, there are no magic foods (chicken soup notwithstanding) that can prevent or cure colds; however, there are a few food groups that you should "lose" or choose during a bout with the not uncommon cold.

FOODS TO LOSE

Avoid foods with a high fat or oil content, such as mayonnaise, ice cream, peanut butter, butter, margarine, most red meats, egg yolks, avocado, cream cheese, sour cream, hard cheese, and dairy products made from whole milk. A high fat intake may further tax an immune system already overworked during viral infection. If you must drink milk or eat milk products, choose skim milk products and limit intake to no more than 2 cups of milk products per day, because milk sugar—lactose—may contribute to diarrhea.

Avoid heavily sweetened foods, such as pure sugar, candy, and sweetened beverages, in order to avoid hypoglycemia (low blood sugar), which can contribute to dizziness, headache, and other undesirable symptoms during illness.

FOODS TO CHOOSE

Select complex carbohydrates such as brown rice, bean or lentil soup, any vegetables or vegetable soup or broth, baked white or sweet potato, citrus fruits, bananas, pasta with plain tomato sauce, whole-grain breads with unsweetened fruit preserves (such as Tree of Life brand, available in health food stores), beverages from the approved fluid list above, whole-grain breakfast cereals (see Chapter Five for Haas-approved cereal list), multivitamin/mineral supplements (see Appendix I), and up to 3 ounces of chicken, turkey, or seafood per day, if desired.

SAMPLE DAILY MENU OF FOODS THAT FIGHT COLDS

BREAKFAST
6 oz. citrus fruit juice
Hot oatmeal (use Equal sweetener, if desired)

LUNCH
Haas recipe hot soup or Haas-approved hot soup (see list above)
1–2 slices of whole-grain toast with *unsweetened* apple butter

DINNER
Small chicken breast (2–3 ounces)
Steamed vegetable of choice or salad with no oil dressing or baked
    potato
        or
Bowl of bean or lentil soup (if you prefer a light dinner)

SNACK
½ cup *unsweetened* applesauce or one banana or one citrus fruit
    (limit to one snack per day)

BEVERAGES
Hot QuickFix or any other beverage from the approved fluid list
    given above (as desired)

A SPECIAL NOTE ABOUT MARINE OILS

Marine oils such as EPA and DHA (eicosapentanoic acid and docosahexanoic acid, respectively), taken in as food or as nutritional supplements, may help to combat fever and inflammation during the common cold. Recent studies have provided evidence suggesting that these oils may help health conditions involving inflammation, and while no positive proof yet exists to determine that marine oils can help reduce the severity of symptoms associated with the common cold, you may wish to try them the next time you catch a cold. To my knowledge, there has been no widespread recommendation of this use of marine oils, yet several of my clients have reported excellent results using marine oil supplements during the common cold. (The most popular brand is MaxEPA, available in health food stores. Follow manufacturer's dosage recommendations on product label.) EPA and DHA also occur in salmon and mackerel, two fish that should be part of your new Maximum Performance Diet. As little as one ounce of salmon per day has been shown to exert beneficial effects on blood clotting (by helping to make blood less sticky and therefore less likely to block an artery), and this amount may also help to keep fever at safe levels.

Eating to succeed during the common cold can help to reduce the aggravating symptoms of a cold and could well reduce the number of days you miss from work and play. Until researchers develop a safe and effective vaccine against common cold viruses, I believe that the *Eat to Succeed* program can help you feed a cold and fight a fever—by using maximum performance nutrition.

TEN

The *Eat to Succeed* Woman

With the publication of *Eat to Win* in 1983, many women discovered, for the first time, that they had different nutritional needs from those of men. The women's nutritional revolution, now in full swing, has stimulated a great deal of scientific research to define the role of nutrition more clearly in helping women enjoy success in health, beauty, and fitness.

Premenstrual syndrome (PMS), toxemia of pregnancy, and a much higher incidence of obesity, osteoporosis, anemia, gallstones, depression, urinary tract infections, and arthritis than in men all demonstrate that women do have unique nutritional needs that long have been overlooked.

As an *Eat to Succeed* woman, you can enjoy maximum protection against these and other health problems that have afflicted women throughout history. Moreover, you will discover the thrill of maximum performance in all areas of your life—at work, at home, and at play.

During the last two years, I have received questions from women all over the world who want to know more about their unique nutritional needs. I have found that the most commonly asked questions concern the following topics: osteoporosis, iron-deficiency anemia, and obesity.

125

OSTEOPOROSIS

Most of us are now aware of the osteoporosis epidemic that affects so many women in our population. Osteoporosis deteriorates the skeleton through loss of calcium, magnesium, and other vital minerals. Since it is a silent disease, it often goes undetected until one-third or more of the skeletal mass has been lost. The average female adult body contains about 1200 grams of calcium, 99 percent of which is in bone tissue. If too little calcium is present, bone fractures can occur as a result of the most minor bumps or jars to the skeletal system—simply walking across a room or bumping against a door, for example.

Women suffer from osteoporosis because:

• They eat high-protein diets, which cause calcium and other skeletal minerals to be excreted in the urine.

• They eat reduced-calorie diets (to lose or maintain ideal weight) and consequently do not consume enough calcium and magnesium.

• They have not been as physically active as they should have been (regular exercise helps to prevent calcium loss from bones).

• Estrogen and related hormones fluctuate throughout life, causing calcium loss from time to time.

• They do not produce sufficient vitamin D (actually a hormone) in their skin from exposure to sunlight (or they are not exposed often enough to sunlight), and/or they do not consume enough vitamin D from dietary sources. (The latter is rare today because vitamin D is added to so many foods, but it can occur in women who remain on unbalanced diets or who receive little or no exposure to sunlight.)

While milk and milk products remain the primary source of calcium in the American diet, many women who cannot digest milk, who have milk allergies, or who do not enjoy these foods have learned that they can obtain their calcium from dietary supplements and vegetables. The RDA for calcium is currently set at 800 milligrams per day, yet many populations around the world thrive and grow—and do not suffer from osteoporosis—on calcium intakes of as little as 200 milligrams per day. Most scientists believe that this is because they eat diets that provide less protein (25 to 40 grams each day, mainly from vegetable sources) than the 50 to 200 grams consumed by American women.

I do not recommend that women eat very-low-protein diets (less than 40 grams each day) because adaptation to low-protein intakes is best initiated in childhood. Adults who suddenly switch to very-low-protein diets begin to lose calcium from their bodies almost immediately. The adaptation process can take many months to years. That's why I always have recommended that women, especially those who are not active, take a calcium-magnesium supplement containing at least 500 to 1000 milligrams of calcium (and half as much magnesium) each day. Many women have been losing calcium from their bodies for decades, and extra calcium and exposure to sunlight (or supplementary vitamin D) can help to *reverse* the mineral losses of a lifetime.

Calcium supplementation at the level recommended above may still be insufficient for women who continue to consume very-high-protein diets (150 or more grams of protein per day). Since female bodybuilding has become popular, I have noticed that many women have begun to take the protein supplements used by bodybuilders and overconsume high-protein foods such as steak and eggs. This is not the way to build better muscles, nor is it the way to prevent osteoporosis. The best advice is to follow a moderate protein diet—generally 40 to 80 grams of protein per day with about two-thirds coming from grains, cereals, legumes, and vegetables and the other one-third from poultry and seafood (and skim milk products if desired).

My calcium recommendations are based on published research that shows that a woman's average daily calcium losses may total 320 milligrams per day or more and that the estimated absorption rate of calcium from the diet is between 20 to 40 percent. Some groups of people, such as those on certain medications or with gastrointestinal diseases, may have an absorption rate of less than 15 percent, resulting in skeletal calcium losses even when intakes reach 800 milligrams per day. Pregnant and lactating women need even more calcium. Stress and worry, commonplace in the high-pressure and fast-paced life-style of today's woman, may also cause calcium losses of up to 900 milligrams per day. Calcium losses in physically active women may be significant, especially during heavy sweating. The RDAs for calcium are:

Infants
0–0.5 year............................... 360 mg.
0.5–1 year............................... 540 mg.

Children
1–10 years............................... 800 mg.
11–18 years.............................. 1000 mg.

Adult women
Not pregnant or lactating.................... 800 mg.
Pregnant................................ 1200 mg.
Lactating................................ 1200 mg.

IRON AND ANEMIA

Men store more iron in their bodies than woman do. A healthy man may store 1000 milligrams of iron, while a healthy woman may only store 200 milligrams prior to menopause and even less if she eats an iron-deficient diet. Pregnancy and menstrual blood losses can deplete these iron stores at a rate of 10 to 40 milligrams per day.

Women are thus predisposed to suffer from iron-deficiency anemia, a condition in which red blood cells contain less than the normal amount of hemoglobin (which carries oxygen to all parts of the body). The reduced iron and oxygen supply to the tissues can decrease energy production and cause lethargy, tiredness, reduced brain function, apathy, headache, spoon-shaped nails, and pallor.

Iron deficiency affects women of childbearing years, the elderly, low-income groups, and minorities, although nearly every sector of the U.S. population (including males) is a potential candidate for iron-deficiency anemia. Studies have shown that approximately one in every four college women has depleted iron stores. Monthly blood losses from menstruation, on the average, amount to 28 milligrams of iron. This loss, if combined with a diet already deficient in iron, may double a woman's supplemental iron needs.

Women absorb iron from their diets at various rates, so we can only estimate how much iron the "average" woman absorbs daily. The amount of iron absorbed from foods each day is a function of how much iron is carried in the blood, the type of iron ingested (whether it is heme iron, which comes from animal products, or non-heme iron, which comes from grains, fruits, and vegetables), and the presence or absence of enhancing or blocking substances (e.g., vitamin C, an enhancer, and/or oxalic acid, a blocker). Additionally, absorption rates increase during times of growth, during pregnancy, and when iron stores become depleted.

Substances that convert iron to its most readily absorbable form include stomach acid and ascorbic acid (vitamin C). In fact, vitamin C is frequently added to iron preparations for this reason. Antacids, which reduce the stomach's acidity may block the effects of vitamin C if used on a regular basis and actually cause iron-deficiency anemia.

The RDA for iron for women assumes an average absorption of 10 percent per day and is based on the average iron content of the normal American diet, which provides about 6 milligrams of iron for each 1000 kilocalories. This means that a woman must eat about 2800 kilocalories each day to meet the RDA for iron if she depends only on unsupplemented food sources. For most women, consuming that amount of kilocalories daily would doom them to obesity. The RDA for pregnant and lactating women, set at 40 to 70 milligrams per day, would require an enormous daily caloric intake.

The RDAs for iron are:

Infants
    0–0.5 year .... 10 mg.
    0.5–1 year .... 15 mg.

Children
    1–3 years .... 15 mg.
    4–6 years .... 10 mg.
    7–10 years .... 10 mg.

Young adults and adults
    General average .... 18 mg.
    Females 11–50 years .... 18 mg.

Females 51 + years .... 10 mg.
Pregnant women .... 40–70 mg.
Lactating women (up to 3 months post partum). 40–70 mg.

Short of obesity, how can today's woman insure that she gets all the iron she needs each day to prevent anemia? By choosing maximum performance iron-rich foods and by judiciously supplementing her diet with iron-containing supplements.

MAXIMUM PERFORMANCE IRON-RICH FOODS

I recommend avoiding the traditionally recommended food sources of iron such as liver, peanut butter, eggs, and red meats. These foods contain too much fat and/or cholesterol for optimal health. Instead, I recommend the following foods for all women who want to enjoy maximum performance and better health:

Beans	Brussels sprouts
Peas	Broccoli
Lentils	Potatoes
Dark green leafy vegetables	Unsweetened applesauce
Whole grains and cereals	Corn
Winter squash	Peaches
Strawberries	Pears

Two additional hints for increasing iron intake without increasing calories:

• Cook in iron pots and pans (which may increase the iron content of certain foods by as much as 3000 percent).
• Consume vitamin C–rich foods or a combination of supplements and foods from the above list.

A woman's RDA for iron can easily be met by following these maximum performance suggestions. In cases where recommended foods cannot be consumed on a regular basis, iron supplements can help prevent iron-deficiency anemia.

OBESITY

Being thin is more important to a woman's health than previously supposed. Today, we know that women suffer from *twice* the incidence of diabetes than men. Most female diabetics are overweight, and obesity contributes to the occurrence of this disease. Even if you have a family history of diabetes, you are by no means doomed to suffer from this disease. Nearly every case of adult-onset (Type II) diabetes is preventable, and *maintaining a normal body weight is one important way of preventing diabetes.*

Chapter Six contains the *Eat to Succeed* Maximum Weight-Loss Program, ideal for women (and men) who want to shed unwanted body fat safely and successfully. The recommended maximum performance foods and food supplements in Chapter Six will provide women with a powerful nutrition program that addresses their unique feminine nutritional needs.

ELEVEN

Fit for the Office

Would you like to eat your way to success in business? You can, just as my clients do, if you follow my maximum performance Fit for the Office plan. This is the same plan that top executives of some of this country's largest and most powerful companies—e.g., Walter Kidde, Inc., and Carter, Hawley, and Hale—use to help them succeed in business and in health.

This plan has worked for businessmen and women in large and small companies alike, because staying fit for the office means performing at your highest level of creativity and work output, regardless of your corporate position or responsibilities. It can boost your energy during board meetings, sales conferences, presentations, and during stressful periods of both mental and physical labor. Just as importantly, staying fit for the office means protecting yourself against hidden hazards of the workplace that can cause serious health problems.

BEATING OFFICE FATIGUE

Working in a relatively confined area for eight or more hours per day under the normal stresses and strains of routine office work (which may involve meetings, telephone work, computer work, etc.) can cause mental and physical fatigue by late morning to early afternoon. This is the period when office productivity and general office efficiency usually decline and employees make costly mistakes. Most office workers almost instinctively reach for sugar-laden foods and coffee to boost their sagging energy. *This is precisely what they should not do for more energy.* In the end, sugar and caffeine will increase fatigue and inefficiency.

Whatever goes up must come down, and in this case, your blood sugar performs like a roller coaster. At first, sugar and caffeine will cause blood sugar levels to rise dramatically, but after a few hours, blood sugar will plunge, often to levels even lower than those that originally caused fatigue and decreased productivity. The common "executive" breakfast of jelly donuts, a Danish, or a muffin and coffee is exactly what you should *not* eat for maximum office performance.

Granted, most offices contain candy and donut machines alongside the ubiquitous coffee pot, so employees are constantly tempted to reach for these handy foods and beverages. Avoid them. Instead, bring Maximum Performance Diet snacks from home in your purse or briefcase, to help you sustain a smooth blood sugar level throughout the day and thereby avoid fatigue. These snacks include:

- Puffed brown rice cakes
- Unsalted Dutch pretzels (available in most supermarkets)
- Whole-grain breads with unsweetened apple butter
- Popcorn (preferably hot-air-popped)
- Crunchy dry whole grain cereal (see the approved cereal list in Chapter Five)
- Any Haas recipe for muffins or bread (one serving)
- QuickFix beverage mix (hot or cold) instead of coffee

DOWN WITH COFFEE, UP WITH QUICKFIX

I would like to see sugar-free energy drinks replace coffee as the national office drink. I particularly recommend QuickFix. Unlike coffee, QuickFix contains substantial energy nutrients such as B-complex vitamins, potassium and magnesium aspartates, and vitamin C, and it does not contain caffeine, sugar, or artificial ingredients (see Appendix I for complete nutritional information on QuickFix). Corporations would be wise to provide sugar-free beverages for their employees instead of coffee, especially in light of recent research that clearly shows an association of caffeine intake with increased serum cholesterol levels.

THE EXECUTIVE LUNCH

Lunch is perhaps the most dangerous time of day for every office worker and executive. The traditional executive lunch can contain more fat, cholesterol, and calories than many people consume in an entire day. Here's what I order whenever I'm invited to a business lunch:

6 ounces tomato juice or vegetable juice cocktail
Large garden salad or salad bar with a dressing made from vinegar, Equal sweetener, and a teaspoon of grated Parmesan cheese

and one of the following

1 cup of soup (bean, pea, lentil, vegetable, or minestrone)

or

Baked potato with a low-fat topping such as cottage cheese or yogurt

or

Seafood cocktail (lobster preferred) with red cocktail sauce

or

Half a chicken or turkey sandwich (no more than 2 ounces poultry) made with mustard only

Forget the two-martini lunch. Choose beverages made with NutraSweet, low-sodium carbonated water (such as Perrier) with a splash of lemon or lime juice, or plain tap water. (Check to see if your local tap water contains a high level of sodium. If it does, use bottled water that has had most of the sodium removed instead.)

OZONE, FLUORESCENT LIGHTS, AND CIGARETTE SMOKE

Three of the most harmful substances office workers encounter each day in their work environment are ozone, fluorescent lights, and secondhand or passive cigarette smoke. They are the silent assassins in the office that rob workers of energy and good health. Moreover, chronic exposure to these toxic substances may lead to serious disease and disability. Here's why.

Ozone (three atoms of oxygen bonded together) is normally produced from the interaction of ordinary oxygen (two atoms of oxygen bonded together) with an electrical charge. Electrical storms are a natural source of ozone. Electronic machinery, e.g. office and home typewriters and computers and photocopying machines, also generate varying amounts of ozone (see ozone chart in Chapter Seven). Chronic exposure to ozone in a confined office space may jeopardize the health of workers because ozone can destroy lung tissue; it may be related to lung diseases such as cancer and emphysema. It may also aggravate medical problems such as bronchitis, pneumonia, and asthma in susceptible individuals.

Fluorescent lighting has been associated with increased risk of malignant melanoma, a particularly lethal form of skin cancer if not caught in time. Fluorescent lighting emits a different wavelength of light from that of the sun. Scientists are currently investigating how artificial light from fluorescent light tubes affects the body. Some researchers believe that chronic exposure to fluorescent light while avoiding sunlight (something most office workers are forced to do at least five days each week) may account for fatigue, irritability on the job, and unexplained headaches and eyestrain. Fluorescent light tubes also contain several gases that leak from the fixtures as they age; the effects of these gases on human health have not yet been fully evaluated. However, preliminary evidence suggests that chronic exposure to these noxious gases may pose health risks for office workers, but more research is needed before we can establish their long-term health effects.

PASSIVE CIGARETTE SMOKE

Nonsmoking office workers actually smoke up to one pack of cigarettes each day if they work in a closed office environment where coworkers are permitted to smoke. Sidestream or secondhand smoke, like smoke inhaled directly from the end of a cigarette, can cause emphysema, lung cancer, and cardiovascular disease. Sidestream smoke contains about twice as much tar and nicotine and five times the carbon monoxide (which deprives the heart of oxygen) as the secondary smoke that enters a smoker's lungs. Secondary smoke passes through tobacco and filter before entering the lungs; sidestream smoke remains unfiltered and is therefore more toxic to smoker and nonsmoker alike.

If you work in a room in which seven cigarettes are smoked within an hour (not unusual in many offices), the carbon monoxide level in the room reaches half the maximum limit allowed by standards set by governmental health agencies. The poor office worker sitting next to a single smoker may inhale over twice the upper limit set for industry. Nonsmoking office workers who inhale sidestream smoke can quadruple their blood levels of carbon monoxide in just two hours. If you are a nonsmoker and you work in a smoke-filled environment, *you become a smoker too,* like it or not.

The political and economic issues relative to nonsmoking office employees being forced to inhale the deadly gases and toxic substances given off by others' cigarettes are debatable. The nutritional protection you can use to guard against damage from cigarette smoke is not.

THE FIT FOR THE OFFICE NUTRITIONAL PROTECTION PLAN

My Fit for the Office Nutritional Protection Plan consists of two simple rules designed to help protect you against unavoidable exposure to ozone, fluorescent light and associated gases emitted from fluorescent tubes, and cigarette smoke—the hidden health hazards in the office.

Rule One. Protect your body with a balanced formula of antioxidants. Any multivitamin that contains vitamins C, E, beta carotene, selenium, molybdenum, and B-complex vitamins in a clear, hard gelatin capsule will provide the basic nutrients you need to provide the extra nutritional protection you need against toxic office hazards. Antioxidants help prevent free radicals and cancer-causing chemicals from doing their damage by rendering them ineffective. (See Appendix I for formulas I recommend.)

Rule Two. Avoid vegetable oils (diunsaturated oils) such as corn oil and safflower oil, because they possess a high free radical potential—something you should avoid if you work in an office that already promotes free radical formation. People who eat low-fat and low-cholesterol diets are less susceptible to the harmful effects of cigarette smoke and other toxic substances such as ozone. For example, Japanese smokers who live in Japan and smoke American brands of cigarettes enjoy a much lower rate of lung cancer as long as they eat the traditional low-fat, low-cholesterol diet. Once they migrate to the United States and adopt the high-fat, high-cholesterol diet traditional in America, they suffer from the same rate of lung cancer and other smoking-related lung diseases as American smokers who eat the same way.

Proper diet and nutritional supplements can provide a degree of protection against the hidden hazards in the office, but they can never completely protect against them. The reality of life, however, is that we will probably always suffer exposure to pernicious substances. Rather than throw up our hands in despair, we should take every step possible to protect ourselves from environmental pollution in the office. Maximum performance nutrition should be your first line of defense against hidden office health hazards.

WHAT TO EAT BEFORE A BOARD MEETING OR IMPORTANT PRESENTATION

If you want to reach the top of your profession and stay there, you must turn in a world class performance at board meetings, sales conferences, and other important presentations. To do that, you'll need the energy and confidence that maximum performance nutrition can give you. You'll look better, fitter, and healthier and acquire the commanding presence of leadership as a result. That is what eating to succeed in business is all about.

Aside from following the Maximum Performance Program outlined in Chapter Five, you may want to follow these tips for maximum performance before your next meeting, annual report, or sales conference.

- Get a great night's sleep before your meeting.
- Avoid coffee, tea, and chocolate before a presentation.

A fretful, worrisome, and sleepless night before your meeting will dull your senses and business acumen. More than one executive has lost the confidence of superiors or clients (and perhaps even a raise or promotion) because of poor performance during important presentations. I recommend Lights Out, a nonprescription, non-drug sleep aid, available in health food stores, to help get a good night's sleep before an important meeting. Lights Out contains vitamin B-3, inositol, and other nutrients involved in helping the brain to relax, working much as a prescription sedative or sleep aid does. There is good evidence that this combination of ordinary nutrients binds to brain receptors that help induce sleep, without any trace of the drug hangover that users of prescription sleep aids experience. A high–complex carbohydrate bedtime snack such as are listed on page 73 may also help induce sleep, because carbohydrates help the brain extract compounds from the blood for use as sleep-inducing substances.

When it comes to a wide-awake, alert presentation, any caffeinated substance will only make an already nervous executive appear more jittery and that much less likely to inspire confidence in the audience. Again, a high–complex carbohydrate meal of not more than 300 kilocalories can exert a calming effect while providing plenty of energy to sustain a first-class presentation. Excessive kilocalories can quickly raise blood fat levels, thereby decreasing oxygen to the brain, something an executive cannot afford during a presentation.

Here is a suggested maximum performance snack to use if you want to eat prior to an important conference or meeting:

1 8-ounce glass of any nonfat, noncaffeinated drink sweetened with NutraSweet (e.g., QuickFix)

2 slices of whole-grain toast with unsweetened apple butter
1 medium size banana or apple

This snack provides an optimum ratio of complex to simple carbohydrates for quick and sustained energy and enough kilocalories to sustain an executive for several hours worth of high-stress work. It is also an excellent mid-afternoon pick-me-up alternative to coffee or chocolate candy.

Staying fit for the office is simple, fun, and delicious. Going for a walk during a break or lunch hour also helps office workers avoid a mid-afternoon slump. That's right. Exercise will *increase* your daily energy levels, as long as you follow the program presented in this book and my special nutritional tips for staying fit for the office. In business, maximum performance results from high-energy nutrition. On-the-job success begins with the Maximum Performance Program.

TWELVE

On the Road to Success

EAT TO SUCCEED is your key to success in life because your performance on the job, at play, in school, and during periods of illness at home and in the hospital all depend on maximum performance nutrition.

The *Eat to Succeed* Maximum Performance Program will work for you just as it has for Cher, Don Johnson, Ivan Lendl, and a host of other people from all walks of life who have taken charge of their own health. These people now enjoy the success of better health, high energy, and a new zest for life. They can work, play, think, and perform better because they have embraced a nutrition program that keeps them going long after others have called it quits. The same program that has worked for them will work for you, because it provides nutritional knowledge everyone can use, regardless of age, sex, occupation, or level of physical activity.

There are no excuses for not embracing the program. You can enjoy many of your favorite foods in the home and on the road. The new breed of delicious meal replacers offers a highly nutritious dessert-like treat for dieters bored with the cottage cheese–and–hamburger diet platters they've suffered with while trying to lose weight. Newer nutritional discoveries, such as the effectiveness of dietary supplements like L-carnitine and the branched chain amino acids in promoting weight loss and energy production, now make dieting more effective than ever before.

140

The *Eat to Succeed* woman, no longer a nutritional second-class citizen, can now enjoy the benefits of optimal health and maximum performance by addressing her unique, feminine nutritional needs. The *Eat to Succeed* woman recognizes that her nutritional needs are different enough from those of men to warrant special dietary modifications. These changes can help reduce her risk of osteoporosis, breast and uterine cancer (thought to be linked to too high a consumption of fats), diabetes, high blood pressure, arthritis, and even depression.

For the physically active person, adherence to the Maximum Performance program can help provide a rich supply of energy for a competitive edge through the scientific use of nutritional supplements, including the newest high-tech waters and high-tech protein supplements. Athletes no longer have to drink sugar-laden beverages or consume excessive amounts of protein in order to boost their performance and endurance.

If hospitalized, the Hospital Protection Program detailed in Chapter Eight can help you avoid hospital-induced malnutrition. You will increase your chances of successful recovery from surgery and heal faster and stronger through the use of proper diet and nutritional supplements.

Men and women in business can use the *Eat to Succeed* Fit for the Office program to prevent energy slumps and increase work output while protecting themselves from the hidden hazards of the office. They can, additionally, reduce days lost from the job due to illness and thereby improve productivity and profits while reducing business costs and medical expenses.

If you want the very best life has to offer, if you want to maximize your chances of success in all aspects of your life, I urge you to embrace the same state-of-the-art *Eat to Succeed* dietary principles that some of the most successful and talented people in this country now use. These are the nutritional principles that will help *you* eat to succeed.

Bon appetit!

SECTION II

The
Eat to Succeed
Recipe Book

Cooking and Shopping Tips

• Use Equal brand low-calorie sweetener as a sugar substitute. If you can't find this product or would like more information about it, write to:

> Equal
> Searle Consumer Affairs
> Box 8517
> Chicago, IL 60680

• Use PAM vegetable cooking spray instead of vegetable oil, margarine, or butter whenever possible for tasty, nonstick cooking. If you can't find this product or would like more information about it, write to:

> Boyle-Midway, Inc.
> Consumer Services
> 685 Third Avenue
> New York, NY 10017

• If you are unable to find Kraft American Cheese Food, Sharp Cheddar Flavor, check the section of your grocery store where Parmesan cheese is located or ask the store manager for help. If you still can't find it or would like more information about the product, write to:

> Consumer Service
> Kraft Court
> Glenview, IL 60025

or call (312) 998-3222.

• Look for Butter Buds in the section of the grocery store or drugstore where sugar substitutes or dietetic foods are located. If you are unable to find the product or would like more information about it, write to:

> Butter Buds
> Cumberland Packing Corporation
> 1636 Taylor Avenue
> Racine, WI 53403

• Toasted wheat germ is found in most grocery stores. Kretschmer regular is a good brand of toasted wheat germ. For information on Kretschmer, write to:

> Consumer Communications
> International Multifoods
> P.O. Box 2942
> Minneapolis, MN 55402

or call (612) 340-3493.

• If you are in a hurry to make a dish that calls for homemade tomato sauce, it's okay to use a brand in a jar once in a while. Prego spaghetti sauce is excellent!

• To make whole wheat bread crumbs, tear day-old whole wheat bread into small pieces and drop pieces into a blender or food processor one at a time to chop fine.

• If a recipe calls for toasted nuts, sesame seeds, or coconut:

1. Preheat oven to 350°.
2. Spread nuts, seeds, or coconut on cookie sheet.
3. Bake 5 to 10 minutes or until golden brown. Watch closely. Browning time will vary because of variations in oven temperatures.

• Some recipes call for defatted chicken broth. Here is a simple method for defatting broth:

1. Chill homemade or canned broth in the refrigerator for several hours.
2. Remove broth from the refrigerator and skim off the white solid substance (the chicken fat) that has congealed at the top.
3. Use broth according to recipe directions.

• Because cooking temperatures may vary from oven to oven, check to make sure you are not overcooking or undercooking when trying a recipe for the first time. Adjust cooking time accordingly when next preparing the dish.

Recipe Index

DRINKS

BREAKFAST DISHES

APPETIZERS

SWEET SLAW
TABBOULEH
TANGY HORSERADISH DRESSING
TOMATO DRESSING
TUNA BEAN SALAD
V-8 DRESSING
VEGETABLE POTATO SALAD

SIDE DISHES

CARROT CASSEROLE
CREAMED CORN
SQUASH AMANDINE
SWEET POTATO CASSEROLE
SWEET POTATOES DISCIPIO
SWEET POTATO STUFFING
ZUCCHINI CORN CASSEROLE

POTATOES

HASH BROWN POTATOES
MASHED POTATOES
NEPTUNE'S POTATO
ONION POTATO PIE
POTATO CHEESE BAKE
POTATO PANCAKES
POTATOES PARMESAN
TURKEY-STUFFED POTATOES

ENTRÉES

BAKED BARLEY
BAKED CANNELLINI
BAKED LENTILS
BLACK BEAN AND RICE CASSEROLE
BROCCOLI MACARONI BAKE
BROILED SHRIMP
CHICKEN AND BROCCOLI STIR FRY

DESSERTS

ALL-IN-ONE APPLE PIE
APPLE CAKE
BANANA NUT LOAF CAKE
CAROB NUT LOAF
FRUIT CAKE
MERV'S FAVORITE CHOCOLATE-COVERED CHERRY CAKE
PINEAPPLE PUMPKIN UPSIDE-DOWN CAKE
PUMPKIN BROWN RICE PUDDING
RASPBERRY PRESERVE BARS

Eat to Succeed Recipes

DRINKS*

BANANA FROTHY

Yields 1½ cups

1 scoop TwinSport Endurance
Weight Gain Powder, Vanilla
Flavor
½ cup skim milk

2 packets Equal sweetener
1 ripe banana
1½ cups ice

1. Place all ingredients except ice in a food processor or blender. With machine on, gradually add ice.

2. Keep machine running until mixture is smooth and thick.

NUTRITIONAL INFORMATION PER SERVING

Calories	438	Carbohydrate	69.1 g.
Protein	13.2 g.	Fat	6.0 g.
Sodium	178 mg.	Cholesterol	6 mg.

CHOCOLATE FROTHY

Yields 1–1½ cups

1 scoop TwinSport Endurance Meal
Replacement and Weight
Control Formula, Chocolate
Flavor
¼ scoop cocoa (imported if
possible)

⅓ cup skim milk
2–3 packets Equal sweetener
1–1½ cups ice (the more ice the
thicker the drink)

1. Place all ingredients except ice in a food processor or blender. With machine on, gradually add ice.

*All recipes are for a single serving.

153

2. Keep machine running until mixture is smooth and thick.

NUTRITIONAL INFORMATION PER SERVING

Calories	136	Carbohydrate	23.3 g.
Protein	8.5 g.	Fat	1.0 g.
Sodium	119 mg.	Cholesterol	5 mg.

CHOCOLATE MALTED   *Yields 1–1½ cups*

1 scoop TwinSport Endurance Meal
Replacement and Weight
Control Formula, Chocolate
Flavor
¼ scoop cocoa (imported if
possible)

2 round tablespoons malt
(Carnation puts out a natural
malt; found in hot cocoa section
of grocery store)
1 cup ice

1. Place all ingredients except ice in a food processor or blender. With machine on, gradually add ice.

2. Keep machine running until mixture is smooth and thick.

NUTRITIONAL INFORMATION PER SERVING

Calories	200	Carbohydrate	44.6 g.
Protein	7.2 g.	Fat	0.8 g.
Sodium	100 mg.	Cholesterol	3 mg.

MOCHA FROTHY   *Yields 1–1½ cups*

1 scoop TwinSport Endurance Meal
Replacement and Weight
Control Formula, Vanilla Flavor
½ cup skim milk

1 teaspoon decaffeinated coffee
2 packets Equal sweetener
1½ cups ice

1. Place all ingredients except ice in a food processor or blender. With machine on, gradually add ice.

2. Keep machine running until mixture is smooth and thick.

Calories	145	Carbohydrate	25.1 g.
Protein	9.6 g.	Fat	0.8 g.
Sodium	142 mg.	Cholesterol	5 mg.

NOG FROTHY   Yields 1½ cups

1 scoop TwinSport Endurance Meal Replacement and Weight Control Formula, Vanilla Flavor
⅛ teaspoon nutmeg
1 teaspoon vanilla

⅓ cup skim milk
1 teaspoon Imitation Brandy Flavor (optional)
2 packets Equal sweetener

1. Place all ingredients except ice in a food processor or blender. With machine on, gradually add ice.

2. Keep machine running until mixture is smooth and thick.

Calories	134	Carbohydrate	23.6 g.
Protein	8.0 g.	Fat	0.8 g.
Sodium	119 mg.	Cholesterol	5 mg.

ORANGE DREAM   Yields 1½–2 cups

1 heaping tablespoon TwinSport Endurance QuickFix
1 scoop TwinSport Meal Replacement and Weight Control Formula, Vanilla Flavor

½ cup water
¼ cup mandarin oranges (optional)
3 packets Equal sweetener
1½ cups ice

1. Place all ingredients except ice in a food processor or blender. Mix until smooth.

2. With machine on, gradually add ice. Run machine until mixture is smooth (2–3 minutes).

Calories	159	Carbohydrate	32.7 g.
Protein	5.6 g.	Fat	0.6 g.
Sodium	79 mg.	Cholesterol	3 mg.

STRAWBERRY FROTHY   *Yields 1–1½ cups*

1 scoop TwinSport Endurance
  Weight Gain Powder, Vanilla
  Flavor
½ cup skim milk

1 cup strawberries
3 packets Equal sweetener
1½ cups ice

1. Place all ingredients except ice in a food processor or blender. With machine on, gradually add ice.

2. Keep machine running until mixture is smooth and thick.

NUTRITIONAL INFORMATION PER SERVING

Calories	349	Carbohydrate	44.5 g.
Protein	12.8 g.	Fat	5.9 g.
Sodium	178 mg.	Cholesterol	6 mg.

BREAKFAST DISHES

APPLE AND BROWN RICE CEREAL   *Serves 4*

3½ cups cooked brown rice
1 6-ounce can apple juice
  concentrate (no sugar added)
  plus a 6-ounce can water

1½ cups chopped apple
1 teaspoon cinnamon
Equal sweetener to taste
½ cup chopped walnuts

1. Place first 4 ingredients in a saucepan.

2. Bring to a boil. Reduce heat to medium high. Cook 5–8 minutes or until liquid cooks down and apples are tender. Stir constantly.

3. Pour into 4 bowls. Sprinkle with Equal. Top with walnuts.

NUTRITIONAL INFORMATION PER SERVING

Calories	299	Carbohydrate	57.3 g.
Protein	5.8 g.	Fat	5.8 g.
Sodium	5 mg.	Cholesterol	0 mg.

CHEDDAR SCRAMBLE   Serves 2

4 egg whites
¼ cup Kraft Grated American
  Cheese Food, Sharp Cheddar
  Flavor

¼ cup low-fat cottage cheese
¼ cup skim milk
Pinch of pepper
Pinch of chili powder (optional)

1. Place all ingredients in a bowl. Beat with an electric beater until well blended.

2. Spray a large nonstick frying pan with PAM. Heat skillet to medium high.

3. Pour mixture into frying pan. Using a rubber spatula, stir mixture as it starts to set. Cook egg mixture until completely set, stirring constantly with spatula.

NUTRITIONAL INFORMATION PER SERVING

Calories	98	Carbohydrate	4.0 g.
Protein	12.7 g.	Fat	3.2 g.
Sodium	345 mg.	Cholesterol	11 mg.

CINNAMON FRENCH TOAST   Serves 4–6

4 egg whites
¾ cup evaporated skim milk
1 teaspoon cinnamon
1 teaspoon vanilla

Pinch of nutmeg
8 pieces whole grain bread
Equal sweetener to taste

1. Place first 5 ingredients in a bowl. Beat until frothy.

2. Spray a nonstick pan with PAM. Heat to medium high.

3. Dip bread into egg white mixture. Place bread in prepared pan. Cook, turning with spatula, until golden brown on both sides.

4. Sprinkle with Equal. Serve with Applesauce (page 212).

NUTRITIONAL INFORMATION PER SERVING

Calories	150	Carbohydrate	26.4 g.
Protein	9.4 g.	Fat	1.5 g.
Sodium	311 mg.	Cholesterol	3 mg.

CORN CAKES

Yields 10–12 pancakes
Serving: 2 cakes

1¼ cups whole wheat pastry flour
2 tablespoons granulated fructose
2 teaspoons baking powder
1 cup evaporated skim milk

1 teaspoon cinnamon
2 egg whites, lightly beaten
2 17-ounce cans corn, drained

1. Combine first 5 ingredients. Blend well. Add egg whites and corn. Mix well.

2. Spray a nonstick pan with PAM. Heat to medium high.

3. Pour batter onto frying pan about ¼ cup at a time, making several pancakes at a time.

4. With a rubber spatula turn pancakes when they are bubbly and bubbles burst on top. Cook until underside is golden brown.

5. Place pancakes on heated platter. Repeat cooking process. You may need to wipe the pan out and respray with PAM to avoid a burned look.

6. Serve with Applesauce (page 212).

NUTRITIONAL INFORMATION PER SERVING

Calories	265	Carbohydrate	57.1 g.
Protein	10.0 g.	Fat	1.5 g.
Sodium	69 mg.	Cholesterol	2 mg.

FRUIT SPREAD

Yields 1¼ cups
Serving: 1 tablespoon

1 cup low-fat cottage cheese
1 tablespoon lemon juice
¼ teaspoon allspice

¼ cup dried papaya, chopped
¼ cup dried pineapple, chopped
¼ cup pecans, chopped

1. Place first 3 ingredients in food processor (using mixing blade).

2. Blend until smooth. Add fruit and nuts. Mix for 1 minute.

3. Refrigerate for 1 week. Serve with whole wheat toast, bagels, or muffins.

NUTRITIONAL INFORMATION PER SERVING

Calories	56	Carbohydrate	6.6 g.
Protein	3.3 g.	Fat	2.2 g.
Sodium	93 mg.	Cholesterol	1 mg.

HAWAIIAN PANCAKES   *Yields 10–12 pancakes, 3½ cups syrup*

SYRUP   *Serving: ½ cup*

1 tablespoon cornstarch
2 20-ounce cans crushed pineapple
in natural juice

1. In a saucepan dissolve cornstarch in juice from both cans of pineapple. Heat to medium high, stirring constantly, until sauce thickens. Add pineapple of 1 can to mixture. Heat a little more.

2. Remove from heat and place in refrigerator.

3. When serving, add Equal sweetener to taste.

PANCAKES   *Serving: 2 pancakes*

1¼ cups whole wheat pastry flour
3 tablespoons granulated fructose
2 teaspoons baking powder
1 cup skim milk

2 egg whites, lightly beaten
Remaining pineapple
⅔ cup unsweetened coconut,
toasted

1. Combine first 4 ingredients in a large bowl. Mix well.

2. Add egg whites and pineapple. Blend well.

3. Spray a nonstick frying pan with PAM. Heat to medium high.

4. Pour batter onto frying pan about ¼ cup at a time, making several pancakes at a time.

5. With a rubber spatula turn pancakes when they are bubbly and bubbles burst. Cook until underside is golden brown.

6. Place pancakes on heated platter. Repeat cooking process. You may need to wipe the pan out and respray with PAM to avoid a burned look.

7. Serve pancakes with pineapple syrup and sprinkle top with toasted coconut.

NUTRITIONAL INFORMATION PER SERVING

Calories	242	Carbohydrate	42.3 g.
Protein	5.2 g.	Fat	6.6 g.
Sodium............	40 mg.	Cholesterol	1 mg.

HOT BROWN RICE CEREAL   *Serves 4*

4 cups cooked brown rice   4 tablespoons raisins
2 cups skim milk   Equal sweetener to taste
1 teaspoon cinnamon

1. Place all ingredients except Equal in a saucepan.

2. Bring to a boil. Reduce heat.

3. Simmer 1 minute, stirring constantly.

4. Remove from heat and pour into bowls. Sprinkle with Equal.

NUTRITIONAL INFORMATION PER SERVING

Calories	254	Carbohydrate	52.6 g.
Protein	8.3 g.	Fat	1.2 g.
Sodium............	67 mg.	Cholesterol	2 mg.

MUSHROOM ONION SCRAMBLE   *Serves 4*

8 egg whites   ½ cup low-fat cottage cheese
½ cup skim milk   1 cup finely sliced fresh
4 tablespoons Parmesan cheese   mushrooms
⅛–¼ teaspoon pepper   4 tablespoons chopped onion

1. Place first 4 ingredients in a bowl. Whisk together until mixture is a little frothy. Whisk in cottage cheese.

2. Spray a large nonstick frying pan with PAM. Heat skillet to medium high.

3. Add mushrooms and onions to egg white mixture. Mix.

4. Pour mixture into frying pan. Using a rubber spatula, stir mixture as it starts to set. Cook until completely set, stirring constantly with spatula.

NUTRITIONAL INFORMATION PER SERVING

Calories	98	Carbohydrate	5.4 g.
Protein	13.7 g.	Fat	2.1 g.
Sodium	323 mg.	Cholesterol	6 mg.

NEED-NO-SYRUP BANANA PANCAKES

Yields 12 pancakes
Serving: 2 pancakes

1¼ cups whole wheat flour
2 tablespoons granulated fructose
2 teaspoons baking powder

1 cup skim milk
2 egg whites, lightly beaten
3–4 large bananas, diced

1. Combine first 4 ingredients in a large bowl. Mix well.

2. Add egg whites and blend.

3. Spray a nonstick frying pan with PAM. Heat to medium high.

4. Add banana to mixture (batter should be full of diced bananas).

5. Pour batter onto frying pan about ¼ cup at a time, making several pancakes at a time.

6. With rubber spatula turn pancakes when they are bubbly and bubbles burst. Cook until underside is golden brown.

7. Place pancakes on heated platter. Repeat cooking process. You may need to wipe the pan out and respray with PAM to avoid a burned look.

NUTRITIONAL INFORMATION PER SERVING

Calories	259	Carbohydrate	59.4 g.
Protein	7.2 g.	Fat	1.5 g.
Sodium	39 mg.	Cholesterol	1 mg.

NOVA SCRAMBLE   *Serves 4*

1 small onion, finely diced
2 ounces Nova salmon, diced
6 egg whites

½ cup skim milk
Dash of pepper

1. Spray a nonstick skillet with PAM. Lightly brown onion. Add Nova and cook another minute.

2. In the meantime whisk together the egg whites, skim milk, and pepper.

3. Pour over Nova and onion. Cook on medium heat, stirring constantly, until egg whites are set.

NUTRITIONAL INFORMATION PER SERVING

Calories	64	Carbohydrate	3.1 g.
Protein	8.9 g.	Fat	1.6 g.
Sodium	971 mg.	Cholesterol	6 mg.

APPETIZERS

CRABMEAT DIP   *Yields 2 cups*
                                    Serving: 2 tablespoons

1 pound crabmeat, flaked
⅓ cup dry sherry
¼ cup plain low-fat yogurt
¼ cup low-fat cottage cheese

1 teaspoon Tamari soy sauce
3 tablespoons chopped green onion
⅛ teaspoon pepper
1 tablespoon chopped fresh parsley

1. Place crabmeat and sherry in a bowl. Chill 30 minutes.

2. Place yogurt, cottage cheese, Tamari, 2 tablespoons green onion, and pepper in a food processor or blender. Mix until smooth.

3. Pour mixture over crabmeat and mix. Add remaining green onion and mix. Sprinkle with parsley.

4. Serve with raw vegetables or whole wheat crackers.

NUTRITIONAL INFORMATION PER SERVING

Calories	81	Carbohydrate	2.3 g.
Protein	11.1 g.	Fat	1.6 g.
Sodium	618 mg.	Cholesterol	58 mg.

CUCUMBER AND ONION DIP

Yields 1½ cups
Serving: 2 tablespoons

¾ cup low-fat cottage cheese
1 cup peeled finely chopped
  cucumber
Dash of pepper
¼ teaspoon onion powder

2 tablespoons dried chopped onion
¼ teaspoon paprika
½ teaspoon Worcestershire sauce
1 teaspoon lemon juice

1. Place cottage cheese, ¼ cup chopped cucumber, pepper, onion powder, 1 tablespoon dried onion, paprika, Worcestershire, and lemon juice in a blender or food processor. Mix until smooth.

2. Remove from blender or food processor. Stir in remaining cucumber and onion. Chill several hours.

3. Serve as a dip for fresh vegetables and whole wheat crackers or as a topping for baked potatoes.

NUTRITIONAL INFORMATION PER SERVING

Calories	18	Carbohydrate	2.2 g.
Protein	2.0 g.	Fat	0.2 g.
Sodium	61 mg.	Cholesterol	1 mg.

GARDEN DIP

Yields 1½ cups
Serving: ¼ cup

½ cup chopped cucumber
½ cup chopped radishes
¼ cup chopped onion
¼ cup chopped green onion

½ cup chopped celery
1 cup low-fat cottage cheese
½ teaspoon Tamari soy sauce
½ teaspoon Mrs. Dash

1. Place vegetables in a food processor or blender. Chop with a couple of quick on-and-off turns.

2. Place in bowl. Add rest of ingredients and mix well. Chill for several hours.

3. Serve as a vegetable dip, spread for bread and crackers, or topping for baked potatoes.

NUTRITIONAL INFORMATION PER SERVING

Calories	38	Carbohydrate	3.5 g.
Protein	5.2 g.	Fat	0.4 g.
Sodium	183 mg.	Cholesterol	2 mg.

ONION DIP

Yields 2 cups
Serving: ½ cup

1 16-ounce container plain low-fat yogurt

1 package dry Lipton Onion Soup Mix (package marked 20 percent less salt)

1. Mix ingredients well.

2. Chill for several hours.

3. Serve as a dip for raw vegetables, topping for baked potatoes, or spread on whole wheat bread, bagels, or crackers.

NUTRITIONAL INFORMATION PER SERVING

Calories	65	Carbohydrate	7.4 g.
Protein	4.1 g.	Fat	2.1 g.
Sodium	218 mg.	Cholesterol	9 mg.

SALMON SPREAD

Yields 1½ cups
Serving: 1 tablespoon

½ pound Nova salmon
1 cup low-fat cottage cheese

¼ cup chopped onion
2 teaspoons lemon juice

1. Place all ingredients in a food processor or blender.

2. Blend until smooth. Chill.

3. Serve with bagels, whole wheat English muffins, or whole wheat toast.

Calories	28	Carbohydrate	0.4 g.
Protein	3.3 g.	Fat	1.4 g.
Sodium	45 mg.	Cholesterol	4 mg.

SHRIMP COCKTAIL *Serves 6*

1 cup chili sauce
4 teaspoons horseradish sauce

1½ cups shrimp, cut into small
  pieces
Lettuce

1. Combine first 3 ingredients. Chill 1–2 hours.

2. Arrange lettuce in 6 small cups. Spoon mixture equally into each cup.

NUTRITIONAL INFORMATION PER SERVING

Calories	79	Carbohydrate	3.6 g.
Protein	14.3 g.	Fat	0.7 g.
Sodium	96 mg.	Cholesterol	85 mg.

STUFFED MUSHROOMS *Serves 4*

½ pound mushrooms (rinsed and
  dried)
½ cup whole wheat bread crumbs
½ cup chopped walnuts
1 tablespoon Tamari soy sauce

⅛ teaspoon garlic powder
⅛ teaspoon pepper
¼ cup chopped onion
1 tablespoon chopped fresh parsley
1 egg white

1. Preheat oven to 400°.

2. Break off stems of mushrooms carefully. Discard.

3. Combine all ingredients except mushrooms. Fill mushroom caps with mixture.

4. Spray a shallow baking dish with PAM. Place stuffed caps in baking dish.

5. Bake for 20 minutes. Serve.

Calories	158	Carbohydrate	12.4 g.
Protein	7.3 g.	Fat	10.1 g.
Sodium.	199 mg.	Cholesterol	1 mg.

SOUPS

BLACK BEAN SOUP   *Serves 4–6*

1 large red onion, chopped
¾ cup thinly sliced celery
1 teaspoon dried minced garlic
3 cups defatted chicken broth
1 tablespoon Worcestershire sauce

2 teaspoons Tamari soy sauce
⅛ teaspoon pepper
3 15-ounce cans black beans,
   rinsed and drained

1. Spray a large Dutch oven with PAM. Brown onion. Add celery and garlic. Cook 1 more minute. Add rest of ingredients except 1 can of the black beans.

2. Simmer 15 minutes. Remove from Dutch oven and puree in a food processor or blender. Return to Dutch oven.

3. Add remaining can of beans. Simmer 30 more minutes.

4. Serve over brown rice and top with chopped onion.

Calories	208	Carbohydrate	36.6 g.
Protein	14.4 g.	Fat	0.9 g.
Sodium.	498 mg.	Cholesterol	0 mg.

CHUNKY CHICKEN NOODLE SOUP   *Serves 4–6*

8 cups defatted chicken broth
1 pound chicken fillets, cubed
1 tablespoon Tamari soy sauce
⅛ teaspoon pepper

⅛ teaspoon garlic powder
8 ounces noodles, broken into
   2" pieces

1. Place all ingredients in a large saucepan.
2. Bring to a boil.
3. Simmer 30 minutes.
4. Add water if reheating or soup becomes too thick. (It is a thick, hearty soup!)

NUTRITIONAL INFORMATION PER SERVING

Calories	266	Carbohydrate	28.2 g.
Protein	29.9 g.	Fat	2.8 g.
Sodium	1171 mg.	Cholesterol	59 mg.

CORN CHOWDER   *Serves 4*

1 large potato, peeled and cubed
2½ cups frozen corn
2½ cups water
1 bay leaf
¼ teaspoon sage
1 cup skim milk
⅛ teaspoon garlic powder

Dash of white pepper
⅛ teaspoon dried dill weed
1 tablespoon Parmesan cheese
1 packet Equal sweetener
1–2 green onions, chopped (include part of the green)

1. Place potato, corn, and water in a large saucepan. Bring to a boil. Cook 15 minutes or until potatoes are tender.
2. Remove all of the potatoes and part of the corn with a slotted spoon. Place in a blender or food processor. Puree. Return to saucepan.
3. Add the rest of the ingredients except the Equal and the green onion. Heat through.
4. Let stand a few minutes. Stir in Equal. Garnish with green onion. Remove bay leaf.

NUTRITIONAL INFORMATION PER SERVING

Calories	230	Carbohydrate	49.8 g.
Protein	9.0 g.	Fat	1.7 g.
Sodium	63 mg.	Cholesterol	2 mg.

HEARTY VEGETABLE SOUP
Serves 6–8

¾ cup diced celery
¾ cup chopped onion
1 cup sliced carrots
1 15-ounce can whole tomatoes, drained, rinsed, and chopped
3 cups tomato juice
2 cups water
1 large leek, sliced (include some of the green)
1 medium potato, peeled and cubed
1 17-ounce can peas, drained and rinsed

1 17-ounce can corn, drained and rinsed
2 15-ounce cans navy beans, drained and rinsed
1 cup cooked brown rice
1 tablespoon Tamari soy sauce
¼ teaspoon thyme
½ teaspoon pepper
¼ teaspoon garlic powder
1 teaspoon dried dill weed

1. Place all ingredients in a large pot.
2. Bring to a boil. Reduce heat. Simmer 30 minutes.

NUTRITIONAL INFORMATION PER SERVING

Calories	314	Carbohydrate	63.6 g.
Protein	16.4 g.	Fat	1.7 g.
Sodium	373 mg.	Cholesterol	0 mg.

LENTIL BARLEY SOUP
Serves 6–8

1 cup lentils
1 cup barley
1 16-ounce can tomatoes, chopped
1 cup chopped onion
1 cup sliced celery
¾ cup sliced carrot

2 tablespoons Tamari soy sauce
½ teaspoon pepper
1 teaspoon dried dill weed
1 teaspoon garlic powder
10 cups defatted chicken broth

1. Place all ingredients in a large saucepan. Bring to a boil. Cover and reduce heat to simmer.
2. Cook 50 minutes, stirring occasionally. Add water if soup becomes too thick.

NUTRITIONAL INFORMATION PER SERVING

Calories	241	Carbohydrate	43.8 g.
Protein	15.9 g.	Fat	0.7 g.
Sodium	1214 mg.	Cholesterol	0 mg.

NAVY BEAN SOUP   *Serves 6–8*

12 ounces dry navy beans, rinsed
12 cups water
4 medium celery ribs, finely
  chopped
3 large cloves garlic, minced

1 medium onion, chopped
4 medium carrots, sliced
½ teaspoon dried thyme
2 tablespoons Tamari soy sauce
½ teaspoon pepper

1. Soak beans overnight or boil 2 minutes, cover, and simmer 30 minutes. Drain off liquid.

2. Place beans and remaining ingredients in a large pot.

3. Bring to a boil. Reduce heat to medium and cook 1½–2 hours. Stir occasionally, smashing beans against side of the pot to thicken soup.

4. When reheating, add water to soup if it becomes too thick.

NUTRITIONAL INFORMATION PER SERVING

Calories	171	Carbohydrate	32.0 g.
Protein	10.5 g.	Fat	0.8 g.
Sodium	159 mg.	Cholesterol	0 mg.

PASTA E FAGIOLI   *Serves 4–6*

2 cups dry navy beans
6 cups water
1 medium onion, cut into quarters
  and sliced
2 teaspoons dried minced garlic
1 28-ounce can tomatoes, with
  liquid
½ teaspoon dried basil

½ teaspoon dried oregano
¼ teaspoon dried marjoram
3 teaspoons Tamari soy sauce
¼ teaspoon pepper
½ teaspoon dried dill weed
1 cup pitalini or elbow macaroni
Parmesan cheese

1. Rinse and pick out bad beans. Cover beans with water. Bring to a boil. Boil 2–3 minutes. Cover and turn off heat. Let stand 1–1½ hours.

2. Discard soaking water. Add 6 cups water. Bring to a boil. Reduce heat and simmer 1–1½ hours or until beans are tender.

3. Add remaining ingredients. Cook 15–20 minutes more. If soup becomes too thick, add more water. Serve. Sprinkle top with Parmesan.

NUTRITIONAL INFORMATION PER SERVING

Calories	353	Carbohydrate	62.4 g.
Protein	21.0 g.	Fat	3.1 g.
Sodium	354 mg.	Cholesterol	4 mg.

SPLIT PEA SOUP

Serves 8

1 medium onion, chopped
2 cups dry green split peas
6 cups water
3 tablespoons Tamari soy sauce
1 teaspoon dried dill weed

1 clove garlic, minced
6 dashes Tabasco sauce
4 carrots, sliced
3 ribs celery, sliced

1. Combine all ingredients in a large pot except carrots and celery.

2. Bring to a boil. Simmer for 30 minutes, covered.

3. Add carrots and celery. Simmer 30 more minutes.

4. Add more water if soup becomes too thick.

NUTRITIONAL INFORMATION PER SERVING

Calories	204	Carbohydrate	38.0 g.
Protein	13.6 g.	Fat	0.6 g.
Sodium	233 mg.	Cholesterol	0 mg.

TOMATO RICE SOUP

Serves 4–6

1 large onion, diced
1½ cups cooked brown rice
1 14½-ounce can tomatoes,
  chopped
1 cup tomato puree

4 cups defatted chicken broth
½ cup chopped chives
½ teaspoon dried oregano
1 tablespoon Tamari soy sauce

1. Spray the bottom of a Dutch oven with PAM. Brown onion.
2. Add remaining ingredients. Simmer 25–30 minutes.

NUTRITIONAL INFORMATION PER SERVING

Calories	109	Carbohydrate	20.0 g.
Protein	6.4 g.	Fat	0.6 g.
Sodium	869 mg.	Cholesterol	0 mg.

SALADS AND SALAD DRESSINGS

APPLE RAISIN SALAD

Serves 6

2 medium Red Delicious apples,
  cubed
1 cup raisins
¾ cup chopped walnuts
¼ cup skim milk
¼ cup low-fat cottage cheese

½ teaspoon horseradish sauce
1½ tablespoons lemon juice
⅛ teaspoon pepper
1 packet Equal sweetener
1 head Boston lettuce, separated
  into leaves

1. Place apples, raisins, and walnuts in a large bowl.
2. Place remaining ingredients except lettuce in a blender or food processor. Mix until smooth.
3. Pour over apple mixture. Toss to coat.
4. Arrange lettuce leaves in 6 bowls. Spoon apple mixture into center of bowls.

NUTRITIONAL INFORMATION PER SERVING

Calories	255	Carbohydrate	33.2 g.
Protein	6.1 g.	Fat	9.8 g.
Sodium	51 mg.	Cholesterol	1 mg.

BEAN SALAD   *Serves 8–10*

1 20-ounce can kidney beans, drained and rinsed
1 16-ounce can corn, drained and rinsed
1 16-ounce can chickpeas, drained and rinsed
1 cup finely chopped carrots
2 tablespoons chopped onion

3 medium green onions, chopped
3 tablespoons sweet pickle relish
½ cup no-oil Italian dressing
3 tablespoons red wine vinegar
2 teaspoons Dijon mustard
Pinch of pepper
⅛ teaspoon garlic powder
1 packet Equal sweetener

1. Combine first 7 ingredients in a large bowl.
2. Place remaining ingredients in another bowl. Mix well. Pour over bean mixture. Toss to coat.
3. Chill.

NUTRITIONAL INFORMATION PER SERVING

Calories	210	Carbohydrate	40.3 g.
Protein	10.7 g.	Fat	1.9 g.
Sodium	274 mg.	Cholesterol	0 mg.

CARROT SALAD WALDORF   *Serves 8*

8 cups peeled and shredded carrots
1 cup raisins
½ cup chopped walnuts

2 cups chopped apples
¾ cup plain low-fat yogurt
¾ cup apple juice concentrate

1. Mix first 4 ingredients in a large bowl.
2. Mix yogurt and apple juice concentrate in a separate bowl.
3. Pour yogurt mixture over carrot mixture and toss. Chill.

NUTRITIONAL INFORMATION PER SERVING

Calories	250	Carbohydrate	50.8 g.
Protein	5.0 g.	Fat	5.1 g.
Sodium	108 mg.	Cholesterol	2 mg.

CAULIFLOWER BROCCOLI SALAD   *Serves 4–6*

2 cups chopped florets of cauliflower
2 cups chopped florets of broccoli
¾ cup low-fat buttermilk

½ cup low-fat cottage cheese
1½ teaspoons dried dill weed
⅛ teaspoon pepper
1 teaspoon Tamari soy sauce

1. Place cauliflower and broccoli in a large bowl.

2. Place remaining ingredients in a food processor or blender. Mix until smooth.

3. Pour over cauliflower and broccoli. Toss to coat.

NUTRITIONAL INFORMATION PER SERVING

Calories	52	Carbohydrate	7.2 g.
Protein	6.3 g.	Fat	0.6 g.
Sodium	131 mg.	Cholesterol	1 mg.

CELERY SEED DRESSING   *Yields 1⅓ cups*
Serving: ⅓ cup

½ cup plain low-fat yogurt
½ cup low-fat cottage cheese
1 tablespoon celery seed
⅛ teaspoon pepper

1 teaspoon Tamari soy sauce
½ teaspoon lemon juice
⅛ teaspoon garlic powder
½ cup finely chopped celery

1. Place all ingredients except celery in a blender or food processor. Blend until smooth.

2. Add celery. Chill. Serve over garden-fresh vegetables or as a dip.

NUTRITIONAL INFORMATION PER SERVING

Calories	44	Carbohydrate	3.7 g.
Protein	5.0 g.	Fat	1.2 g.
Sodium	187 mg.	Cholesterol	4 mg.

CHICKEN SALAD SUPREME   *Serves 6*

2 cups cubed cooked chicken
⅔ cup diced celery
½ cup coarsely chopped pecans
2 cups diced apples
½ cup plain low-fat yogurt
¼ cup low-fat cottage cheese

½ teaspoon prepared mustard
2 teaspoons lemon juice
1 teaspoon Tamari soy sauce
12 leaves lettuce
6 slices pineapple

1. Combine first 4 ingredients in a large bowl.

2. Place yogurt, cottage cheese, mustard, lemon juice, and Tamari in a food processor or blender. Mix until smooth.

3. Pour over the chicken mixture. Toss to coat.

4. Arrange lettuce leaves in 6 salad bowls. Place a slice of pineapple in each bowl. Spoon equal amounts of chicken salad into each bowl. Chill before serving.

NUTRITIONAL INFORMATION PER SERVING

Calories	251	Carbohydrate	25.5 g.
Protein	19.3 g.	Fat	9.3 g.
Sodium	130 mg.	Cholesterol	45 mg.

CHICKPEA AND PASTA SALAD   *Serves 6–8*

2 cups pasta shells, cooked
   according to package directions
1 16-ounce can chickpeas, drained
   and rinsed
2 medium tomatoes, chopped
1 package frozen chopped broccoli,
   defrosted

¾ cup no-oil Italian dressing
¼ teaspoon pepper
1½ teaspoons dried oregano
¼ teaspoon garlic powder
6 tablespoons Parmesan cheese

1. Mix pasta, chickpeas, and vegetables in a large bowl.
2. Mix remaining ingredients in a smaller bowl. Pour over pasta mixture. Toss.
3. Chill 2–3 hours.

NUTRITIONAL INFORMATION PER SERVING

Calories	197	Carbohydrate	33.3 g.
Protein	11.7 g.	Fat	3.0 g.
Sodium	414 mg.	Cholesterol	3 mg.

CORN SALAD   Serves 4–6

2 17-ounce cans corn, drained and rinsed
1 medium tomato, diced
1 medium rib celery, diced
¼ cup chopped green onion
¼ cup low-fat cottage cheese

1 tablespoon red wine vinegar
1 teaspoon Tamari soy sauce
¼ teaspoon pepper
1 tablespoon finely chopped fresh parsley
1 packet Equal sweetener

1. Mix first 4 ingredients in a large bowl.
2. Place remaining ingredients in a food processor or blender. Mix until smooth.
3. Pour over corn mixture and toss. Chill.

NUTRITIONAL INFORMATION PER SERVING

Calories	139	Carbohydrate	31.2 g.
Protein	5.6 g.	Fat	1.3 g.
Sodium	75 mg.	Cholesterol	0+ mg.

CREAMY RUSSIAN DRESSING   Yields 1 cup
                                          Serving: ¼ cup

½ cup low-fat cottage cheese
½ cup plain low-fat yogurt
3 tablespoons chili sauce

1 tablespoon dried minced onion
1 teaspoon chili powder

1. Place all ingredients in a blender or food processor.
2. Mix until smooth.
3. Chill. Serve over a fresh green vegetable salad or use as a dip.

NUTRITIONAL INFORMATION PER SERVING

Calories	218.7	Carbohydrate	41.8 g.
Protein	9.3 g.	Fat	2.7 g.
Sodium	95.9 mg.	Cholesterol	0.1 mg.

GARLIC DRESSING

Yields 1 cup
Serving: 2 tablespoons

1¼ cups low-fat cottage cheese
  (1 percent milk fat)
¼ cup plain low-fat yogurt
2 tablespoons chopped fresh
  parsley

3 cloves garlic, minced
2 teaspoons wine vinegar
1½ teaspoons Tamari soy sauce

1. Place all ingredients in a food processor or blender. Blend until completely smooth.
2. Chill.
3. Serve over fresh garden salad or use as a vegetable dip.

NUTRITIONAL INFORMATION PER SERVING

Calories	31	Carbohydrate	1.8 g.
Protein	4.8 g.	Fat	0.5 g.
Sodium	175 mg.	Cholesterol	2 mg.

GARLIC FRENCH DRESSING

Yields 1½ cups
Serving: ¼ cup

1½ cups no-oil vinaigrette dressing
3 tablespoons chili sauce
2 teaspoons Tamari soy sauce
1 packet Equal sweetener
1 teaspoon horseradish

1 teaspoon mustard
½ teaspoon paprika
¼ teaspoon pepper
1 teaspoon dried minced garlic

1. Place all ingredients in a blender or food processor.
2. Mix until smooth.

NUTRITIONAL INFORMATION PER SERVING

Calories	12	Carbohydrate	3.9 g.
Protein	0.3 g.	Fat	0.1 g.
Sodium	62 mg.	Cholesterol	0 mg.

GRAPE AND CHICKEN SALAD   *Serves 4*

2 cups macaroni shells, cooked according to package directions
Cooked chicken cut in strips to make 2 cups
1½ cups seedless green grapes
½ cup chopped celery

1 cup low-fat buttermilk
¼ teaspoon dried dill weed
Pinch of onion powder
Pinch of garlic powder
½ teaspoon Tamari soy sauce

1. Combine first 4 ingredients in a mixing bowl. Toss to mix.
2. In another bowl mix remaining ingredients. Pour over chicken. Toss to coat.
3. Chill. Serve in lettuce bowls.

NUTRITIONAL INFORMATION PER SERVING

Calories	250	Carbohydrate	27.7 g.
Protein	27.3 g.	Fat	3.3 g.
Sodium	112 mg.	Cholesterol	65 mg.

HAAS MAYONNAISE SPREAD   *Yields ¾ cup*
Serving: 2 tablespoons

1 cup low-fat cottage cheese (1% milk fat)
2 teaspoons lemon juice

½ teaspoon Tamari soy sauce
1 teaspoon prepared mustard

1. Combine all ingredients in a food processor or blender. Mix until completely smooth.
2. Chill.

NUTRITIONAL INFORMATION PER SERVING

Calories	28.4	Carbohydrate	1.2 g.
Protein	4.7 g.	Fat	0.4 g.
Sodium.............	176 mg.	Cholesterol	0.2 mg.

LOBSTER SALAD   *Serves 4*

Cooked lobster chopped into small   ¾ cup Haas Mayonnaise Spread
   pieces to make 1 cup   ½ cup chopped celery
2 tablespoons chopped onion   Pinch of pepper

1. Combine all ingredients. Mix well.

2. Place on lettuce leaves or serve in whole wheat pita bread.

NUTRITIONAL INFORMATION PER SERVING

Calories	109	Carbohydrate	5.1 g.
Protein	17.7 g.	Fat	1.9 g.
Sodium.............	410 mg.	Cholesterol	50 mg.

ORIENTAL SALAD   *Serves 4*

1 cup thinly sliced radishes   1 teaspoon dry mustard
5 cups shredded lettuce   ¼ teaspoon ground ginger
½ cup wine vinegar   ¾ teaspoon garlic powder
⅛ cup water   1½ cups cooked cubed chicken
⅛ cup Tamari soy sauce   ¼ cup chopped green onion
3 packets Equal sweetener   ½ cup sliced almonds, toasted

1. Toss radishes and lettuce. Divide into 4 bowls.

2. Mix vinegar, water, Tamari, Equal, mustard, ginger, and garlic powder in a bowl. Whisk together. Place chicken and onion in vinegar mixture. Marinate 30–40 minutes.

3. Remove chicken and onion from marinade with slotted spoon. Place equal portions in each bowl. Top with toasted almonds. Drizzle salads with extra marinade if needed.

NUTRITIONAL INFORMATION PER SERVING

Calories	234	Carbohydrate	10.7 g.
Protein	23.0 g.	Fat	11.9 g.
Sodium	283 mg.	Cholesterol	48 mg.

PARSLEY PARMESAN DRESSING

Yields 1½ cups
Serving: ¼ cup

½ cup plain low-fat yogurt
½ cup low-fat cottage cheese
⅓ cup Parmesan cheese
¼ cup chopped fresh parsley

¼ cup skim milk
2 tablespoons lemon juice
2 teaspoons Italian seasoning
2 teaspoons wine vinegar

1. Place all ingredients in a food processor or blender. Process until smooth.

2. Chill. Serve over fresh garden salad or use as a dip.

NUTRITIONAL INFORMATION PER SERVING

Calories	51	Carbohydrate	3.1 g.
Protein	5.3 g.	Fat	1.9 g.
Sodium	176 mg.	Cholesterol	6 mg.

RED CABBAGE AND APPLE SLAW

Serves 6

¾ pound red cabbage, shredded
2 large carrots, grated
2 medium Red Delicious apples, diced
½ cup raisins
2 ribs celery, sliced

¼ cup lemon juice
2 packets Equal sweetener
1 tablespoon dried onion
2 teaspoons prepared mustard
⅓ cup no-oil vinaigrette dressing

1. Place first 5 ingredients in a large bowl. Toss to mix.

2. Place remaining ingredients in a food processor or blender. Mix until smooth.

3. Pour over cabbage mixture. Toss to coat.

Calories	125	Carbohydrate	31.1 g.
Protein	2.4 g.	Fat	0.6 g.
Sodium	81 mg.	Cholesterol	0 mg.

RED POTATO SALAD   *Serves 4–6*

4 medium red potatoes, quartered
  (should be 6 cups after cooking)
½ cup low-fat cottage cheese
¾ cup plain low-fat yogurt
¼ cup red wine vinegar
3 teaspoons prepared mustard

3 teaspoons lemon juice
1 tablespoon Tamari soy sauce
⅛ teaspoon pepper
½ cup chopped celery
¼ cup chopped onion
½ cup chopped green onion

1. Cover potatoes with water in a saucepan. Bring to a boil and cook 25–35 minutes or until tender.

2. Place cottage cheese, yogurt, vinegar, mustard, lemon juice, Tamari, and pepper in a food processor or blender. Mix until smooth.

3. Mix celery, onion, and green onion with potatoes. Pour dressing over potato mixture and toss to coat. (It is best to toss potato salad while potatoes are still warm.)

4. Chill.

Calories	146	Carbohydrate	28.4 g.
Protein	6.9 g.	Fat	1.0 g.
Sodium	211 mg.	Cholesterol	3 mg.

SHRIMP SALAD   *Serves 4–6*

1 cup low-fat cottage cheese
½ cup skim milk
3 tablespoons lemon juice
½ teaspoon Tamari soy sauce
1 teaspoon prepared mustard
¼ teaspoon pepper

8 ounces elbow macaroni, cooked,
  rinsed, and drained
1 cup chopped celery
¼ cup chopped onion
½ cup chopped scallions
2 cups cooked, deveined, and
  coarsely chopped shrimp

1. Place first 6 ingredients in a food processor or blender. Mix until smooth.

2. Mix remaining ingredients in a large bowl. Pour cottage cheese mixture over macaroni and vegetables. Toss to mix. Chill.

NUTRITIONAL INFORMATION PER SERVING

Calories	274	Carbohydrate	34.0 g.
Protein	28.9 g.	Fat	1.8 g.
Sodium	320 mg.	Cholesterol	116 mg.

SPINACH SALAD   *Serves 4–6*

1 10-ounce package fresh spinach, cleaned, dried, and cut up into small pieces
½ cup coarsely chopped pecans
1 12-ounce container dry curd cottage cheese

1 cup plain low-fat yogurt
3 packets Equal sweetener
3 tablespoons wine vinegar
1¼ teaspoons dry mustard
1 teaspoon Tamari soy sauce
2 teaspoons horseradish sauce

1. Mix spinach, pecans, and cottage cheese. Toss.

2. Combine remaining ingredients in a bowl. Mix well.

3. When ready to serve, pour dressing over spinach and toss.

NUTRITIONAL INFORMATION PER SERVING

Calories	140	Carbohydrate	7.5 g.
Protein	10.9 g.	Fat	8.0 g.
Sodium	309 mg.	Cholesterol	6 mg.

SWEET SLAW   *Serves 6–8*

1 12-ounce can crushed pineapple in natural juice, drained
1 small head of cabbage, shredded
½ cup raisins
¾ cup finely chopped walnuts

¾ cup low-fat cottage cheese
½ cup plain low-fat yogurt
2 tablespoons lemon juice
3 packets Equal sweetener

1. Combine first 4 ingredients in a large bowl. Toss to mix.

2. Place remaining ingredients in a food processor or blender. Mix until smooth. Pour over cabbage mixture. Toss until slaw is coated.

3. Chill.

NUTRITIONAL INFORMATION PER SERVING

Calories	145	Carbohydrate	18.4 g.
Protein	5.3 g.	Fat	6.6 g.
Sodium	97 mg.	Cholesterol	2 mg.

TABBOULEH   *Serves 4*

1 cup raw bulgur
1¾ cup defatted chicken stock
¼ cup lemon juice
¼ teaspoon garlic powder
½ cup chopped onion
½ cup chopped green onion
¼ cup chopped fresh parsley

½ cup chopped cucumber
1 cup chopped tomato
1 teaspoon dried mint
¼ cup no-oil vinaigrette dressing
⅛ cup lemon juice
Pepper to taste

1. Place bulgur, chicken stock, ¼ cup lemon juice, and garlic powder in a bowl. Let stand 30–45 minutes or until bulgur has softened.

2. Drain well and squeeze out excess liquid. Add remaining ingredients and toss. Chill before serving.

NUTRITIONAL INFORMATION PER SERVING

Calories	204	Carbohydrate	44.1 g.
Protein	7.3 g.	Fat	0.8 g.
Sodium	357 mg.	Cholesterol	0 mg.

TANGY HORSERADISH DRESSING   *Yields 1 cup*
Serving: ¼ cup

3 tablespoons lemon juice
2 tablespoons red wine vinegar
1 tablespoon Dijon mustard
1 tablespoon dried minced garlic
1 tablespoon chopped fresh parsley

1 tablespoon horseradish
1 teaspoon Tamari soy sauce
¼ teaspoon pepper
6 tablespoons no-oil vinaigrette
    dressing

1. Place all ingredients in a blender or food processor.
2. Mix until smooth.

NUTRITIONAL INFORMATION PER SERVING

Calories	141	Carbohydrate	35.4 g.
Protein	0.7 g.	Fat	0.6 g.
Sodium	3 mg.	Cholesterol	0 mg.

TOMATO DRESSING

Yields 2 cups
Serving: ¼ cup

2 medium tomatoes, chopped
(approximately 1 cup)
½ green pepper, chopped
(approximately ½ cup)
1 rib celery, chopped
(approximately ½ cup)

¾ cup low-fat cottage cheese
¼ cup plain low-fat yogurt
2 tablespoons Parmesan cheese
1 teaspoon dry mustard

1. Place all ingredients in a food processor or blender. Process until smooth.
2. Chill. Serve over fresh garden salad or use as a vegetable dip.

NUTRITIONAL INFORMATION PER SERVING

Calories	35	Carbohydrate	3.0 g.
Protein	3.9 g.	Fat	0.9 g.
Sodium	124 mg.	Cholesterol	3 mg.

TUNA BEAN SALAD

Serves 6

¼ cup finely chopped celery
3 tablespoons chopped fresh
parsley
3 tablespoons chopped onion
2 tablespoons lemon juice
1 tablespoon wine vinegar
3 tablespoons pale dry sherry

1 teaspoon Tamari soy sauce
1 teaspoon dried basil
1 19-ounce can cannellini, drained
1 6½-ounce can tuna packed in
water, drained and flaked
¼ cup pitted sliced olives
Lettuce

1. Combine first 8 ingredients in a screw-top jar. Shake to mix. Chill.

2. Combine cannellini, tuna, and olives. Chill several hours.

3. When ready to serve, arrange lettuce in 6 salad bowls. Pour dressing over tuna mixture and toss. Spoon in equal portions into salad bowls.

NUTRITIONAL INFORMATION PER SERVING

Calories	197	Carbohydrate	24.9 g.
Protein	18.3 g.	Fat	2.3 g.
Sodium	305 mg.	Cholesterol	22 mg.

V-8 DRESSING

Yields 1½ cups
Serving: ¼ cup

1 cup V-8 vegetable juice
½ cup red wine vinegar
½ teaspoon garlic powder
1 teaspoon dried basil
1 teaspoon dried oregano

¼ teaspoon dried marjoram
¼ teaspoon dried thyme
¼ teaspoon dry mustard
1 teaspoon cornstarch
1 packet Equal sweetener

1. Place all ingredients except Equal in a saucepan. Stir until cornstarch is dissolved.

2. Turn heat to medium high. Heat, stirring constantly until dressing thickens.

3. Remove from heat. Add Equal and chill.

4. Serve over a fresh vegetable salad.

NUTRITIONAL INFORMATION PER SERVING

Calories	17	Carbohydrate	4.1 g.
Protein	0.4 g.	Fat	0.1 g.
Sodium	11 mg.	Cholesterol	0 mg.

VEGETABLE POTATO SALAD   *Serves 4–6*

6 cups cooked, peeled, and cubed
  potatoes
¾ cup chopped carrots
½ cup chopped celery
1 17-ounce can sweet peas, drained
  and rinsed
¼ cup chopped green onion
¼ cup chopped onion
¾ cup low-fat cottage cheese

¼ cup plain low-fat yogurt
3 tablespoons skim milk
2 teaspoons prepared mustard
2 teaspoons lemon juice
1 packet Equal sweetener
½ teaspoon garlic powder
1 tablespoon red wine vinegar
⅛ teaspoon pepper
1 teaspoon dried dill weed

1. Place potatoes and rest of vegetables in a large bowl.

2. Place remaining ingredients in a food processor or blender. Mix until smooth.

3. Pour over potato mixture and toss to coat.

NUTRITIONAL INFORMATION PER SERVING

Calories	193	Carbohydrate	36.5 g.
Protein	11.6 g.	Fat	1.0 g.
Sodium	455 mg.	Cholesterol	2 mg.

SIDE DISHES

CARROT CASSEROLE   *Serves 6*

1 cup peeled and shredded carrot
1 cup peeled and shredded potato
¾ cup peeled and shredded sweet
  potato
2 tablespoons chopped onion

1½ cups cooked brown rice
⅓ cup skim milk
1 teaspoon Mrs. Dash seasoning
⅓ cup Parmesan cheese
1 tablespoon Tamari soy sauce

1. Preheat oven to 350°. Spray a 1½-quart casserole dish with PAM.

2. Bring 1 cup water to a boil. Add vegetables. Cover and cook 5 minutes.

3. Add ½ cup water to vegetables plus remaining ingredients. Mix well.

4. Pour into casserole dish. Bake 25–30 minutes.

NUTRITIONAL INFORMATION PER SERVING

Calories	125	Carbohydrate	22.9 g.
Protein	4.6 g.	Fat	1.8 g.
Sodium	180 mg.	Cholesterol	4 mg.

CREAMED CORN

Yields 3 cups
Serving: ½ cup

2 17-ounce cans corn, drained
⅓ cup evaporated skim milk

1. Place half the corn in a food processor. Add skim milk. Blend until smooth.

2. Pour into a saucepan. Add remaining corn. Heat until warmed.

3. Serve as a side dish or over brown rice.

NUTRITIONAL INFORMATION PER SERVING

Calories	133	Carbohydrate	30.5 g.
Protein	5.1 g.	Fat	1.2 g.
Sodium	20 mg.	Cholesterol	1 mg.

SQUASH AMANDINE

Serves 4

4 cups rinsed and sliced yellow
  squash
½ cup chopped onion
2 tablespoons flour
1 cup skim milk

⅛ teaspoon hot pepper sauce
2 teaspoons Tamari soy sauce
½ cup Parmesan cheese
½ cup sliced almonds

1. Preheat oven to 350°. Spray a 1½-quart casserole dish with PAM.

2. Place squash and onion in a saucepan and cover with water. Boil 5 minutes. Drain well. Pour into casserole dish.

3. Place remaining ingredients except almonds in a saucepan. Heat and stir until mixture thickens a little.

4. Pour over squash mixture. Sprinkle top with almonds.

5. Bake 40–45 minutes or until almonds are golden and casserole is hot and bubbly.

NUTRITIONAL INFORMATION PER SERVING

Calories	221	Carbohydrate	16.9 g.
Protein	11.7 g.	Fat	13.1 g.
Sodium	294 mg.	Cholesterol	9 mg.

SWEET POTATO CASSEROLE   *Serves 6–8*

4 cups cooked sweet potato
1 20-ounce can pineapple chunks,
   drained
½ cup raisins
2 cups peeled cubed apple

¾ cup granulated fructose
3 egg whites
½ cup evaporated skim milk
1 teaspoon cinnamon

1. Preheat oven to 350°. Spray a 2-quart casserole dish with PAM.

2. Combine sweet potato, fruit, and fructose. Mix well.

3. Beat together egg whites, skim milk, and cinnamon. Fold into sweet potato mixture.

4. Pour into prepared casserole dish. Bake 30–35 minutes.

NUTRITIONAL INFORMATION PER SERVING

Calories	228	Carbohydrate	54.5 g.
Protein	3.1 g.	Fat	0.8 g.
Sodium	33 mg.	Cholesterol	0+ mg.

SWEET POTATOES DISCIPIO   *Serves 1*

1 medium sweet potato, cooked   1 packet Equal sweetener
1 tablespoon plain low-fat yogurt   1 tablespoon raisins
¼ teaspoon cinnamon

1. Cut potato open and mash with fork. Add yogurt and mix.
Sprinkle with cinnamon and Equal.

2. Add raisins. Mix.

NUTRITIONAL INFORMATION PER SERVING

Calories	297	Carbohydrate	67.6 g.
Protein	4.7 g.	Fat	1.2 g.
Sodium	31 mg.	Cholesterol	1 mg.

SWEET POTATO STUFFING   *Serves 8–10*

3 cups chopped onion   1½ teaspoons dried marjoram
2 cups chopped celery   ½ teaspoon sage
4 cups mashed sweet potato   ½ teaspoon pepper
8 cups cubed whole wheat bread   ½ cup skim milk
1½ cups chopped pecans   2 egg whites, lightly beaten
1½ teaspoons dried thyme   1 tablespoon Tamari soy sauce

1. Spray a nonstick frying pan with PAM. Sauté onion and celery
until onion is lightly browned.

2. In a large bowl mix sweet potato, bread cubes, pecans, thyme,
marjoram, sage, and pepper. Mix well.

3. Add onion and celery. Toss to mix.

4. In a separate bowl mix skim milk, egg whites, and Tamari.
Beat lightly. Pour over rest of ingredients. Toss.

5. Stuff turkey or chicken. There is enough for a 12-pound bird.
If not stuffing a bird, spray a large casserole dish with PAM. Pour
mixture into casserole. Bake in a preheated 350° oven 30–35 minutes, covered.

NUTRITIONAL INFORMATION PER SERVING

Calories	235	Carbohydrate	28.1 g.
Protein	6.3 g.	Fat	12.5 g.
Sodium	239 mg.	Cholesterol	1 mg.

ZUCCHINI CORN CASSEROLE   *Serves 4*

1 teaspoon dried minced garlic
¼ teaspoon crushed red pepper
½ cup Kraft Grated American Cheese Food, Sharp Cheddar Flavor
¾ cup low-fat cottage cheese
4 egg whites

1 tablespoon chopped fresh parsley
1 teaspoon Tamarai soy sauce
3 cups Creamed Corn (page 186)
1 large onion, chopped
4 cups sliced zucchini, steamed to tender crisp
1 tablespoon Parmesan cheese

1. Preheat oven to 350°. Spray a 1½-quart casserole dish with PAM.

2. Place garlic, pepper, Kraft Cheese Food, cottage cheese, egg whites, parsley, and Tamari in a food processor or blender. Mix until smooth.

3. Place cheese mixture, creamed corn, onion, and zucchini in a large bowl. Toss gently to mix.

4. Pour into prepared casserole dish. Sprinkle with Parmesan.

5. Bake 45–50 minutes or until casserole is golden brown on top and set.

NUTRITIONAL INFORMATION PER SERVING

Calories	328	Carbohydrate	57.6 g.
Protein	20.6 g.	Fat	5.4 g.
Sodium	432 mg.	Cholesterol	13 mg.

POTATOES

HASH BROWN POTATOES   Serves 2

1 medium potato, shredded   ¼ cup water
¼ cup chopped onion   Dash of pepper
2 teaspoons Tamari soy sauce

1. Spray a nonstick frying pan with PAM.

2. Place all ingredients in the pan on medium high heat. Cook until crispy brown, stirring constantly with a rubber spatula.

NUTRITIONAL INFORMATION PER SERVING

Calories	121	Carbohydrate	26.4 g.
Protein	3.6 g.	Fat	0.6 g.
Sodium	150 mg.	Cholesterol	0 mg.

MASHED POTATOES   Serves 4

4 medium potatoes, peeled and   Dash of pepper
  quartered   2 teaspoons Tamari soy sauce
¾–1 cup skim milk   4 teaspoons Parmesan cheese

1. Boil potatoes 20–25 minutes or until very soft. Drain.

2. Place in large bowl. Gradually add skim milk, using electric beater or fork to blend. Mix until smooth.

3. Add remaining ingredients and mix well.

NUTRITIONAL INFORMATION PER SERVING

Calories	188	Carbohydrate	38.4 g.
Protein	7.5 g.	Fat	0.9 g.
Sodium	139 mg.	Cholesterol	3 mg.

NEPTUNE'S POTATO   *Serves 4*

2 large baking potatoes, baked and cooled
½ teaspoon garlic powder
3 tablespoons skim milk
¼ cup plain low-fat yogurt
½ teaspoon lemon juice
½ teaspoon Worcestershire sauce
2 tablespoons chopped green onion

2 tablespoons chopped green pepper
2 tablespoons chopped celery
1 tablespoon chopped onion
¾ cup coarsely chopped fresh shrimp
Parmesan cheese

1. Cut each potato in half and scoop out centers, leaving ¼-inch shell.

2. Place potatoes, garlic powder, skim milk, yogurt, lemon juice, and Worcestershire in a large mixing bowl. Using an electric beater, mix until smooth.

3. Fold in remaining ingredients except Parmesan.

4. Preheat oven to 350°.

5. Fill potato shells with mixture. Place in a baking dish. Sprinkle with Parmesan.

6. Bake 25–30 minutes or until lightly browned on top.

NUTRITIONAL INFORMATION PER SERVING

Calories	277	Carbohydrate	52.3 g.
Protein	13.7 g.	Fat	1.8 g.
Sodium	117 mg.	Cholesterol	36 mg.

ONION POTATO PIE   *Serves 4–6*

3 cups shredded potato
1 medium onion, chopped
½ cup chopped green onion
1 cup low-fat cottage cheese
½ cup plain low-fat yogurt

4 egg whites
½ cup Parmesan cheese
¼ teaspoon pepper
1 tablespoon Tamari soy sauce
¼ teaspoon garlic powder

1. Preheat oven to 350°. Spray a 10″ deep-dish pie plate with PAM.

2. Mix potato, onion, and green onion. Arrange in pie plate.

3. Place remaining ingredients in a food processor or blender. Mix until smooth. Pour over potato mixture.

4. Bake 45–50 minutes or until pie is set and golden brown on top.

NUTRITIONAL INFORMATION PER SERVING

Calories	144	Carbohydrate	17.1 g.
Protein	12.2 g.	Fat	3.0 g.
Sodium	465 mg.	Cholesterol	9 mg.

POTATO CHEESE BAKE   *Serves 4–6*

10 egg whites
1 cup low-fat cottage cheese
⅓ cup Kraft Grated American
  Cheese Food, Sharp Cheddar
  Flavor

½ teaspoon dried dill weed
Pinch of cayenne pepper
½ cup chopped onion
2 medium potatoes, cooked and
  chopped into small pieces

1. Preheat oven to 350°. Spray an 8″ × 8″ baking pan with PAM.

2. Place egg whites, cottage cheese, Kraft Cheese Food, dill weed, and cayenne pepper in a bowl. Beat with an electric mixer until well blended and frothy.

3. Fold in onion and potatoes. Pour into baking pan.

4. Bake 35–40 minutes or until golden brown on top.

NUTRITIONAL INFORMATION PER SERVING

Calories	146	Carbohydrate	19.6 g.
Protein	12.9 g.	Fat	1.7 g.
Sodium	289 mg.	Cholesterol	6 mg.

POTATO PANCAKES   *Yields 6–8 patties*
                                      Serving: 2 patties

⅓ cup chopped onion
2 cups Mashed Potatoes (page 190)
2–3 tablespoons flour

2 egg whites
1 teaspoon Tamari soy sauce

1. Spray a nonstick frying pan with PAM. Brown onion. Add onion to potatoes. Mix.

2. Add flour to potatoes 1 tablespoon at a time. Mixture should be dry. Form mixture into patties.

3. Whisk together egg whites and Tamari.

4. Wipe out frying pan with paper towel and respray with PAM. Dip potato patties in egg white mixture. Place in frying pan and cook on medium heat until lightly browned on both sides.

NUTRITIONAL INFORMATION PER SERVING

Calories	125	Carbohydrate	24.0 g.
Protein	6.0 g.	Fat	0.7 g.
Sodium	130 mg.	Cholesterol	1 mg.

POTATOES PARMESAN   *Serves 4*

1½ cups skim milk
½ teaspoon garlic powder
¼ teaspoon pepper
5 tablespoons Parmesan cheese

4 large potatoes, peeled and sliced
⅛" thick
Paprika

1. Preheat oven to 400°. Spray an 8" × 12" baking dish with PAM.

2. Mix skim milk, garlic powder, pepper, and 4 tablespoons Parmesan in a bowl. Whisk together to blend.

3. Arrange one-third of the potatoes in the baking dish. Pour part of milk mixture over potatoes. Make 2 more layers.

4. Sprinkle top with paprika and remaining Parmesan.

5. Bake covered for 40 minutes. Remove cover and bake 20 more minutes or until top is golden brown and potatoes are tender.

NUTRITIONAL INFORMATION PER SERVING

Calories	282	Carbohydrate	54.2 g.
Protein	11.9 g.	Fat	2.6 g.
Sodium	172 g.	Cholesterol	7 mg.

TURKEY-STUFFED POTATOES   *Serves 4*

2 large baking potatoes, baked and
cooled
⅔ cup plain low-fat yogurt
⅔ cup low-fat cottage cheese
½ cup Parmesan cheese
½ cup finely chopped onion

¼ teaspoon pepper
1 teaspoon Tamari soy sauce
½ teaspoon dried dill weed
2 cups cubed cooked turkey
Paprika

1. Cut each potato in half and scoop out centers, leaving ¼" shell.

2. Place potatoes and remaining ingredients except turkey and paprika in a bowl. Using an electric beater, mix until smooth. Fold in turkey.

3. Preheat oven to 350°.

4. Fill potato shells with mixture. Sprinkle tops with paprika. Place in a baking dish.

5. Bake 25–30 minutes or until lightly browned on top.

NUTRITIONAL INFORMATION PER SERVING

Calories	466	Carbohydrate	54.9 g.
Protein	41.6 g.	Fat	8.7 g.
Sodium	465 mg.	Cholesterol	77 mg.

ENTRÉES

BAKED BARLEY   *Serves 6*

1 large onion, finely chopped
½ pound mushrooms, sliced
2 cups defatted chicken broth

2 tablespoons Tamari soy sauce
⅛ teaspoon pepper
1 cup dry barley

1. Spray a nonstick pan with PAM. Brown onion in pan. Add mushrooms and cook 2–3 more minutes.

2. Preheat oven to 350°. Spray a 2-quart casserole dish with PAM.

3. Mix chicken broth, Tamari, and pepper in a large bowl. Add barley, onion, and mushrooms. Pour into casserole.

4. Cover and bake 50 minutes or until liquid is absorbed.

NUTRITIONAL INFORMATION PER SERVING

Calories	149	Carbohydrate	31.0 g.
Protein	6.1 g.	Fat	0.5 g.
Sodium	418 mg.	Cholesterol	0 mg.

BAKED CANNELLINI   *Serves 6–8*

1 28-ounce can whole tomatoes, cut up (include liquid)
½ cup chopped onion
2 19-ounce cans cannellini, drained and rinsed
¾ cup whole wheat bread crumbs
3 tablespoons Romano cheese

1 teaspoon Tamari soy sauce
¼ teaspoon dried oregano
⅛ teaspoon dried thyme
1 teaspoon dried minced garlic
½ teaspoon dried basil
Pinch of pepper
3 tablespoons Parmesan cheese

1. Preheat oven to 350°. Spray a 2-quart casserole dish with PAM.

2. Combine all ingredients except Parmesan in a large bowl. Mix well. Turn into prepared casserole dish.

3. Bake covered for 50 minutes. Remove cover and sprinkle with the Parmesan. Bake 5–10 more minutes or until cheese is melted.

NUTRITIONAL INFORMATION PER SERVING

Calories	235	Carbohydrate	41.0 g.
Protein	14.3 g.	Fat	2.5 g.
Sodium	263 mg.	Cholesterol	3 mg.

BAKED LENTILS   *Serves 4–6*

1 cup lentils
1 cup finely chopped carrot
1 large onion, finely chopped
1 teaspoon garlic powder

2 teaspoons Tamari soy sauce
2½ cups defatted chicken broth
2 cups cooked brown rice
⅔ cup Parmesan cheese

1. Place all ingredients except rice and Parmesan in a large saucepan. Bring to a boil. Reduce heat and simmer 1–1½ hours.

2. Preheat oven to 400°. Spray a 3-quart casserole dish with PAM.

3. Add rice and Parmesan to lentils. Blend well.

4. Pour mixture into casserole dish. Bake 10 minutes or until heated through.

NUTRITIONAL INFORMATION PER SERVING

Calories	252	Carbohydrate	39.6 g.
Protein	16.1 g.	Fat	3.5 g.
Sodium	573 mg.	Cholesterol	7 mg.

BLACK BEAN AND RICE CASSEROLE   *Serves 6–8*

1½ cups chopped onion
1½ cups evaporated skim milk
1 cup low-fat cottage cheese
  (1 percent milk fat)
¾ cup Kraft Grated American
  Cheese Food, Sharp Cheddar
  Flavor
1 teaspoon Tamari soy sauce

½ teaspoon dried tarragon
¼ teaspoon pepper
1 teaspoon Worcestershire sauce
1 cup cooked brown rice
2 cups cooked black beans, rinsed
  well
5 egg whites, beaten until stiff

1. Preheat oven to 350°.

2. Steam the onion in a small amount of water until soft.

3. Place skim milk, cottage cheese, Kraft Cheese Food, Tamari, tarragon, pepper, and Worcestershire in a blender or food processor and mix until completely smooth.

4. Place rice and beans in a large bowl. Pour cheese mixture over the rice and beans.

5. Fold in egg whites. Spray a 10″ deep-dish pie plate with PAM.

6. Pour mixture into pie dish. Bake 35–45 minutes until edges are lightly browned.

7. Let sit 10 minutes.

NUTRITIONAL INFORMATION PER SERVING

Calories	179	Carbohydrate	25.2 g.
Protein	13.9 g.	Fat	2.7 g.
Sodium	296 mg.	Cholesterol	10 mg.

BROCCOLI MACARONI BAKE   *Serves 6–8*

¼ cup toasted wheat germ
1¼ cups low-fat cottage cheese
4 egg whites
½ teaspoon pepper
¼ teaspoon paprika
¼ teaspoon dry mustard
½ cup plus 2 tablespoons Parmesan
  cheese

2 tablespoons Tamari soy sauce
2 10-ounce packages frozen
  broccoli spears, cooked and
  cut up
1 pound macaroni, cooked
  according to package directions

1. Preheat oven to 350°. Spray a 12″ × 7½″ baking dish with PAM. Sprinkle with toasted wheat germ.

2. Place cottage cheese, egg whites, pepper, paprika, mustard, ½ cup Parmesan, and Tamari in a blender or food processor. Mix until smooth.

3. Mix broccoli, macaroni, and cheese mixture in a large bowl. Turn into baking dish. Sprinkle top with remaining Parmesan.

4. Bake 25–30 minutes or until top is golden brown.

NUTRITIONAL INFORMATION PER SERVING

Calories	311	Carbohydrate	50.1 g.
Protein	19.3 g.	Fat	3.8 g.
Sodium	403 mg.	Cholesterol	7 mg.

BROILED SHRIMP   *Serves 4*

¾ cup finely chopped onion
½ cup sliced mushrooms
1½ cups coarsely chopped cooked
  shrimp
½ teaspoon tarragon vinegar
¼ cup plain low-fat yogurt
¼ teaspoon dry mustard
1 teaspoon Tamari soy sauce
¾ teaspoon garlic powder

3 tablespoons Parmesan cheese
1 egg white
¾ cup whole wheat bread crumbs
½ teaspoon dried basil
1 tablespoon chopped fresh parsley
⅛ teaspoon dried marjoram
Pinch of pepper
Paprika

1. Preheat oven broiler. Spray a nonstick frying pan with PAM.

Brown onion. Add mushrooms and shrimp. Cook 2–3 more minutes. Set aside.

2. Whisk together vinegar, yogurt, mustard, Tamari, ½ teaspoon garlic powder, 1 tablespoon Parmesan, and egg white. Add shrimp, onion, and mushrooms to sauce. Spoon into 4 ramekins.

3. Mix bread crumbs, basil, parsley, marjoram, pepper, 2 tablespoons Parmesan, and ¼ teaspoon garlic powder. Sprinkle on top of shrimp equally. Sprinkle with paprika.

4. Place under broiler 3–4 minutes or until hot and bubbly.

NUTRITIONAL INFORMATION PER SERVING

Calories	230	Carbohydrate	17.9 g.
Protein	30.0 g.	Fat	3.6 g.
Sodium	390 mg.	Cholesterol	154 mg.

CHICKEN AND BROCCOLI STIR FRY   *Serves 4*

½ cup water
4 teaspoons Tamari soy sauce
3 cups cooked brown rice
1 cup cubed cooked chicken
Pinch of pepper

Pinch of garlic powder
1 10-ounce package broccoli spears, cooked according to package directions and drained well
Chopped scallions

1. Spray a nonstick frying pan with PAM.

2. Place water, Tamari, and rice in pan. Heat to medium high. Stir constantly.

3. Add chicken, pepper, and garlic. Heat through. Add broccoli. Stir until hot.

4. Serve in bowls immediately. Garnish with scallions.

NUTRITIONAL INFORMATION PER SERVING

Calories	225	Carbohydrate	34.0 g.
Protein	17.1 g.	Fat	2.4 g.
Sodium	181 mg.	Cholesterol	32 mg.

CHICKEN BROWN RICE PIE   Serves 4–6

½ cup Kraft Grated American Cheese Food, Sharp Cheddar Flavor
1½ cups skim milk
½ cup low-fat cottage cheese
½ cup flour
¼ teaspoon baking powder
¼ teaspoon baking soda
4 egg whites
1 cup cubed cooked chicken
1½ cups cooked brown rice
½ cup sliced fresh mushrooms
2 green onions, sliced

1. Preheat oven to 350°. Spray a 9″ deep-dish pie plate with PAM.

2. Place first 7 ingredients in a blender or food processor. Mix until smooth.

3. Mix chicken and rice. Place in pie plate. Pour cheese mixture on top. Arrange mushrooms and green onion on top of pie.

4. Bake 45 minutes or until pie is set. Let stand 10 minutes before serving.

NUTRITIONAL INFORMATION PER SERVING

Calories	192	Carbohydrate	21.8 g.
Protein	17.8 g.	Fat	3.3 g.
Sodium	271 mg.	Cholesterol	29 mg.

CHICKEN FRIED RICE   Serves 4

½ cup water
¼ cup finely chopped onion
½ cup finely chopped celery
½ cup finely chopped carrot
½ cup finely chopped cooked chicken
3 cups cooked brown rice
Dash of garlic powder
Dash of pepper
1½ tablespoons Tamari soy sauce
¼ cup chopped green onion (include part of green portion)

1. Spray a large nonstick frying pan with PAM. Place first 4 ingredients in pan. Cook on medium high heat for 5 minutes.

2. Add remaining ingredients except green onion. Continue to cook on medium high heat, stirring constantly, for another 5–8 minutes.

3. Remove from heat. Mix in green onion. Serve.

NUTRITIONAL INFORMATION PER SERVING

Calories	189	Carbohydrate	33.6 g.
Protein	9.6 g.	Fat	1.6 g.
Sodium	208 mg.	Cholesterol	16 mg.

CHICKEN TETRAZZINI   *Serves 8*

1 16-ounce package spaghetti,
cooked according to package
directions
2 pounds chicken breast fillets,
cubed
2 small onions, chopped
2 tablespoons Tamari soy sauce
Water
¼ teaspoon pepper

½ pound mushrooms, sliced
1 tablespoon lemon juice
½ cup flour
Pinch of nutmeg
½ teaspoon paprika
¼ cup dry sherry
1 cup skim milk
4 tablespoons Parmesan cheese

1. Spray a 13″ × 9″ baking dish with PAM. Spread cooked spaghetti evenly in dish.

2. Place chicken, onions, and Tamari in a large nonstick frying pan. Pour enough water in pan to cover chicken. Cook on medium high heat 15–20 minutes.

3. Remove chicken and onion from pan with slotted spoon. Add 1 cup water, pepper, mushrooms, and lemon juice to remaining liquid. Cook 5 minutes on high heat. Set aside.

4. Preheat oven to 350°.

5. Place flour, nutmeg, paprika, sherry, 2½ cups water, and skim milk in a blender or food processor. Mix until smooth. Pour into a 4-quart saucepan. Heat mixture on medium high, stirring constantly, until sauce thickens.

6. Add chicken and mushroom mixtures. Cook until heated through. Spoon over spaghetti. Sprinkle top with Parmesan.

7. Bake 30 minutes or until bubbly and top is golden brown.

NUTRITIONAL INFORMATION PER SERVING

Calories	209	Carbohydrate	26.6 g.
Protein	18.9 g.	Fat	1.9 g.
Sodium	118 mg.	Cholesterol	46 mg.

CHILI   Serves 8–10

1 pound ground veal
2 large onions, finely chopped
2 teaspoons dried minced garlic
1 29-ounce can tomato sauce
1 16-ounce can whole tomatoes,
  drained, rinsed, and chopped

1 40- and 1 15-ounce can kidney
  beans, drained and rinsed
4 tablespoons chili powder
¾ teaspoon hot pepper sauce
Pinch of cumin

1. Brown veal and drain. Add onion and garlic. Cook a few minutes.

2. Place remaining ingredients in a large saucepan. Add veal, onion, and garlic. Simmer 30–35 minutes.

NUTRITIONAL INFORMATION PER SERVING

Calories	343	Carbohydrate	34.7 g.
Protein	28.2 g.	Fat	10.5 g.
Sodium	577 mg.	Cholesterol	69 mg.

CORN AND BROWN RICE STIR FRY   Serves 4

1 17-ounce can corn, drained and
  rinsed
¼ cup water

3 cups cooked brown rice
1 tablespoon Tamari soy sauce
½ cup chopped green onion

1. Spray a nonstick pan with PAM. Place corn in pan on medium high heat. Cook 4–5 minutes.

2. Add water, rice, and Tamari. Continue cooking, stirring constantly, until liquid has evaporated.

3. Remove from heat and add green onion.

NUTRITIONAL INFORMATION PER SERVING

Calories	234	Carbohydrate	51.8 g.
Protein	6.1 g.	Fat	1.7 g.
Sodium	113 mg.	Cholesterol	0 mg.

CORNISH HENS   *Serves 4*

1 cup cooked brown rice
3 green onions, chopped
2 ribs celery, finely chopped
1 medium Red Delicious apple,
  finely chopped
¼ cup raisins
¼ cup chopped dried papaya
¼ cup chopped pecans

½ teaspoon sage
3 teaspoons Tamari soy sauce
½ cup plus 2 tablespoons apple
  juice concentrate
4 Rock Cornish hens, rinsed and
  patted dry
⅛ teaspoon pepper
½ cup water

1. Combine first 8 ingredients, 2 teaspoons Tamari, and 2 table-spoons apple juice concentrate in a large bowl.

2. Preheat oven to 350°.

3. Stuff birds with filling. Tie legs together. Arrange birds in a baking dish breast side up. Sprinkle with pepper.

4. Mix together ½ cup apple juice concentrate, water, and remaining Tamari.

5. Bake 1–1¼ hours, basting frequently with juices.

NUTRITIONAL INFORMATION PER SERVING

Calories	488	Carbohydrate	44.2 g.
Protein	45.5 g.	Fat	14.4 g.
Sodium	242 mg.	Cholesterol	101 mg.

CREAMY LASAGNA   *Serves 8–10*

1 pound ground veal
2 teaspoons dried minced garlic
2 large onions, chopped
3 cups skim milk
¼ cup white wine
⅓ cup flour
¼ teaspoon white pepper

Pinch of nutmeg
1 16-ounce package lasagna
  noodles, cooked according to
  package directions
1½ pounds low-fat cottage cheese
Parmesan cheese

1. Place veal, garlic, and onion in a nonstick frying pan. Brown veal.

2. Place milk, white wine, flour, pepper, and nutmeg in a sauce-

pan. Stir until flour has dissolved. Heat on medium high, stirring constantly, until sauce thickens a little.

3. Add veal and onion. Keep stirring and mix well. Heat through.

4. Spray a 13″ × 9″ pan with PAM. Preheat oven to 350°.

5. Place noodles crosswise on bottom of pan. Spoon veal mixture over noodles. Place half the cottage cheese on top and sprinkle with 2 tablespoons Parmesan.

6. Repeat. End with veal mixture on top. Sprinkle with 2 tablespoons Parmesan.

7. Cover and bake 25 minutes. Uncover and bake 30–35 more minutes or until golden brown on top.

NUTRITIONAL INFORMATION PER SERVING

Calories	405	Carbohydrate	43.8 g.
Protein	32.3 g.	Fat	10.2 g.
Sodium	442 mg.	Cholesterol	55 mg.

INDIAN RICE CASSEROLE   Serves 6

1 medium onion, chopped
2 cups cooked brown rice
2 medium apples, chopped
2⅔ cups plain low-fat yogurt

2 teaspoons curry powder
¼ teaspoon cinnamon
3 teaspoons granulated fructose
Paprika

1. Preheat oven to 350°. Spray a 2-quart casserole dish with PAM.

2. Spray a nonstick frying pan with PAM. Sauté onion until lightly browned.

3. Mix onion and remaining ingredients except paprika in a large bowl. Pour into prepared baking dish. Sprinkle with paprika.

4. Bake covered 45 minutes.

NUTRITIONAL INFORMATION PER SERVING

Calories	158	Carbohydrate	29.6 g.
Protein	5.1 g.	Fat	2.5 g.
Sodium	55 mg.	Cholesterol	8 mg.

MEXICAN RICE

Serves 4–6

1 14½-ounce can tomatoes, chopped
½ cup chopped green pepper
1 large onion, finely chopped
½ teaspoon dried minced garlic

3 teaspoons Tamari soy sauce
2 teaspoons hot chili powder
1 tablespoon tomato paste
4 cups cooked brown rice
1 cup cubed cooked chicken

1. Place all ingredients except rice and chicken in a large non-stick frying pan on medium high. Heat 5–10 minutes.

2. Add rice and chicken. Cook 5 more minutes or until heated through.

NUTRITIONAL INFORMATION PER SERVING

Calories	192	Carbohydrate	32.3 g.
Protein	11.8 g.	Fat	1.8 g.
Sodium	214 mg.	Cholesterol	21 mg.

NOODLES ROMANOFF

Serves 6–8
Serving: 1 cup

1½ tablespoons Vogue Chicken Flavor Base
4 cups water
8 ounces linguine (broken in half)
1½ cups low-fat cottage cheese
1 cup plain low-fat yogurt

½ teaspoon Tamari soy sauce
¼ teaspoon dried thyme
¼ teaspoon garlic powder
6 tablespoons Parmesan cheese
½ cup whole wheat bread crumbs

1. Dissolve Vogue in water. Bring to a boil.

2. Add linguine to water. Cook 8–10 minutes or until tender. Remove from heat.

3. Preheat oven to 350°. Spray a 3-quart casserole dish with PAM.

4. Add cottage cheese, yogurt, Tamari, thyme, garlic powder, and 5 tablespoons Parmesan to the linguine and water. Mix well.

5. Pour mixture into casserole dish. Sprinkle top with whole wheat bread crumbs and the remaining tablespoon of Parmesan.

6. Bake 25–30 minutes or until bubbly and top is golden brown.

NUTRITIONAL INFORMATION PER SERVING

Calories	263	Carbohydrate	37.1 g.
Protein	19.4 g.	Fat	3.6 g.
Sodium	931 mg.	Cholesterol	10 mg.

POACHED SALMON   *Serves 4*

4 small salmon steaks, sprinkled
lightly with garlic powder
½ cup water
½ cup dry sherry

2 teaspoons Tamari soy sauce
2 lemons, thinly sliced
4 green onions, chopped

1. Preheat oven to 350°. Spray a baking pan with PAM. Arrange salmon steaks in pan.

2. Combine water, sherry, and Tamari. Pour over salmon steaks.

3. Lay lemon slices on top of steaks. Cover.

4. Bake 45 minutes to 1 hour. The last 10 minutes uncover and sprinkle with green onions.

NUTRITIONAL INFORMATION PER SERVING

Calories	247	Carbohydrate	8.9 g.
Protein	27.7 g.	Fat	7.7 g.
Sodium	190 mg.	Cholesterol	47 mg.

RICE-STUFFED GREEN PEPPERS   *Serves 4–6*

6 large green peppers
1 large onion, finely chopped
1 cup diced celery
½ cup sliced mushrooms
¾ cup low-fat cottage cheese
¼ cup Kraft Grated American

Cheese Food, Sharp Cheddar
Flavor
2 tablespoons Parmesan cheese
4 cups cooked brown rice
½ cup chopped walnuts
1 egg white

1. Cut a thin slice off top of peppers and clean centers. Parboil 2–3 minutes. Drain.

2. Preheat oven to 350°. Line a 13″ × 9″ pan with aluminum foil. Arrange peppers in pan.

3. Spray a nonstick frying pan with PAM. Brown onion. Add celery and mushrooms. Cook 2–3 more minutes.

4. Place cottage cheese, Kraft Cheese Food, and Parmesan in a food processor or blender. Mix until smooth.

5. In a large bowl mix rice, onion, celery, mushrooms, walnuts, cottage cheese mixture, and egg white. Blend well.

6. Fill peppers with mixture. Bake 30 minutes.

NUTRITIONAL INFORMATION PER SERVING

Calories	253	Carbohydrate	33.7 g.
Protein	11.4 g.	Fat	8.7 g.
Sodium	231 mg.	Cholesterol	6 mg.

ROLLED STUFFED EGGPLANT   *Serves 4–6*

1 egg white
⅔ cup skim milk
1 teaspoon Tamari soy sauce
½ cup flour
1 medium eggplant, peeled and sliced lengthwise into 10 ¼"-thick slices

1 cup low-fat cottage cheese
½ cup Romano cheese
2 tablespoons chopped fresh parsley
2 cups Quick Tomato Sauce (page 214)

1. Spray a nonstick pan with PAM.

2. Whisk together egg white, skim milk, and Tamari. Gradually add flour and mix until blended.

3. Dip eggplant into batter a few at a time. Cook on medium heat in frying pan until tender. Set aside.

4. Combine cottage cheese, Romano cheese, and parsley. Mix well.

5. Preheat oven to 375°. Spray a 10" × 6" × 2" pan with PAM.

6. Place 1 heaping tablespoon of cheese mixture in center of each eggplant slice. Roll up jelly-roll style.

7. Place seam down in baking dish. Pour sauce over eggplant rolls.

8. Bake 25–35 minutes or until hot and bubbly.

NUTRITIONAL INFORMATION PER SERVING

Calories	202	Carbohydrate	31.5 g.
Protein	13.3 g.	Fat	3.2 g.
Sodium	950 mg.	Cholesterol	9 mg.

STUFFED SHELLS   *Serves 6–8*

4 cups low-fat cottage cheese
¼ cup Kraft Grated American Cheese Food, Sharp Cheddar Flavor
¼ cup plus 4 tablespoons Parmesan cheese
2 egg whites
⅓ cup whole wheat bread crumbs

¼ cup chopped fresh parsley
¼ teaspoon pepper
4 cups Quick Tomato Sauce (page 214)
1 16-ounce package jumbo macaroni shells, cooked according to package directions

1. Preheat oven to 350°. Spray two 9″ × 13″ pans with PAM.

2. Combine cottage cheese, Kraft Cheese Food, ¼ cup Parmesan, egg whites, bread crumbs, parsley, and pepper. Mix well.

3. Pour part of tomato sauce over bottom of prepared pans.

4. Fill shells with cheese mixture. Arrange in pans.

5. Pour streams of remaining sauce over shells. Sprinkle with remaining Parmesan.

6. Bake 30 minutes.

NUTRITIONAL INFORMATION PER SERVING

Calories	462	Carbohydrate	72.4 g.
Protein	30.0 g.	Fat	5.6 g.
Sodium	1657 mg.	Cholesterol	15 mg.

TOMATO BROCCOLI PIE   *Serves 4–6*

1 cup low-fat cottage cheese
1 cup plain low-fat yogurt
¼ cup flour
¼ teaspoon baking powder
½ teaspoon baking soda
Pinch of white pepper

3 egg whites
⅓ cup plus 2 tablespoons Parmesan
 cheese
2 medium tomatoes, thinly sliced
1 10-ounce package frozen chopped
 broccoli

1. Preheat oven to 350°. Spray a 9″ deep-dish pie plate with PAM.

2. Place cottage cheese, yogurt, flour, baking powder, baking soda, pepper, egg whites, and ⅓ cup Parmesan in a blender or food processor and pureé.

3. Arrange half the tomatoes on the bottom of the pie dish. Place broccoli on top of tomatoes. Pour half the cottage cheese mixture on top of broccoli.

4. Arrange remaining tomatoes on top of mixture. Pour remaining cottage cheese mixture on top. Sprinkle with 2 tablespoons Parmesan.

5. Bake 30–35 minutes or until golden brown on top.

6. Let stand 10 minutes before serving.

NUTRITIONAL INFORMATION PER SERVING

Calories	125	Carbohydrate	11.8 g.
Protein	12.7 g.	Fat	3.3 g.
Sodium	387 mg.	Cholesterol	10 mg.

VEAL LASAGNA   *Serves 8–10*

¾ pound ground veal
4 cups Quick Tomato Sauce
 (page 214)
⅔ of a 16-ounce package lasagna

noodles, cooked according to
 package directions
2 pounds low-fat cottage cheese
Parmesan cheese

1. Brown veal in nonstick frying pan and drain. Add to tomato sauce.

2. Preheat oven to 350°. Spray a 13" × 9" pan with PAM.

3. Spoon small amount of sauce on bottom of baking dish. Arrange part of lasagna noodles widthwise to cover bottom of baking dish. Spoon half the cottage cheese over noodles. Sprinkle with 2 tablespoons Parmesan. Spoon sauce over cheese. Repeat layers, finishing with noodles and sauce on top. Sprinkle top layer with 2 tablespoons Parmesan.

4. Bake 45 minutes. Remove and let stand for 10 minutes.

NUTRITIONAL INFORMATION PER SERVING

Calories	330	Carbohydrate	38.7 g.
Protein	27.2 g.	Fat	7.1 g.
Sodium	1230 g.	Cholesterol	42 mg.

VEAL-STUFFED EGGPLANT   *Serves 6–8*

½ pound ground veal
1 medium onion, chopped
1 teaspoon dried minced garlic
4 small eggplants
1 cup cooked brown rice
1 cup canned tomatoes, well
  drained and chopped
½ teaspoon allspice

¼ cup pine nuts, toasted
2 tablespoons chopped fresh
  parsley
⅓ cup whole wheat bread crumbs
2 teaspoons Tamari soy sauce
1 egg white, lightly beaten
Pinch of pepper

1. Brown veal, onion, and garlic in a nonstick frying pan. Set aside.

2. Cut eggplants in half lengthwise. Scoop out pulp, chop, and place in a saucepan. Set shells aside for stuffing. Add enough water in pan to cover eggplant pulp. Cook on medium high until pulp changes color. Drain.

3. Preheat oven to 350°. Add eggplant pulp, rice, tomatoes, allspice, pine nuts, parsley, bread crumbs, Tamari, egg white, and pepper to veal. Mix well.

4. Spray a baking dish with PAM. Arrange eggplant shells in dish. Spoon filling into eggplant shells.

5. Bake 30 minutes.

NUTRITIONAL INFORMATION PER SERVING

Calories	188	Carbohydrate	21.6 g.
Protein	12.4 g.	Fat	6.9 g.
Sodium	129 mg.	Cholesterol	29 mg.

VEGETABLE RICE CASSEROLE   *Serves 4*

2 cups cooked brown rice
1 10-ounce package frozen Le Seur
    peas, cooked and drained
1 cup plain low-fat yogurt
1 cup diced celery

2 tablespoons dried minced onion
1 tablespoon Tamari soy sauce
½ teaspoon dry mustard
½ teaspoon curry powder

1. Preheat oven to 350°. Spray a 1-quart casserole dish with PAM.

2. Mix all ingredients in a large bowl. Pour into prepared casserole.

3. Bake covered 20–25 minutes or until heated through.

NUTRITIONAL INFORMATION PER SERVING

Calories	190	Carbohydrate	36.1 g.
Protein	8.4 g.	Fat	2.1 g.
Sodium	430 mg.	Cholesterol	5 mg.

ZITI CASSEROLE   *Serves 8*

1 pound ziti noodles, freshly
    cooked and drained
1 pound low-fat cottage cheese
2 15½-ounce jars marinara sauce
    (low-fat, low-sodium)
4 egg whites, lightly beaten

⅔ cup Parmesan cheese
½ teaspoon pepper
2 tablespoons Tamari soy sauce
⅛ teaspoon garlic powder
2 teaspoons Italian seasoning

1. Preheat oven to 350°. Spray a 3-quart casserole dish with PAM.

2. Combine all ingredients in a large bowl. Mix well.

3. Pour into casserole dish. Bake 25–30 minutes or until top is lightly browned and sauce is bubbly.

NUTRITIONAL INFORMATION PER SERVING

Calories	320	Carbohydrate	48.0 g.
Protein	20.9 g.	Fat	5.1 g.
Sodium	683 mg.	Cholesterol	8 mg.

ZUCCHINI AND CAULIFLOWER ITALIAN   *Serves 4–6*

1 teaspoon dried minced garlic
1 14½-ounce can tomatoes
1 tablespoon chopped fresh parsley
1 tablespoon tomato paste
1 teaspoon Tamari soy sauce
½ teaspoon dried oregano

¼ teaspoon pepper
½ cup water
2 cups cauliflowerets
2 medium zucchini, sliced ½″ thick
2 tablespoons Parmesan cheese

1. Spray a large nonstick frying pan with PAM. Place garlic, tomatoes, parsley, tomato paste, Tamari, oregano, pepper, and water in pan on medium high heat. Cook 2–3 minutes.

2. In the meantime steam the cauliflowerets and zucchini to tender crisp. Add to frying pan. Cook, stirring constantly and cutting tomatoes with a wooden spoon, about 5 minutes.

3. Sprinkle with Parmesan. Serve over brown rice or freshly cooked spaghetti. Can also be served as a side dish.

NUTRITIONAL INFORMATION PER SERVING

Calories	48	Carbohydrate	8.0 g.
Protein	3.4 g.	Fat	0.9 g.
Sodium	176 mg.	Cholesterol	1 mg.

SAUCES AND SPREADS

APPLE CRANBERRY SAUCE

Yields 5 cups
Serving: 1 tablespoon

1 12-ounce package cranberries
3 cups peeled and cubed apple
⅔ cup apple juice concentrate
(no sugar added)

1½ cups water
½ teaspoon cinnamon
25–35 packets Equal sweetener

1. Place all ingredients except Equal into a saucepan. Bring to a boil.

2. Reduce heat immediately. Simmer 10 minutes on low heat.

3. Let cool. Add Equal to taste.

NUTRITIONAL INFORMATION PER SERVING

Calories	20	Carbohydrate	4.3 g.
Protein	0.2 g.	Fat	0.1 g.
Sodium	0+ mg.	Cholesterol	0 mg.

APPLESAUCE

Yields 3 cups
Serving: ½ cup

6 cups peeled and cubed apple
(Rome or McIntosh)
1 6-fluid-ounce can apple juice
concentrate (no sugar added)

plus 1 can water
⅛ teaspoon cinnamon
Equal sweetener to taste

1. Place all ingredients except Equal in saucepan.

2. Bring to a boil. Reduce to medium high.

3. Cook 8–10 minutes for chunky applesauce. Cook 10–15 minutes for smoother applesauce.

4. Cool in refrigerator. Add Equal.

NUTRITIONAL INFORMATION PER SERVING

Calories	218.7	Carbohydrate	41.8 g.
Protein	9.3 g.	Fat	2.7 g.
Sodium	95.9 mg.	Cholesterol	0.1 mg.

EGGPLANT SAUCE   *Serves 4–6*

1 28-ounce can tomato puree
3 cups peeled and cubed eggplant
1 medium onion, chopped
1 4½-ounce can mushrooms, drained
1 teaspoon dried minced garlic
⅓ cup burgundy

¼ cup sliced pitted black olives
2 teaspoons granulated fructose
1 teaspoon dried oregano
½ teaspoon dried basil
1 tablespoon Tamari soy sauce
⅛ teaspoon pepper

1. Place all ingredients in a large saucepan.
2. Bring to a boil. Reduce heat to medium. Cook 30 minutes or until sauce is desired consistency.
3. Serve over pasta.

NUTRITIONAL INFORMATION PER SERVING

Calories	142	Carbohydrate	23.1 g.
Protein	4.6 g.	Fat	4.3 g.
Sodium	950 mg.	Cholesterol	0 mg.

PESTO   *Yields 1 cup*
Serving: ½ cup

1½ cups fresh basil leaves, rinsed and stems removed
½ cup chopped fresh parsley
¼ cup pine nuts

2½ teaspoons dried minced garlic
½ cup plus 2 tablespoons Parmesan cheese
½ cup no-oil Italian salad dressing

1. Combine basil, parsley, pine nuts, and garlic in food processor. Chop fine.
2. Add Parmesan and blend well.

3. Slowly add the Italian dressing while blending. Blend until fine paste forms.

4. Toss with hot pasta (approximately ½ cup pesto to 8 ounces pasta).

NUTRITIONAL INFORMATION PER SERVING

Calories	155	Carbohydrate	11.0 g.
Protein	5.7 g.	Fat	10.9 g.
Sodium	592 mg.	Cholesterol	4 mg.

QUICK TOMATO SAUCE

Yields 4 cups
Serving: ½ cup

2 16-ounce cans tomato sauce
1 cup finely chopped onion
1 12-ounce can tomato paste
¾ teaspoon dried minced garlic
3 tablespoons granulated fructose
2 tablespoons finely chopped fresh parsley
1 teaspoon dried oregano

Pinch of dried thyme
2 teaspoons Tamari soy sauce
⅛ teaspoon pepper
1 anchovy fillet
¼ cup peeled and finely chopped apple
1 bay leaf

1. Place all ingredients in a large saucepan.

2. Bring to a boil. Reduce heat to medium low. Simmer 30 minutes. Remove bay leaf.

3. Serve over freshly cooked pasta.

NUTRITIONAL INFORMATION PER SERVING

Calories	114	Carbohydrate	23.9 g.
Protein	4.1 g.	Fat	0.8 g.
Sodium	1002 mg.	Cholesterol	2 mg.

BREADS AND MUFFINS *

BANANA DATE MUFFINS

Yields 16–18 muffins

1½ cups whole wheat pastry flour
½ cup bran
½ cup granulated fructose
½ cup chopped dates
1 cup peeled and shredded apple
(pack firmly in cup)

1 tablespoon baking powder
3 large very ripe bananas, mashed
(approximately 1½ cups)
2 egg whites
½ cup skim milk

1. Preheat oven to 350 °. Spray muffin tin with PAM.

2. Mix all ingredients except skim milk and egg whites in a large bowl.

3. Lightly beat egg whites. Gradually add skim milk while beating eggs.

4. Add to the rest of the ingredients. Blend well.

5. Fill muffin tins ⅔ full.

6. Bake 20–25 minutes or until a wooden pick inserted in center of a muffin comes out clean.

NUTRITIONAL INFORMATION PER SERVING

Calories	105	Carbohydrate	25.1 g.
Protein	1.8 g.	Fat	0.3 g.
Sodium	10 mg.	Cholesterol	0+ mg.

BRAN DATE BREAD

1 loaf

1 cup chopped dates
2½ cups whole wheat pastry flour
1 cup bran
2 teaspoons baking powder
½ teaspoon baking soda

¾ cup granulated fructose
1 cup chopped walnuts
1 cup peeled and shredded apple
3 egg whites
1 cup evaporated skim milk

1. Preheat oven to 375°. Spray a 9″×5″×3″ loaf pan with PAM.

*Serving size on all breads is a ½-inch slice; one muffin equals a single serving for all muffin recipes.

2. Place dates in a saucepan with enough water to cover them. Bring to a boil. Remove from heat and cover.

3. Combine flour, bran, baking powder, baking soda, and fructose. Add date-water mixture, walnuts, and apple. Mix well.

4. Mix egg whites and milk in a separate bowl. Add to dry ingredients and blend.

5. Pour into loaf pan. Bake 50–60 minutes or until a wooden pick inserted into middle of loaf comes out clean.

NUTRITIONAL INFORMATION PER SERVING

Calories	178	Carbohydrate	31.5 g.
Protein	4.5 g.	Fat	4.4 g.
Sodium	48 mg.	Cholesterol	1 mg.

CHERRY ALMOND MUFFINS *Yields 12–18 muffins*

2 cups whole wheat pastry flour
1 cup granulated fructose
4 teaspoons baking powder
1 egg white
1 cup evaporated skim milk

1 teaspoon almond extract
1 cup peeled and shredded apple
1 cup cherries, cut in half (use frozen if fresh are out of season)
⅔ cup chopped almonds

1. Preheat oven to 400°. Spray a muffin tin with PAM.

2. Combine flour, fructose, and baking powder. In a separate bowl combine egg white, milk, and almond extract. Add to dry ingredients and mix well.

3. Add apple, cherries, and nuts. Mix well.

4. Spoon batter into muffin tin approximately ¾ full.

5. Bake 20–25 minutes until they are golden brown or until a wooden pick inserted in middle of a muffin comes out clean.

NUTRITIONAL INFORMATION PER SERVING

Calories	146	Carbohydrate	26.7 g.
Protein	3.3 g.	Fat	3.1 g.
Sodium	20 mg.	Cholesterol	1 mg.

CHICKEN CURRY MUFFINS

Yields 6 muffins

2 cups cooked brown rice
1 cup finely chopped cooked
chicken
1 tablespoon chopped fresh parsley
½ cup chopped celery
¼ cup plus 1 tablespoon chopped
onion

1½ teaspoons curry powder
8 heaping tablespoons plain low-fat
yogurt
2 teaspoons Tamari soy sauce
1 tablespoon lemon juice
3 egg whites

1. Preheat oven to 375°. Spray a muffin tin with PAM.

2. Combine all ingredients except egg whites. Blend well. Beat egg whites until stiff peaks form. Fold into batter.

3. Fill muffin tin with mixture. Make mounds with mixture in the shape of a muffin.

4. Bake 35–40 minutes or until golden brown on top. Run knife around edge of each muffin to loosen.

NUTRITIONAL INFORMATION PER SERVING

Calories	130	Carbohydrate	15.9 g.
Protein	12.0 g.	Fat	1.9 g.
Sodium	117 mg.	Cholesterol	24 mg.

PECAN CRANBERRY BREAD

Yields 1 loaf

1½ cups chopped cranberries (fresh
or frozen)
½ cups chopped pecans
2 cups whole wheat pastry flour
1 cup granulated fructose
1½ teaspoons baking powder
1½ teaspoons baking soda

¾ cup plus 2 tablespoons apple
juice concentrate (natural)
1 egg white, beaten until stiff peaks
form
½ cup peeled and shredded apple
(pack firmly in cup)
1 tablespoon grated orange rind

1. Preheat oven to 350°. Spray an 8″ × 5″ × 3″ loaf pan with PAM.

2. Combine all ingredients in a large bowl and mix well.

3. Pour into loaf pan. Bake 45–50 minutes or until a wooden pick inserted into middle of loaf comes out clean.

NUTRITIONAL INFORMATION PER SERVING

Calories	148	Carbohydrate	29.6 g.
Protein	1.8 g.	Fat	2.6 g.
Sodium...........	81 mg.	Cholesterol	0 mg.

PUMPKIN APPLE BREAD   *Yields 1 loaf*

1½ cups whole wheat flour
¾ cup granulated fructose
1 teaspoon baking soda
1 teaspoon baking powder
1 teaspoon cinnamon
½ teaspoon allspice

3 egg whites, well beaten
½ cup evaporated skim milk
1½ cups raisins, plumped
1 cup peeled and shredded apples
1½ cups canned pure pumpkin

1. Preheat oven to 350°. Spray a 9″×5″ loaf pan with PAM.

2. Combine flour, fructose, baking soda, baking powder, cinnamon, and allspice in a large bowl. Combine egg whites and milk in another bowl. Add to dry ingredients. Mix well.

3. Add raisins and apple. Blend well. Pour into loaf pan.

4. Bake 50–60 minutes or until a wooden pick inserted into middle of bread comes out clean. Cool for 20 minutes on wire rack.

NUTRITIONAL INFORMATION PER SERVING

Calories	92	Carbohydrate	21.3 g.
Protein	3.0 g.	Fat	0.4 g.
Sodium...........	64 mg.	Cholesterol	0+ mg.

SESAME SWEET BREAD   *Yields 1 loaf*

2 cups whole wheat pastry flour
½ cup bran
½ cup granulated fructose
1 tablespoon baking powder
1 teaspoon cinnamon

1 cup skim milk
½ cup plain low-fat yogurt
¾ cup peeled and shredded apple
4 tablespoons toasted sesame
  seeds*

1. Preheat oven to 350°.

2. Spray an 8″×4″×2″ loaf pan with PAM.

3. Combine all ingredients in a large bowl except 1 tablespoon sesame seeds. Mix well.

4. Pour mixture into loaf pan. Sprinkle remaining sesame seeds on top of loaf.

5. Bake for 1 hour or until a wooden pick inserted in middle of loaf comes out clean

*If using untoasted sesame seeds, spread seeds in a shallow pan and bake 8–10 minutes in a 350° oven until brown.

NUTRITIONAL INFORMATION PER SERVING

Calories	110	Carbohydrate	20.5 g.
Protein	2.7 g.	Fat	2.1 g.
Sodium	13 mg.	Cholesterol	1 mg.

SWEET POTATO MUFFINS   *Yields 16–18 muffins*

1 cup peeled and shredded apple
1⅜ cups granulated fructose
1¼ cups mashed cooked sweet
  potatoes
2 large egg whites
1 cup evaporated skim milk
1½ cups whole wheat pastry flour

2 teaspoons baking powder
1 teaspoon cinnamon
Pinch of nutmeg
½ cup raisins
¼ cup chopped walnuts
¼ teaspoon cinnamon

1. Preheat oven to 375°. Spray a muffin tin with PAM.

2. Combine apple, 1¼ cups fructose, sweet potatoes, egg whites, and milk. Beat together with an electric mixer.

3. Add rest of ingredients except cinnamon and ⅛ cup fructose. Blend well.

4. Combine fructose and cinnamon and set aside.

5. Spoon mixture into prepared muffin tin. Fill each tin about ¾ full. Sprinkle top with fructose and cinnamon mixture. Bake 25–30 minutes or until wooden pick inserted into middle of muffin comes out clean.

Calories	140	Carbohydrate	30.7 g.
Protein	2.1 g.	Fat	1.3 g.
Sodium	14 mg.	Cholesterol	0+ mg.

DESSERTS

ALL-IN-ONE APPLE PIE   *Serves 8*

6½–7 cups cored, peeled, and sliced apples
¾ cup granulated fructose
½ cup whole wheat flour
¼ teaspoon baking powder
¼ teaspoon baking soda

1 13-ounce can evaporated skim milk
2 egg whites
2 teaspoons cinnamon
1 tablespoon lemon juice

1. Spray a 9″ pie pan with PAM. Place apples in pan.

2. Preheat oven to 350°. Place remaining ingredients in a food processor or blender. Mix until smooth.

3. Pour over apples. Bake 45–50 minutes or until top is golden.

Calories	226	Carbohydrate	51.7 g.
Protein	5.4 g.	Fat	0.8 g.
Sodium	118 mg.	Cholesterol	2 mg.

APPLE CAKE   *Yields 24 servings*

2 cups whole wheat flour
2 teaspoons baking soda
2 teaspoons cinnamon
1 cup granulated fructose
2 egg whites
2 teaspoons vanilla

2 cups peeled and cubed apple
2½ cups peeled and shredded apple
1 cup raisins
1 cup chopped walnuts

1. Preheat oven to 350°. Spray a 13″×9″×2″ baking pan with PAM.

2. Mix all the dry ingredients. Add the egg whites, vanilla, apples, and raisins. Blend well.

3. Spread mixture in baking pan. Sprinkle nuts on top of mixture. Bake 35–45 minutes. Cool in pan. Cut into 2″ squares.

NUTRITIONAL INFORMATION PER SERVING

Calories	142	Carbohydrate	27.1 g.
Protein	2.3 g.	Fat	3.3 g.
Sodium	74 mg.	Cholesterol	0 mg.

BANANA NUT LOAF CAKE   *Yields 2 loaves*

1 cup granulated fructose
1 cup peeled and shredded apple
5 ripe bananas
3 egg whites
2 cups whole wheat pastry flour

1 teaspoon baking soda in 3
   tablespoons warm water
1 teaspoon vanilla extract
1 teaspoon natural banana flavor
1 cup chopped pecans

1. Preheat oven to 350°. Spray two 8″×2″×4″ loaf pans with PAM.

2. Mix all ingredients except pecans with a hand mixer until well blended. Add pecans and mix well.

3. Pour into loaf pans. Bake 50–60 minutes or until a wooden pick inserted into middle of loaves comes out clean. Cool and cut into slices.

NUTRITIONAL INFORMATION PER SERVING

Calories	101	Carbohydrate	18.7 g.
Protein	1.4 g.	Fat	2.6 g.
Sodium	31 mg.	Cholesterol	0 mg.

CAROB NUT LOAF
Yields 1 loaf

1¼ cups chopped pitted dates
¾ cup water
1½ cups carob chips
¾ cup peeled and shredded apple
2¾ cups whole wheat pastry flour
¾ cup granulated fructose

1 teaspoon baking powder
1 teaspoon baking soda
2 cups coarsely chopped walnuts
1 egg white
1 teaspoon vanilla extract
¾ cup evaporated skim milk

1. Combine dates, water, and ¾ cup of the carob chips in a saucepan. Warm over medium heat, stirring constantly, until chips have melted. Let cool.

2. Preheat oven to 350°. Spray a 9″ × 5″ loaf pan with PAM.

3. Combine apple, flour, fructose, baking powder, baking soda, and 1⅓ cup walnuts. Mix well.

4. In a separate bowl lightly beat egg white, vanilla, and milk. Add date mixture to flour mixture. Blend well. Add rest of carob chips and mix.

5. Pour mixture into loaf pan. Sprinkle top with remaining ⅔ cup walnuts.

6. Bake for 1 hour and 10–20 minutes or until a wooden pick inserted in middle of loaf comes out clean.

NUTRITIONAL INFORMATION PER SERVING

Calories	298	Carbohydrate	42.5 g.
Protein	6.2 g.	Fat	12.5 g.
Sodium	64 mg.	Cholesterol	0 + mg.

FRUITCAKE
Yields 1 loaf

¾ cup granulated fructose
¾ cup whole wheat flour
¼ teaspoon baking powder
¼ teaspoon baking soda
1 cup pitted dates, cut in half

1½ cups dried papaya, cubed
1½ cups dried pineapple, cubed
1 cup chopped macadamia nuts
5 egg whites
½ teaspoon rum

1. Preheat oven to 300°. Spray a 9″ × 5″ × 3″ loaf pan with PAM.

2. Combine all the dry ingredients. Add the fruit and nuts and mix.

3. Beat egg whites lightly with rum. Add to the fruit mixture. Blend well.

4. Pour mixture into loaf pan. Bake 1¼–1½ hours. Turn out of pan and let cool.

NUTRITIONAL INFORMATION PER SERVING

Calories	203	Carbohydrate	37.8 g.
Protein	2.8 g.	Fat	6.0 g.
Sodium	29 mg.	Cholesterol	0 mg.

MERV'S FAVORITE CHOCOLATE-COVERED CHERRY CAKE

Serves 12

FILLING

16 ounces frozen whole dark sweet pitted cherries, defrosted
¼ cup water

3 tablespoons granulated fructose
1½ tablespoons cornstarch
1½ teaspoons almond flavor

1. Drain juice from cherries into saucepan. Set cherries aside.

2. Add water, fructose, and cornstarch to cherry juice. Stir until fructose and cornstarch have dissolved. Turn heat on medium high. Stir constantly until sauce thickens and turns clear.

3. Remove from heat and add cherries and almond flavor. Place in refrigerator to cool.

CAKE

⅔ cup whole wheat pastry flour
¼ cup cocoa
¼ cup carob powder
¾ cup peeled and shredded apple (pack firmly in cup)

1½ cups chopped walnuts
1 cup granulated fructose
3 egg whites
3 teaspoons vanilla extract

1. Preheat oven to 350°. Spray an 8″ cake pan with PAM.

2. Combine all ingredients except egg whites and vanilla in a large bowl.

3. Beat egg whites and vanilla together lightly. Add to dry ingredients and mix well.

4. Pour half of mixture into cake pan. Spoon cherry mixture over cake mixture. Pour rest of cake mixture on top of cherries. Spread to cover cherries.

5. Bake 45–50 minutes or until a wooden pick inserted into middle of cake comes out clean.

NUTRITIONAL INFORMATION PER SERVING

Calories	244	Carbohydrate	39.5 g.
Protein	4.0 g.	Fat	8.7 g.
Sodium	13 mg.	Cholesterol	0 mg.

PINEAPPLE PUMPKIN UPSIDE-DOWN CAKE   *Serves 24*

2 cups granulated fructose
2 16-ounce cans pineapple rings, drained
3 cups whole wheat pastry flour
1½ cups peeled and shredded apple (pack firmly in cup)

1 16-ounce can pure pumpkin
4 egg whites
2 teaspoons baking powder
2 teaspoons baking soda
2 teaspoons cinnamon
2 cups raisins

1. Preheat oven to 350°. Spray a 13″ × 9″ pan with PAM. Sprinkle the pan with 2 tablespoons of the fructose. Shake pan to spread fructose evenly.

2. Arrange pineapple rings on bottom and sides of pan. Cut some of the rings in half to arrange on the sides.

3. Combine remaining ingredients in a large bowl. Mix well. Pour into prepared pan.

4. Bake 1 hour and 15 minutes or until a wooden pick inserted into middle of cake comes out clean.

5. Let cake cool in pan. After cooled, turn pan upside down on platter to release cake. Cut into 2″ squares.

Calories	191	Carbohydrate	46.2 g.
Protein	2.4 g.	Fat	0.4 g.
Sodium	79 mg.	Cholesterol	0 mg.

PUMPKIN BROWN RICE PUDDING   *Serves 6*

2 cups canned pure pumpkin
2 cups cooked brown rice
1 cup evaporated skim milk
1 teaspoon cinnamon

½ teaspoon allspice
3 egg whites
⅔ cup raisins, plumped
8–10 packages Equal sweetener

1. Preheat oven to 350°. Spray a 1½-quart casserole dish with PAM.

2. Combine all ingredients except raisins and Equal in a large bowl. Blend with hand mixer for 3–5 minutes. Add raisins.

3. Pour into casserole dish. Place casserole in a pan of hot water. Bake 55 minutes.

4. Remove from oven and let cool at least 30 minutes. Add Equal to taste. Blend well and smooth top with back of spoon. Serve warm or chilled.

Calories	179	Carbohydrate	36.6 g.
Protein	7.4 g.	Fat	0.7 g.
Sodium	77 mg.	Cholesterol	2 mg.

RASPBERRY PRESERVE BARS   *Yields 16 bars*

½ cup whole wheat pastry flour
¼ cup wheat germ
½ cup granulated fructose
⅔ cup peeled and shredded apple
2 teaspoons cocoa powder

2 egg whites
1½ cups chopped almonds
½ cup unsweetened raspberry
  preserves
1 teaspoon almond extract

1. Preheat oven to 350°. Spray an 8″ × 8″ pan with PAM.

2. Combine all ingredients and mix well. Spread mixture in pan and press down with back of spoon.

3. Bake 30–35 minutes. Cut into 2″ square bars.

NUTRITIONAL INFORMATION PER SERVING

Calories	162	Carbohydrate	21.2 g.
Protein	4.0 g.	Fat	7.6 g.
Sodium	8 mg.	Cholesterol	0 mg.

SECTION III

The
Eat to Succeed
Food Composition
Tables

The Haas Maximum
Performance Food Tables

I've designed the following food composition tables to provide you with the most up-to-date nutritional information on ordinary foods and Haas recipes from *Eat to Win* and *Eat to Succeed*. The tables contain the most important nutritional information about foods you ever will need to know—the six vital values that will help you eat to succeed: calories, protein, fat, carbohydrate, cholesterol, and sodium. You don't need to be overly concerned with the vitamin and mineral content of foods because you receive a plentiful supply from the recommended foods, meal replacers, and nutritional supplements on the Haas Maximum Performance Program. Even if your orange or baked potato has lost most of its vitamin C content (as is often the case after these and other foods have been processed, cooked, or stored), you will still get plenty of vitamin C and other essential nutrients from the other foods and food supplements on the program.

The most unusual feature (and bonus) of these food composition tables is that, unlike most other food composition books and tables, *there are no missing values*. With these new tables, dieters and health-care professionals are no longer forced to guess or merely estimate the total cholesterol in a daily menu plan or recipe.

Another unusual feature of these tables is that they contain the latest nutritional information from the United States Department of Agriculture's National Technical Information Service (NTIS). Through a special agreement, the USDA/NTIS has granted me the right to provide this information to you in this book and in my *Eat to Win* computer programs (see Appendix IV for details). This vital information can be used by anyone on any dietary program to accurately determine the six vital nutrient values of their favorite foods (including fast foods) and recipes.

Use the following food composition information to help you enjoy foods and recipes that fall within the level of the Maximum Performance Program that's right for you, based on your blood chemistry values. By using these tables, you will become a food composition expert. Soon you will automatically know, for example, how much cholesterol an egg contains, or how much fat you ate in your last Big Mac. These tables are as much an education in food composition as they are a guide to healthful eating. (Where "ETS Recipe" is indicated, the reference is to a recipe contained in this book's Section II. Where "ETW Recipe" is indicated, the reference is to a recipe contained in *Eat to Win*.)

	Weight (oz.)	Calories	Carbo-hydrates (g.)	Protein (g.)	Fat (g.)	Cholesterol (mg.)	Sodium (mg.)
APPETIZERS							
Crabmeat Dip, ETS recipe (1 serving)	3.0	81.5	2.3	11.1	1.6	58.2	617.9
Cucumber and Onion Dip, ETS recipe (1 serving)	0.9	17.9	2.2	2.0	0.2	0.7	61.5
Garden Dip, ETS recipe (1 serving)	3.0	38.4	3.5	5.2	0.4	1.8	182.9
Onion Dip, ETS recipe (1 serving)	4.3	65.4	7.4	4.1	2.1	9.1	217.8
Salmon Spread, ETS recipe (1 serving)	5.9	193.7	3.6	25.9	7.8	32.4	5018.0
Shrimp Cocktail, ETS recipe (1 serving)	4.4	79.4	3.6	14.3	0.7	85.0	95.6
Stuffed Mushrooms, ETS recipe (1 serving)	3.5	157.6	12.4	7.3	10.1	0.6	198.5
BEVERAGES							
Banana Frothy, ETS recipe (12 fluid ounces)	17.4	437.7	69.1	13.2	6.0	6.4	178.1
Beer, light (12 fluid ounces)	12.7	100.0	6.0	0.4	0	0	25.0
Beer, 3.6% alcohol by weight (12 fluid ounces)	12.7	151.2	13.7	1.1	0	0	25.2
Brandy (1 fluid ounce)	1.0	42.9	2.3	0+	0	0	1.1
Burgundy (1 fluid ounce)	1.0	24.3	1.2	0+	0	0	1.4
Chocolate Drink, commercial, w/skim milk (12 fluid ounces)	13.0	264.6	38.2	11.8	7.4	25.7	221.2
Chocolate Drink, commercial, w/whole milk (12 fluid ounces)	12.9	303.8	37.7	11.7	12.4	43.9	218.1
Chocolate Frothy, ETS recipe (12 fluid ounces)	10.3	136.0	23.3	8.5	1.0	4.6	119.3
Chocolate Malted, ETS recipe (12 fluid ounces)	12.5	299.3	66.9	10.8	1.2	4.5	150.1
Club Soda, unsweetened (12 fluid ounces)	12.7	0	0	0	0	0	88.5
Coca-Cola (12 fluid ounces)	12.7	144.0	36.0	0	0	0	1.0
Cocoa Powder, dry form, low–medium fat, plain (1 tablespoon)	0.2	11.0	2.7	1.0	0.6	0	0.3
Coconut Milk (12 fluid ounces)	6.8	484.0	10.0	6.1	47.8	0	48.0
Coffee, ground, beverage (8 fluid ounces)	8.3	2.0	0.5	0	0	0	26.0
Coffee, instant, beverage (8 fluid ounces)	8.5	2.0	1.2	0	0	0	2.0

	Weight (oz.)	Calories	Carbo-hydrates (g.)	Protein (g.)	Fat (g.)	Cholesterol (mg.)	Sodium (mg.)
Coffee, instant, decaf., dry form (⅓ tablespoon)	0.1	4.0	1.1	0.3	0.1	0	2.0
Coffee, Sanka, instant, decaf. beverage (8 fluid ounces)	8.3	5.0	1.2	0	0	0	0
Cointreau (3½ ounces)	3.5	347.3	32.7	0	0	0	0
Cream Soda (12 fluid ounces)	12.7	154.8	39.6	0	0	0	0
Gatorade, citrus (12 fluid ounces)	12.2	58.5	15.8	0	0	0	184.5
Gatorade, cola (12 fluid ounces)	12.2	58.5	13.8	0	0	0	162.0
Gin, 80 proof, 33.4% alcohol by weight (1 fluid ounce)	1.1	69.3	0	0	0	0	0.3
Ginger Ale, pale dry, golden (12 fluid ounces)	12.7	111.6	28.8	0	0	0	4.0
Ginger Ale, sugar-free (12 fluid ounces)	12.7	4.0	1.5	0	0	0	32.0
Hawaiian Punch (12 fluid ounces)	13.2	180.0	43.9	0.1	0	0	75.0
Hot Cocoa, homemade (8 fluid ounces)	8.5	208.8	24.7	8.6	8.6	31.2	117.8
Kool-Aid, all flavors (12 fluid ounces)	12.7	150.0	37.5	0	0	0	1.5
Liquor, almond-flavored (1 serving)	5.6	560.0	52.8	0	0	0	0
Mocha Frothy, ETS recipe (12 fluid ounces)	14.0	173.6	30.1	11.6	1.0	6.5	170.5
Mountain Dew (12 fluid ounces)	12.7	171.0	42.8	0	0	0	31.0
Mr Pibb (12 fluid ounces)	12.7	140.0	37.5	0	0	0	17.0
Nog Frothy, ETS recipe (12 fluid ounces)	15.6	200.9	35.5	12.0	1.1	6.9	178.7
Orange Dream, ETS recipe (12 fluid ounces)	13.7	159.5	32.7	5.6	0.6	3.0	78.7
Orange Soda (12 fluid ounces)	12.7	167.0	45.4	0.1	0	0	18.0
Pepsi-Cola (12 fluid ounces)	12.7	156.0	39.4	0	0	0	18.0
Pepsi-Cola, sugar-free (12 fluid ounces)	12.7	1.0	0.2	0	0	0	63.0
Pepsi Light (12 fluid ounces)	12.7	71.0	17.6	0	0	0	12.0
Postum, instant powder (⅓ tablespoon)	0.1	10.0	2.5	0.2	0	0	2.0
Quinine Soda, sweetened (12 fluid ounces)	12.7	111.6	28.8	0	0	0	0

	Weight (oz.)	Calories	Carbo-hydrates (g.)	Protein (g.)	Fat (g.)	Cholesterol (mg.)	Sodium (mg.)
Root Beer, Hires (12 fluid ounces)	12.7	146.0	39.8	0	0	0	4.0
Root Beer, Hires, sugar-free (12 fluid ounces)	12.7	2.0	0.4	0	0	0	53.0
Royal Crown Cola (12 fluid ounces)	12.7	156.0	39.0	0	0	0	1.0
Rum, 80 proof, 33.4% alcohol by weight (1 fluid ounce)	1.1	69.3	0	0	0	0	0
Seven-Up (12 fluid ounces)	12.7	144.0	36.0	0	0	0	4.0
Sherry, dry (1 fluid ounce)	1.1	42.0	2.4	0.1	0	0	1.0
Sprite (12 fluid ounces)	12.7	144.0	62.3	0	0	0	47.0
Sprite, sugar-free (12 fluid ounces)	12.7	5.0	0	0	0	0	48.0
Strawberry Frothy, ETS recipe (12 fluid ounces)	17.4	348.7	44.5	12.8	5.9	6.4	177.6
Tab, sugar-free (12 fluid ounces)	12.7	1.0	0.1	0	0	0	27.0
Tang, orange, beverage (12 fluid ounces)	12.7	202.5	50.7	0	0.1	0	25.5
Tang, orange, dry powder (½ ounce)	0.5	51.5	12.6	0	0+	0	6.5
Tea, instant, beverage (8 fluid ounces)	8.5	4.8	1.0	0	0	0	1.6
Tea, instant, dry powder (⅓ tablespoon)	0.1	5.9	1.6	0	0	0	1.0
Tom Collins Mixer, 10–13% sugar (6 fluid ounces)	6.6	86.2	22.5	0	0	0	0
Vodka, 80 proof, 33.4% alcohol by weight (1 fluid ounce)	1.1	69.30	0	0	0	0	0.3
Water (12 fluid ounces)	12.5	0	0	0	0	0	4.5
Whiskey, 80 proof, 36.4% alcohol by weight (1 fluid ounce)	1.1	69.3	0	0	0	0	0.3
Whiskey Sour Mix (6 fluid ounces)	6.3	71.4	17.7	0	0	0	12.0
Wine, dessert, 15.3% alcohol by weight (6 fluid ounces)	6.3	246.6	13.9	0.2	0	0	7.2
Wine, table, 9.9% alcohol by weight (6 fluid ounces)	6.3	153.0	7.6	0.2	0	0	9.0

BREADS/ROLLS/CRACKERS

	Weight (oz.)	Calories	Carbo-hydrates (g.)	Protein (g.)	Fat (g.)	Cholesterol (mg.)	Sodium (mg.)
Apple Bread, ETW recipe (1 slice)	1.6	110.4	23.1	3.9	1.0	0	58.3
Apple Muffins, ETW recipe (1 average)	2.6	178.8	40.3	5.0	1.0	0.3	69.3

	Weight (oz.)	Calories	Carbo-hydrates (g.)	Protein (g.)	Fat (g.)	Cholesterol (mg.)	Sodium (mg.)
Bagel, whole wheat (1 average)							
	1.6	102.0	22.0	4.8	1.4	0	242.0
Banana Bread, ETW recipe (1 slice)							
	2.2	153.8	35.0	4.4	1.1	0	59.5
Banana Date Muffins, ETS recipe (1 average)							
	2.2	105.4	25.1	1.8	0.3	0.1	9.6
Biscuit, from mix, w/milk (1 average)							
	1.0	92.1	14.8	2.0	2.6	0.3	275.8
Blueberry Bran Muffins, ETW recipe (1 average)							
	1.7	97.3	20.2	3.5	0.8	0.3	68.6
Boston Brown Bread (1 serving)							
	1.0	59.8	12.9	1.6	0.4	0.3	71.2
Bran Date Bread, ETS recipe (1 average)							
	2.3	177.9	31.5	4.5	4.4	0.6	48.0
Bread Crumbs, dry, grated (3½ ounces)							
	3.5	389.0	72.8	12.5	4.6	5.0	730.3
Bread Crumbs, whole wheat (3½ ounces)							
	3.5	287.1	56.4	12.5	3.7	5.0	621.3
Bun, hamburger or hot dog (1 average)							
	1.4	119.0	21.2	3.3	2.2	0	202.0
Cherry Almond Muffins, ETS recipe (1 average)							
	1.9	146.1	26.7	3.3	3.1	0.6	19.9
Corn Bread, from mix, w/egg, milk (1 slice)							
	1.6	104.9	14.8	2.7	3.8	31.1	334.8
Corn Fritters (1 average)							
	3.5	377.0	39.7	7.8	21.5	88.0	477.0
Corn Muffins, ETW recipe (1 average)							
	2.9	116.9	24.1	4.8	0.9	0.6	113.6
Cracked Wheat Bread (1 slice)							
	0.8	60.5	12.0	2.0	0.5	0.5	121.7
Crackers, sandwich type, peanut-cheese (3½ ounces)							
	3.5	487.2	55.7	15.1	23.7	15.9	984.3
Earth Bread, ETW recipe (2 slices)							
	2.5	160.1	32.9	6.3	1.4	0	73.7
French or Vienna Bread (2 slices)							
	1.4	116.0	22.2	3.6	1.2	1.2	232.0
Graham Crackers, plain (2 average)							
	0.5	53.8	10.3	1.1	1.3	0	93.8
Italian Bread (2 slices)							
	1.4	110.4	22.6	3.6	0.3	0.4	234.0
Matzo, unsalted (1 slice)							
	1.1	117.0	25.4	3.0	0.3	0	1.0
Muffins, blueberry, home recipe (1 average)							
	1.6	126.5	18.9	3.3	4.2	37.3	284.4
Muffins, bran, home recipe (1 average)							
	1.4	104.4	17.2	3.1	3.9	41.2	179.2
Muffins, corn, w/whole ground meal, vegetable shortening (1 average)							
	1.6	129.6	19.1	3.2	4.6	24.8	222.8

	Weight (oz.)	Calories	Carbo-hydrates (g.)	Protein (g.)	Fat (g.)	Cholesterol (mg.)	Sodium (mg.)
Muffins, plain, home recipe (1 average) 1.6		132.3	19.0	3.5	4.5	23.9	198.5
Orange Muffins, ETW recipe (1 average) 1.7		127.6	26.2	5.3	1.0	0.4	114.4
Pecan Cranberry Bread, ETS recipe (1 slice) 1.5		148.3	29.6	1.8	2.6	0	80.6
Pumpernickel Bread (2 slices) 2.3		157.4	34.0	5.8	0.8	0.6	364.2
Pumpkin Apple Bread, ETS recipe (1 slice) 1.6		92.4	21.3	3.0	0.4	0.3	63.9
Raisin Bread (2 slices) 1.6		120.5	24.7	3.0	1.3	1.4	167.9
Raisin Bread, toasted (1 slice) 0.7		60.0	12.3	1.5	0.6	0.6	83.6
Rice Cakes (1 average) 0.3		35.0	7.6	0.7	0.2	0	14.1
Rice Crackers (3 average) 0.4		31.0	6.7	0.8	0	0	8.0
Rolls, brown-and-serve, browned (1 average) 1.4		131.2	21.9	3.5	3.1	3.2	224.8
Rolls, Danish pastry, commercial, ready-to-serve (1 average) 1.4		164.6	17.8	2.9	9.2	25.4	142.7
Rolls, from mix (1 average) 1.2		104.6	19.1	3.1	1.6	1.4	109.5
Rolls, hard, commercial (1 average) 1.2		109.2	20.8	3.4	1.1	1.1	218.8
Rolls, sweet (1 small) 1.2		110.6	17.3	3.0	3.2	3.1	136.1
Rolls, whole wheat (1 average) 1.2		89.9	18.3	3.5	1.0	1.1	197.4
Rusk (1 slice) 0.4		41.9	7.1	1.4	0.9	0.9	24.6
Rye Bread, American (2 slices) 1.6		112.0	24.0	4.2	0.6	1.0	256.0
Saltines (2 average) 0.2		26.0	4.3	0.5	0.7	0	66.0
Sesame Sweet Bread, ETS recipe (1 slice) 1.7		110.0	20.5	2.7	2.1	0.9	13.2
Soda Crackers (2 average) 0.5		61.5	9.9	1.3	1.8	0	154.0
Sweet Potato Muffins, ETS recipe (1 average) 2.1		140.5	30.7	2.1	1.3	0.3	13.9
White Bread (2 slices) 1.6		124.2	23.2	4.0	1.5	1.4	233.2
Whole Wheat Bread (2 slices) 1.6		111.8	21.9	4.8	1.4	1.4	242.4
Whole Wheat Bread, ETW recipe (1 slice) 1.6		107.8	23.2	4.0	0.6	0.1	3.1

	Weight (oz.)	Calories	Carbo-hydrates (g.)	Protein (g.)	Fat (g.)	Cholesterol (mg.)	Sodium (mg.)
Whole Wheat Raisin Bread, ETW recipe (1 slice)	1.2	110.4	22.4	4.7	1.0	0.5	73.0
Zweiback (3½ ounces)	3.5	419.7	73.7	10.6	8.7	8.9	248.1

CASSEROLES/COMBINATIONS

	Weight (oz.)	Calories	Carbo-hydrates (g.)	Protein (g.)	Fat (g.)	Cholesterol (mg.)	Sodium (mg.)
Baked Cannellini, ETS recipe (1 serving)	8.7	235.4	41.0	14.3	2.5	3.4	262.9
Baked Lentils, ETS recipe (1 serving)	8.3	251.7	39.6	16.1	3.5	7.0	573.4
Basic Brown Rice and Chicken, ETW recipe (1 serving)	7.8	305.1	39.0	24.0	5.2	53.1	276.4
Beans and Frankfurters, canned (1 serving)	9.0	367.3	32.1	19.4	18.1	33.2	1375.0
Beef Pot Pie, commercial, frozen, unheated (1 average)	8.0	435.8	40.9	16.6	22.5	40.9	830.8
Black Bean and Rice Casserole, ETS recipe (1 serving)	6.1	178.7	25.2	13.9	2.7	9.8	295.7
Broccoli Brown Rice Hollandaise, ETW recipe (1 serving)	7.7	140.6	20.3	10.8	2.4	4.8	180.3
Broccoli Macaroni Bake, ETS recipe (1 serving)	8.5	311.3	50.1	19.3	3.8	6.7	403.4
Brown Rice and Cottage Cheese, ETW recipe (1 serving)	6.7	181.8	24.7	12.9	3.2	9.7	370.0
Cannellini-Stuffed Zucchini, ETW recipe (1 serving)	10.8	358.3	64.4	20.4	3.3	4.5	196.6
Carrot Casserole, ETS recipe (1 serving)	4.5	124.6	22.9	4.6	1.8	3.8	180.4
Chicken and Broccoli Stir Fry, ETS recipe (1 serving)	8.7	225.4	34.0	17.1	2.4	32.2	180.9
Chicken Brown Rice Pie, ETS recipe (1 serving)	6.8	192.1	21.8	17.8	3.3	29.5	270.8
Chicken Casserole, ETW recipe (1 serving)	6.7	340.7	42.8	26.4	6.0	42.4	300.8
Chicken Chow Mein, w/o noodles, canned (1 serving)	8.0	86.4	16.1	5.9	0.2	6.8	659.1
Chicken Curry, ETW recipe (1 serving)	13.7	464.8	80.1	28.6	4.5	53.6	582.9
Chicken Curry Muffins, ETS recipe (1 average)	4.7	130.4	15.9	12.0	1.9	23.8	116.8
Chicken Fried Rice, ETS recipe (1 serving)	7.2	188.8	33.6	9.6	1.6	16.1	208.3
Chicken Pot Pie, commercial, frozen (1 average)	8.0	497.1	50.4	15.2	26.1	29.5	933.0
Chik 'n' Chili, ETW recipe (1 serving)	7.2	148.5	26.4	9.2	1.8	12.5	444.5
Chili Pie, ETW recipe (1 serving)	8.1	247.1	48.4	12.9	1.6	0.3	305.4
Chop Suey, w/meat, canned (1 serving)	8.8	155.0	10.5	11.0	8.0	30.0	1377.5

	Weight (oz.)	Calories	Carbo-hydrates (g.)	Protein (g.)	Fat (g.)	Cholesterol (mg.)	Sodium (mg.)
Coq au Vin Casserole, ETW recipe (1 serving)	7.2	257.2	29.1	17.4	3.0	25.9	180.7
Corn and Brown Rice Stir Fry, ETS recipe (1 serving)	8.7	234.0	51.8	6.1	1.7	0	112.7
Corn and Chicken Frittata, ETW recipe (1 serving)	5.7	160.6	13.8	20.9	2.7	35.3	179.6
Corned Beef Hash with Potatoes, canned (1 serving)	7.8	398.7	23.6	19.4	24.9	72.7	1189.4
Crabmeat au Gratin, ETW recipe (1 serving)	13.5	439.7	45.2	35.8	10.1	108.2	812.9
Creamy Lasagna, ETS recipe (1 serving)	9.7	404.7	43.8	32.3	10.2	54.6	442.0
Eggplant Moussaka, ETW recipe (1 serving)	13.7	380.9	53.6	27.9	4.5	15.0	692.7
Frozen Dinner, beef pot roast, w/potatoes, peas, corn (1 average)	11.0	330.7	19.0	40.9	10.0	156.0	808.1
Frozen Dinner, fried chicken, w/potatoes, vegetables (1 average)	11.0	539.8	35.3	39.9	26.5	152.9	1073.3
Frozen Dinner, meat loaf, w/tomato sauce, vegetables (1 average)	11.0	407.4	30.5	24.9	20.8	96.4	1222.2
Frozen Dinner, sliced turkey, w/potatoes, peas (1 average)	11.0	349.4	39.6	26.2	9.4	99.8	1248.0
Glazed Ratatouille, ETW recipe (1 serving)	6.5	109.0	17.6	5.5	2.1	5.2	153.8
Imam Bayeldi, ETW recipe (1 serving)	5.7	121.7	22.4	4.2	1.3	2.0	388.8
Indian Rice Casserole, ETS recipe (1 serving)	7.5	157.7	29.6	5.1	2.5	8.1	55.0
Indian Vegetable and Rice Casserole, ETW recipe (1 serving)	9.2	206.6	34.7	10.9	3.3	8.8	464.2
Italian Macaroni and Beans, ETW recipe (1 serving)	7.0	112.9	19.9	5.3	1.6	2.6	324.0
Italian Stuffed Peppers, ETW recipe (1 large)	15.0	420.1	76.4	22.8	3.3	3.9	910.0
Italian Vegetable Bake, ETW recipe (1 serving)	7.5	94.9	14.9	5.1	2.1	3.9	658.6
Italian White Beans, ETW recipe (1 serving)	7.0	112.9	19.9	5.3	1.6	2.6	324.0
Macaroni and Cheese, canned (1 serving)	7.1	190.0	21.4	7.8	8.0	20.0	608.0
Melanzane al Forno (Baked Eggplant), ETW recipe (1 serving)	9.7	131.2	24.7	7.6	1.9	3.0	355.5
Mexican Rice, ETS recipe (1 serving)	8.2	192.5	32.3	11.8	1.8	21.5	214.4
Onion Potato Pie, ETS recipe (1 serving)	6.3	143.6	17.1	12.2	3.0	8.6	465.5
Potato Casserole, ETW recipe (1 serving)	12.0	283.1	55.4	13.2	1.5	5.5	208.3
Potato Cheese Bake, ETS recipe (1 serving)	7.1	146.4	19.6	12.9	1.7	5.7	288.7

	Weight (oz.)	Calories	Carbo-hydrates (g.)	Protein (g.)	Fat (g.)	Cholesterol (mg.)	Sodium (mg.)
Rice-Stuffed Green Peppers, ETS recipe (1 large)							
	8.3	252.8	33.7	11.4	8.7	5.6	230.7
Rolled Stuffed Eggplant, ETS recipe (1 serving)							
	10.0	202.1	31.5	13.3	3.2	9.0	950.2
Salmon Rice Loaf (1 serving)							
	3.5	122.0	7.3	12.0	4.5	21.0	275.0
Spaghetti in Tomato Sauce, w/cheese, canned (1 serving)							
	7.8	168.1	34.1	4.9	1.3	6.6	845.1
Spaghetti with Meat Balls in Tomato Sauce, canned (1 serving)							
	7.8	227.9	25.2	10.8	9.1	19.9	1079.6
Spinach Cheese Pie, ETW recipe (1 serving)							
	7.5	132.8	7.7	19.3	2.8	8.6	582.4
Spinach Noodle Casserole, ETW recipe (1 serving)							
	6.8	234.3	33.4	17.4	3.3	7.1	520.8
Stuffed Cabbage, ETW recipe (1 serving)							
	9.4	163.6	31.8	5.7	1.8	3.0	697.3
Stuffed Green Peppers, w/beef and bread crumbs (1 average)							
	6.7	324.7	32.1	24.8	10.5	72.6	599.7
Stuffed Tomatoes, ETW recipe (1 serving)							
	11.0	276.0	56.5	12.2	3.5	3.5	380.9
Sweet Potato Casserole, ETS recipe (1 serving)							
	7.6	227.5	54.5	3.1	0.8	0.3	32.8
Sweet Potato Stuffing, ETS recipe (1 serving)							
	5.8	235.3	28.1	6.3	12.5	0.8	239.2
Tabbouleh, ETS recipe (1 serving)							
	9.7	204.0	44.1	7.3	0.8	0	357.5
Tomato Broccoli Pie, ETS recipe (1 slice)							
	6.5	124.5	11.8	12.7	3.3	9.7	386.6
Tomato Salmon Casserole, ETW recipe (1 serving)							
	6.0	206.4	29.7	14.3	3.7	13.8	348.0
Tuna Casserole Supreme, ETW recipe (1 serving)							
	7.0	253.7	30.9	20.1	4.6	31.6	207.2
Tuna Muffins, ETW recipe (1 average)							
	4.2	129.4	14.8	13.4	1.5	22.8	147.0
Turkey Pot Pie, commercial, frozen (1 average)							
	8.0	227.0	23.2	6.7	12.0	10.4	425.2
Turkey-Stuffed Potato, ETS recipe (1 average)							
	14.5	465.7	54.9	41.6	8.7	77.4	465.3
Veal-Stuffed Eggplant, ETS recipe (1 serving)							
	8.1	187.6	21.6	12.4	6.9	28.8	128.9
Vegetable Rice Casserole, ETS recipe (1 serving)							
	7.7	190.2	36.1	8.4	2.1	4.5	430.3
Welsh Rarebit (1 serving)							
	8.2	415.3	14.6	18.8	31.6	99.8	770.3
Ziti Casserole, ETS recipe (1 serving)							
	9.7	320.4	48.0	20.9	5.1	8.0	682.7
Zucchini Corn Casserole, ETS recipe (1 serving)							
	16.2	328.4	57.6	20.6	5.4	12.7	431.7

	Weight (oz.)	Calories	Carbo-hydrates (g.)	Protein (g.)	Fat (g.)	Cholesterol (mg.)	Sodium (mg.)
Zucchini Squares, ETW recipe (1 average)							
	1.0	28.7	3.9	2.2	0.6	1.1	84.3
CEREALS/GRAINS							
Apples and Brown Rice Cereal, ETS recipe (1 serving)							
	10.4	298.6	57.3	5.8	5.8	0	5.1
Baked Barley, ETS recipe (1 serving)							
	6.7	148.6	31.0	6.1	0.5	0	417.5
Barley, pearled, light, dry (3½ ounces)							
	3.5	346.3	78.2	8.1	1.0	0	3.0
Barley, pearled, pot or Scotch (3½ ounces)							
	3.5	345.3	76.6	9.5	1.1	0	4.0
Bran, All-Bran (1 serving)							
	1.0	70.6	21.1	4.1	0.5	0	319.8
Bran, wheat (1 serving)							
	0.3	1.7	0.5	0.1	0+	0	0.1
Bran Buds Cereal (1 serving)							
	1.0	73.1	21.5	3.9	0.7	0	174.1
Bran Cereal, All-Bran (1 serving)							
	1.0	70.6	21.1	4.1	0.5	0	319.8
Bran Cereal, 100% Bran (1 serving)							
	1.0	76.3	20.7	3.5	1.4	0	196.5
Bran Cereal, 40% Bran Flakes (1 serving)							
	1.0	92.4	22.2	3.6	0.5	0	263.9
Bran Flakes with Raisins (1 serving)							
	1.0	88.5	21.4	3.1	0.6	0	207.0
Brown Rice, cooked w/o salt (1 serving)							
	5.3	178.5	38.3	3.8	0.9	0	3.0
Brown Rice, cooked w/salt (1 serving)							
	5.3	178.5	38.3	3.8	0.9	0	423.0
Brown Rice, raw (1 serving)							
	1.7	176.4	37.9	3.7	0.9	0	4.4
Buckwheat, whole grain (3½ ounces)							
	3.5	332.4	72.3	11.6	2.4	0	2.0
Bulgur, dry, commercial, from club wheat (3½ ounces)							
	3.5	356.2	78.9	8.6	1.4	0	4.0
Corn Chex, shredded corn cereal (1 serving)							
	1.0	111.1	24.9	2.0	0.1	0	271.0
Corn Flakes (1 serving)							
	1.0	110.3	24.4	2.3	0.1	0	351.0
Corn Flakes, low-sodium (1 serving)							
	1.0	113.1	25.2	2.2	0.1	0	2.8
Corn Flakes, sugar-covered (1 serving)							
	1.0	108.0	25.7	1.4	0.1	0	229.6
Corn Grits, cooked w/o salt (1 serving)							
	8.5	145.3	31.5	3.4	0.5	0	0
Corn Grits, cooked w/salt (1 serving)							
	8.5	145.3	31.5	3.4	0.5	0	540.0

	Weight (oz.)	Calories	Carbo-hydrates (g.)	Protein (g.)	Fat (g.)	Cholesterol (mg.)	Sodium (mg.)
Corn Grits, dry form (1 serving)							
	1.4	148.4	31.8	3.5	0.5	0	0.4
Cream of Wheat, cooked (1 serving)							
	7.1	108.0	22.4	3.0	0.4	0	116.0
Cream of Wheat, instant, dry form (1 serving)							
	1.3	139.1	28.7	4.0	0.5	0	5.7
Farina, quick-cooking, cooked w/o salt (1 serving)							
	8.6	122.5	26.0	3.4	0.2	0	0
Farina, quick-cooking, dry form (1 serving)							
	1.3	140.2	29.6	4.0	0.2	0	1.1
Grape Nuts Cereal (1 serving)							
	1.0	100.0	23.0	3.7	0.3	0	174.0
Hot Brown Rice Cereal, ETS recipe (1 serving)							
	10.0	253.7	52.6	8.3	1.2	2.4	67.3
Millet, whole grain (1 serving)							
	1.8	163.5	36.4	4.9	1.4	0	0.5
Oat Cereal, plain (1 serving)							
	1.5	155.0	30.1	7.7	0.8	0	218.9
Oat Cereal, puffed (1 serving)							
	0.9	97.7	17.3	3.8	1.6	0	270.8
Oat Cereal, puffed, sugar-coated (1 serving)							
	0.9	98.0	21.6	1.9	0.6	0	193.0
Oat Flakes (1 serving)							
	1.6	166.2	32.6	8.4	0.7	0	402.7
Oatmeal Royale, ETW recipe (1 serving)							
	13.3	281.1	63.5	6.5	2.5	0	7.8
Oats, rolled, cooked w/o salt (1 serving)							
	8.3	146.6	25.5	6.1	2.4	0	2.4
Oats, rolled, dry form (1 serving)							
	1.0	108.7	19.0	4.5	1.8	0	1.1
Rice Bran (1 serving)							
	0.4	27.6	5.1	1.3	1.6	0	0
Rice Cereal, Cream of, cooked w/o salt (1 serving)							
	8.6	127.5	28.2	2.2	0.2	0	2.5
Rice Cereal, Cream of, dry form (3½ ounces)							
	3.5	367.1	81.8	6.3	0.5	0	6.0
Rice Cereal, puffed (1 serving)							
	0.5	56.3	12.6	0.9	0.1	0	0.4
Rice Chex Cereal (1 serving)							
	1.0	112.0	25.3	1.5	0.1	0	237.0
Rice Krispies Cereal (1 serving)							
	1.0	110.9	24.8	1.8	0.1	0	205.6
Rie Krispies Cereal, low-sodium (1 serving)							
	1.0	112.6	25.5	1.5	0.1	0	2.8
Rice Polish (3½ ounces)							
	3.5	262.9	57.3	12.0	12.7	0	0
Rye, whole grain, raw (3½ ounces)							
	3.5	331.4	72.8	12.0	1.7	0	1.0

	Weight (oz.)	Calories	Carbo-hydrates (g.)	Protein (g.)	Fat (g.)	Cholesterol (mg.)	Sodium (mg.)
Sorgum Grain, all types (3½ ounces)	3.5	329.4	72.4	10.9	3.3	0	1.0
Tapioca, dry (1 serving)	0.4	35.2	8.6	0.1	0+	0	0.3
Wheat, Malted Barley Cereal, cooked w/o salt (1 serving)	7.1	144.0	31.8	4.6	0.8	0	8.0
Wheat, Malted Barley Cereal, dry form (1 serving)	1.8	176.0	38.6	5.6	1.0	0	8.5
Wheat, Malted Barley Flakes Cereal (1 serving)	1.0	101.5	23.2	3.0	0.3	0	217.7
Wheat, Malted Barley Granules Cereal (1 serving)	1.0	101.2	23.2	3.3	0.1	0	197.0
Wheat, Puffed Cereal, w/o sugar, salt (1 serving)	1.0	103.2	22.6	4.2	0.3	0	1.1
Wheat, Shredded Wheat Cereal, w/o salt (1 serving)	1.6	158.4	35.9	4.9	0.6	0	0.9
Wheat, whole grain, dry (3½ ounces)	3.5	329.4	69.6	12.6	2.5	0	3.0
Wheat Chex Cereal, w/malt, salt, sugar (1 serving)	1.4	146.8	32.9	4.0	1.0	0	268.0
Wheat Flakes Cereal (1 serving)	1.0	97.8	22.3	2.7	0.5	0	350.1
Wheat Germ, crude, commercially milled (1 serving)	0.4	36.3	4.7	2.7	1.1	0	0.3
Wheat Germ Cereal, toasted (3½ ounces)	3.5	379.0	49.2	28.9	10.6	0	4.0
Wheat Meal Cereal, cooked w/o salt (3½ ounces)	3.5	52.6	11.1	2.2	0.3	0	2.0
Wheat Meal Cereal, dry (1 serving)	1.0	96.7	20.4	4.0	0.6	0	3.1
White Rice, cooked w/o salt (1 serving)	5.3	163.4	36.3	3.0	0.1	0	0
White Rice, raw (1 serving)	1.1	112.6	24.9	2.1	0.1	0	1.6
Whole Wheat Cereal, cooked w/o salt (1 serving)	4.0	69.5	15.4	2.2	0.4	0	0
Whole Wheat Cereal, dry form (1 serving)	1.0	97.0	21.3	3.2	0.6	0	0.6
Wild Rice, raw (1 serving)	1.0	100.1	21.3	4.0	0.2	0	2.0

CHEESE

	Weight (oz.)	Calories	Carbo-hydrates (g.)	Protein (g.)	Fat (g.)	Cholesterol (mg.)	Sodium (mg.)
American Cheese, past. process (1 ounce)	1.0	106.3	0.5	6.3	8.9	26.6	405.4
American Cheese Food, grated (1 ounce)	1.0	93.0	2.1	5.6	7.0	25.0	337.0
American Cheese Food, past. process (1 ounce)	1.0	93.0	2.1	5.6	7.0	18.1	452.5

	Weight (oz.)	Calories	Carbo-hydrates (g.)	Protein (g.)	Fat (g.)	Cholesterol (mg.)	Sodium (mg.)
American Cheese Spread, past. process (1 ounce)	1.0	82.2	2.5	4.6	6.0	15.6	460.7
Blue Cheese (1 ounce)	1.0	100.1	0.7	6.1	8.1	21.3	395.6
Brick Cheese (1 ounce)	1.0	105.2	0.8	6.6	8.4	26.6	158.6
Camembert Cheese, domestic (1 ounce)	1.0	85.0	0.1	5.6	6.9	20.4	238.4
Cheddar Cheese (1 ounce)	1.0	114.2	0.4	7.1	9.4	29.8	175.9
Cottage Cheese, creamed (1 ounce)	1.0	29.2	0.8	3.5	1.3	4.3	114.8
Cottage Cheese, dry curd (1 ounce)	1.0	24.1	0.5	4.9	0.1	2.0	3.6
Cottage Cheese, 1% fat (1 ounce)	1.0	20.4	0.8	3.5	0.3	1.4	115.2
Cottage Cheese, 2% fat (1 ounce)	1.0	25.5	1.0	3.9	0.5	2.4	115.2
Cream Cheese (1 ounce)	1.0	98.9	0.8	2.2	9.9	31.2	83.8
Limburger Cheese (1 ounce)	1.0	92.7	0.1	5.7	7.7	25.5	226.8
Mozzarella Cheese, part skim, low-moisture (1 ounce)	1.0	79.0	0.9	7.8	4.8	15.0	150.0
Parmesan Cheese, grated (1 ounce)	1.0	129.3	1.0	11.8	8.5	22.4	527.7
Parmesan Cheese, hard (1 ounce)	1.0	111.1	0.9	10.1	7.3	19.3	454.0
Romano Cheese, grated (1 ounce)	1.0	110.0	1.0	9.0	7.6	22.4	340.0
Roquefort Cheese (1 ounce)	1.0	100.1	0.7	6.1	8.1	21.3	395.6
Swiss Cheese, domestic (1 ounce)	1.0	106.6	1.0	8.1	7.8	26.1	73.7
Swiss Cheese, past. process, w/o AD2 phosphate (1 ounce)	1.0	94.7	0.6	7.0	7.1	24.1	193.1
Swiss Cheese, past. process, w/1.5% AD2 Phosphate (1 ounce)	1.0	94.7	0.6	7.0	7.1	24.1	388.5

COOKIES/CANDY/SNACKS

Animal Crackers (3½ ounces)	3.5	425.7	79.3	6.5	9.3	29.8	300.6
Apricots, candied (3½ ounces)	3.5	335.4	85.8	0.6	0.2	0	1.0
Butter Cookies, thin, rich (4 average)	0.8	100.5	15.6	1.3	3.7	16.7	92.0
Butterscotch Candy (3½ ounces)	3.5	393.9	94.1	0	3.4	9.9	65.5

	Weight (oz.)	Calories	Carbo-hydrates (g.)	Protein (g.)	Fat (g.)	Cholesterol (mg.)	Sodium (mg.)
Caramels, chocolate-flavored roll (3½ ounces)							
	3.5	392.9	82.1	2.2	8.1	1.0	195.5
Caramels, plain or chocolate (3½ ounces)							
	3.5	395.9	76.0	4.0	10.1	2.0	224.2
Caramels, plain or chocolate, w/nuts (3½ ounces)							
	3.5	424.7	70.0	4.5	16.2	2.0	201.4
Cheese Crackers (3½ ounces)							
	3.5	475.3	59.9	11.1	21.1	31.8	1030.9
Cheese Straws, w/lard (3½ ounces)							
	3.5	449.5	34.2	11.1	29.7	53.6	715.4
Cheese Straws, w/veg. shortening (3½ ounces)							
	3.5	449.5	34.2	11.1	29.7	31.8	715.4
Cherries, candied (3½ ounces)							
	3.5	336.4	86.0	0.5	0.2	0	2.0
Chewing gum (3½ ounces)							
	3.5	314.5	94.5	0	0	0	0
Chocolate Candy, bittersweet (3½ ounces)							
	3.5	473.3	46.4	7.8	39.4	0	3.0
Chocolate Candy, semisweet (3½ ounces)							
	3.5	503.1	56.6	4.2	35.4	0	2.0
Chocolate Candy, sweet (3½ ounces)							
	3.5	523.9	57.5	4.4	34.8	1.0	32.7
Chocolate Chip Cookies, commercial (1 serving)							
	0.8	103.6	15.3	1.2	4.6	8.6	88.2
Chocolate-Coated Almonds (3½ ounces)							
	3.5	564.6	39.3	12.2	43.4	1.0	58.5
Chocolate-Coated Chocolate Fudge Candy (3½ ounces)							
	3.5	426.7	72.5	3.8	15.9	2.0	226.2
Chocolate-Coated Chocolate Fudge Candy, w/nuts (3½ ounces)							
	3.5	448.5	66.8	4.9	20.6	2.0	203.4
Chocolate-Coated Coconut Center Candy (3½ ounces)							
	3.5	434.6	71.4	2.8	17.5	1.0	195.5
Chocolate-Coated Fondant (3½ ounces)							
	3.5	406.8	80.4	1.7	10.4	1.0	183.6
Chocolate-Coated Fudge, Caramel, and Peanuts Candy (3½ ounces)							
	3.5	429.6	63.6	7.6	18.0	3.0	202.4
Chocolate-Coated Honeycombed Candy, w/peanut butter (3½ ounces)							
	3.5	459.4	70.1	6.5	19.3	1.0	161.7
Chocolate-Coated Nougat and Caramel Candy (3½ ounces)							
	3.5	412.8	72.2	4.0	13.8	5.0	171.7
Chocolate-Coated Peanuts (3½ ounces)							
	3.5	556.6	38.8	16.3	41.0	1.0	59.5
Chocolate-Coated Raisins (3½ ounces)							
	3.5	421.7	70.0	5.4	17.0	9.9	63.5
Chocolate-Coated Vanilla Creams (3½ ounces)							
	3.5	431.6	69.8	3.8	17.0	2.0	180.6
Chocolate Fudge Candy (3½ ounces)							
	3.5	396.9	74.4	2.7	12.1	1.0	188.5

	Weight (oz.)	Calories	Carbo-hydrates (g.)	Protein (g.)	Fat (g.)	Cholesterol (mg.)	Sodium (mg.)
Chocolate Fudge Candy, w/nuts (3½ ounces)							
	3.5	422.7	68.5	3.9	17.3	1.0	169.7
Citron, candied (3½ ounces)							
	3.5	311.6	79.6	0.2	0.3	0	287.7
Coconut Bar (3½ ounces)							
	3.5	490.2	63.4	6.2	24.3	108.2	146.9
Cookies, from dough chilled in roll (2 average)							
	0.8	119.0	15.6	0.9	6.0	9.4	131.5
Crackers, w/whole wheat (4 average)							
	0.5	56.4	9.5	1.2	1.9	0	76.6
Fig Bars (2 average)							
	1.0	100.2	21.1	1.1	1.6	10.9	70.6
Figs, candied (3½ ounces)							
	3.5	296.7	73.1	3.5	0.2	0	33.7
Fondant Candy (3½ ounces)							
	3.5	361.2	88.9	0.1	2.0	0	210.4
Ginger Root, crystallized, candied (3½ ounces)							
	3.5	337.4	86.4	0.3	0.2	0	59.5
Gingersnap Cookies (6 small)							
	0.8	100.8	19.2	1.3	2.1	9.4	137.0
Graham Crackers, chocolate-coated (2 average)							
	0.9	123.5	17.7	1.3	6.1	0	105.8
Graham Crackers, sugar-honey-coated (2 average)							
	0.9	106.9	19.9	1.7	3.0	0	131.0
Grapefruit Peel, candied (3½ ounces)							
	3.5	313.5	80.0	0.4	0.3	0	0
Gumdrops, starch jelly pieces (3½ ounces)							
	3.5	344.3	86.7	0.1	0.7	0	34.7
Hard Candy (3½ ounces)							
	3.5	383.0	96.4	0	1.1	0	31.8
Jelly Beans (3½ ounces)							
	3.5	364.1	92.4	0	0.5	0	11.9
Ladyfingers (2 large)							
	1.0	100.8	18.1	2.2	2.2	99.7	19.9
Lemon Peel, candied (3½ ounces)							
	3.5	313.5	80.0	0.4	0.3	0	0
Macaroons (2 average)							
	1.0	133.0	18.5	1.5	6.5	30.5	9.5
Marshmallow Cookies (1 average)							
	1.0	114.5	20.2	1.1	3.7	21.3	58.5
Marshmallows (3½ ounces)							
	3.5	316.5	79.8	2.0	0	1.0	38.7
Milk Chocolate Candy, plain (3½ ounces)							
	3.5	516.0	56.5	7.6	32.0	19.8	93.3
Milk Chocolate Candy, w/almonds (3½ ounces)							
	3.5	527.9	50.9	9.2	35.3	16.9	79.4
Milk Chocolate Candy, w/peanuts (3½ ounces)							
	3.5	538.8	44.3	14.0	37.8	12.9	65.5

	Weight (oz.)	Calories	Carbo-hydrates (g.)	Protein (g.)	Fat (g.)	Cholesterol (mg.)	Sodium (mg.)
Molasses Cookies (2 average)							
	1.1	126.6	22.8	1.9	3.2	11.7	115.8
Oatmeal Cookies, w/raisins (2 average)							
	1.0	126.3	20.6	1.7	4.3	10.9	45.4
Oatmeal Fruit Bars, ETW recipe (2 average)							
	8.0	628.6	141.6	14.6	3.8	2.9	72.6
Orange Peel, candied (3½ ounces)							
	3.5	313.5	80.0	0.4	0.3	0	0
Peanut Bar (3½ ounces)							
	3.5	511.0	46.8	17.4	31.9	0	9.9
Peanut Brittle (3½ ounces)							
	3.5	417.7	80.4	5.7	10.3	0	30.8
Peanut Cookies (2 average)							
	0.8	113.5	16.1	2.4	4.6	9.4	41.5
Pears, candied (3½ ounces)							
	3.5	300.6	75.3	1.3	0.6	0	6.9
Popcorn, popped, plain (1 serving)							
	0.5	54.1	10.7	1.8	0.7	0	0.4
Popcorn, popped, w/butter, salt (1 serving)							
	0.5	63.9	8.3	1.4	3.1	6.3	271.7
Popcorn, sugar-coated (3½ ounces)							
	3.5	380.0	84.3	6.1	3.5	0	1.0
Popcorn, unpopped (3½ ounces)							
	3.5	359.2	71.5	11.8	4.7	0	3.0
Potato Chips (50 average)							
	3.5	568.0	50.0	5.3	39.8	0	340.0
Potato Sticks (1 serving)							
	3.5	544.0	50.8	6.4	36.4	0	340.0
Pretzels, salted (10 average)							
	4.8	526.5	102.5	13.2	6.1	0	2268.0
Pretzels, unsalted (2 average)							
	1.0	110.0	22.0	4.0	1.0	0	10.0
Raisin Cookies (2 average)							
	1.1	113.7	24.2	1.3	1.6	11.7	15.6
Salt Sticks, regular type, w/o salt coating (3½ ounces)							
	3.5	381.0	74.7	11.9	2.9	3.0	694.6
Salt Sticks, regular type, w/salt coating (3½ ounces)							
	3.5	381.0	74.7	11.9	2.9	3.0	1661.0
Shortbread Cookies (4 average)							
	1.0	139.4	18.2	2.0	6.5	10.9	16.8
Sugar-Coated Almonds (3½ ounces)							
	3.5	452.5	69.7	7.7	18.5	0	19.8
Sugar-Coated Chocolate Discs (3½ ounces)							
	3.5	462.4	72.1	5.2	19.5	11.9	71.4
Sugar Cookies, thick, home recipe, w/butter (1 average)							
	0.7	85.2	13.4	1.2	3.0	15.2	93.8
Sugar Cookies, thick, home recipe, w/veg. shortening (1 average)							
	0.7	88.8	13.6	1.2	3.4	7.8	63.6

	Weight (oz.)	Calories	Carbo-hydrates (g.)	Protein (g.)	Fat (g.)	Cholesterol (mg.)	Sodium (mg.)
Sugar Wafers (4 average)							
	0.8	106.7	16.1	1.1	4.3	8.6	41.6
Vanilla Fudge Candy (3½ ounces)							
	3.5	394.9	74.2	3.0	11.0	2.0	206.4
Vanilla Fudge Candy, w/nuts (3½ ounces)							
	3.5	420.7	68.3	4.2	16.3	2.0	185.5
Vanilla Wafers (4 average)							
	0.8	101.6	16.4	1.2	3.5	8.6	55.4

DESSERTS/DESSERT SAUCES

	Weight (oz.)	Calories	Carbo-hydrates (g.)	Protein (g.)	Fat (g.)	Cholesterol (mg.)	Sodium (mg.)
All-in-One Apple Pie, ETS recipe (1 slice)							
	8.1	225.9	51.7	5.4	0.8	1.8	118.3
Angel Food Cake (1 slice)							
	1.6	116.5	26.7	2.6	0.1	0	65.7
Apple Brown Betty (1 serving)							
	7.6	324.7	63.9	3.4	7.5	17.2	329.0
Apple Cake, ETS recipe (1 slice)							
	2.4	141.8	27.1	2.3	3.3	0	74.0
Apple Pie, w/lard (1 slice)							
	5.6	409.6	61.0	3.5	17.8	17.6	481.6
Applie Pie, w/veg. shortening (1 slice)							
	5.6	409.6	61.0	3.5	17.8	0	481.6
Baked Apple, ETW recipe (1 average)							
	10.5	302.6	77.3	2.5	1.1	0	9.2
Baked Plantains, ETW recipe (1 serving)							
	5.3	155.0	39.7	1.4	0.6	0	5.2
Banana Custard Pie, w/lard, no salt in filling (1 slice)							
	5.6	353.6	49.1	7.2	14.9	102.4	310.4
Banana Custard Pie, w/veg. short, no salt in filling (1 slice)							
	5.6	353.6	49.1	7.2	14.9	92.8	310.4
Banana Noodle Custard, ETW recipe (1 slice)							
	9.1	324.0	65.9	14.5	1.5	4.0	154.7
Banana Nut Loaf Cake, ETS recipe (½ slice)							
	1.8	101.0	18.7	1.4	2.6		30.6
Blackberry Pie, w/lard, no salt in filling (1 slice)							
	5.6	388.8	55.0	4.2	17.6	17.6	428.8
Blackberry Pie, w/veg. shortening, no salt in filling (1 slice)							
	5.6	388.8	55.0	4.2	17.6	0	428.8
Blueberry Pie, w/lard, no salt in filling (1 slice)							
	5.6	387.2	55.8	3.8	17.3	17.6	428.8
Blueberry Pie, w/veg. shortening, no salt in filling (1 slice)							
	5.6	387.2	55.8	3.8	17.3	0	428.8
Boston Cream Pie, w/butter (1 slice)							
	3.5	294.0	49.4	5.0	8.8	101.0	315.0
Boston Cream Pie, w/veg. shortening (1 slice)							
	3.5	302.0	49.9	5.0	9.4	86.0	186.0
Bread Pudding, w/raisins (1 serving)							
	5.8	308.6	46.9	9.2	10.1	112.2	331.6

	Weight (oz.)	Calories	Carbo-hydrates (g.)	Protein (g.)	Fat (g.)	Cholesterol (mg.)	Sodium (mg.)
Brownie, from mix, w/water, nuts (1 large)	1.8	201.5	29.9	2.4	9.3	32.0	109.0
Brownie, from mix, w/water, nuts, eggs (1 large)	1.8.	214.0	31.5	2.5	10.0	21.5	83.0
Brownie, w/nuts, chocolate icing, commercial (1 serving)	1.8	209.5	30.3	2.4	10.3	19.5	100.0
Brown Rice Fruit Custard, ETW recipe (1 serving)	8.7	258.2	51.9	12.0	0.8	4.1	157.2
Butterscotch Pie, w/lard, no salt in filling (1 slice)	3.5	267.0	38.3	4.4	11.0	57.0	321.0
Butterscotch Pie, w/veg. shortening, no salt in filling (1 slice)	3.5	267.0	38.3	4.4	11.0	52.0	214.0
Cane Syrup (3½ ounces)	3.5	260.7	67.4	0	0	0	5.0
Caramel Cake, no icing, w/butter (1 slice)	1.6	162.9	23.3	2.0	7.1	51.7	207.0
Caramel Cake, w/caramel icing, butter (1 slice)	1.9	198.6	31.6	2.0	7.5	51.2	204.1
Carob Chips (3½ ounces)	3.5	511.0	60.2	5.9	28.7	0	17.5
Carob Nut Loaf, ETS recipe (1 slice)	3.0	297.8	42.5	6.2	12.5	0.4	64.3
Cherry Pie, w/lard (1 slice)	5.6	417.6	61.4	4.2	18.1	17.6	486.4
Cherry Pie, w/veg. shortening (1 slice)	5.6	417.6	61.4	4.2	18.1	0	486.4
Chocolate, bitter or baking (3½)	3.5	501.1	28.7	10.6	52.6	0	4.0
Chocolate Cake, no icing, w/butter (1 slice)	1.8	174.5	25.3	2.4	8.0	41.5	201.0
Chocolate Cake, no icing, w/veg. shortening (1 slice)	1.8	183.0	26.0	2.4	8.6	29.0	147.0
Chocolate Cake, w/chocolate icing, butter (1 slice)	1.8	179.5	27.7	2.2	7.7	33.0	158.0
Chocolate Cake, w/chocolate icing, veg. shortening (1 slice)	1.8	184.5	27.9	2.2	8.2	24.0	117.5
Chocolate Cake Icing (1 serving)	0.4	36.0	7.7	0.1	0.7	2.2	8.3
Chocolate Chiffon Pie, w/lard, no salt in filling (1 slice)	2.8	262.4	35.0	5.4	12.2	112.0	201.6
Chocolate Chiffon Pie, w/veg. shortening, no salt in filling (1 slice)	2.8	262.4	35.0	5.4	12.2	105.6	201.6
Chocolate Cookies (1 average)	0.8	97.9	15.7	1.6	3.5	8.6	30.1
Chocolate Meringue Pie, w/lard (1 slice)	3.5	252.0	33.5	4.8	12.0	62.0	256.0
Chocolate Meringue Pie, w/veg. shortening (1 slice)	3.5	250.0	33.2	4.8	11.9	55.6	254.0

	Weight (oz.)	Calories	Carbo- hydrates (g.)	Protein (g.)	Fat (g.)	Cholesterol (mg.)	Sodium (mg.)
Chocolate Pudding, from mix, w/milk, cooked (1 serving)							
	4.6	161.2	29.6	4.4	3.9	15.6	167.7
Coffee Cake, from mix, w/eggs, milk (1 slice)							
	2.1	193.2	31.4	3.8	5.8	37.2	258.6
Cone, for ice cream (1 average)							
	0.4	45.2	9.3	1.2	0.3	0	27.8
Cookie Dough, plain, chilled in roll (3½ ounces)							
	3.5	445.5	58.3	3.5	22.4	32.7	492.1
Cranberry Relish, ETW recipe (1 serving)							
	1.5	51.4	13.1	0.3	0.1	0	1.1
Cream Puff, w/custard filling (1 average)							
	3.7	244.7	21.5	6.8	14.6	151.2	87.2
Crustless Pumpkin Pie, ETW recipe (1 slice)							
	5.0	163.0	34.0	6.2	0.5	1.8	104.3
Cupcakes, no icing, from mix, w/eggs, milk (1 average)							
	0.9	87.5	13.9	1.2	3.0	15.0	113.2
Cupcakes, w/chocolate icing, from mix, w/eggs, milk (1 average)							
	1.4	143.2	23.7	1.8	5.0	18.8	134.0
Custard, baked (1 serving)							
	4.6	149.5	14.4	7.0	7.2	136.5	102.7
Custard Pie (1 slice)							
	5.3	327.0	35.1	9.1	16.6	162.0	430.5
Devil's Food Cake, w/chocolate icing, cream-filled (1 slice)							
	3.0	315.3	37.2	3.0	18.6	44.2	161.5
Doughnuts, cake type (1 average)							
	1.1	125.1	16.4	1.5	6.0	19.2	160.3
Dougnuts, glazed (1 average)							
	1.3	149.9	16.5	2.0	8.5	9.3	74.0
Doughnuts, plain (1 average)							
	1.1	132.5	12.1	2.0	8.5	8.0	74.9
Eclair, w/custard filling, chocolate icing (1 average)							
	3.9	262.9	25.5	6.8	15.0	149.6	90.2
French Apple Bake, ETW recipe (1 serving)							
	7.0	261.5	58.2	6.3	1.5	0.5	43.7
Frozen Yogurt, soft-serve (1 serving)							
	4.0	149.9	30.8	4.4	1.7	11.3	117.2
Fruitcake, dark, w/butter (1 slice)							
	1.4	145.2	23.9	1.9	5.5	26.4	94.0
Fruitcake, dark, w/veg. shortening (1 slice)							
	1.4	151.6	23.9	1.9	6.1	18.0	63.2
Fruitcake, ETS recipe (1 slice)							
	2.0	203.4	37.8	2.8	6.0	0	29.2
Gelatin Dessert, plain, from powder, w/water (1 serving)							
	4.2	70.9	16.9	1.8	0	0	61.3
Gelatin Dessert, w/fruit, from powder, w/water (1 serving)							
	4.4	83.7	20.5	1.6	0.1	0	42.5
Gingerbread Cake, w/butter (1 slice)							
	1.8	148.5	25.7	1.9	4.9	33.0	169.5

	Weight (oz.)	Calories	Carbo-hydrates (g.)	Protein (g.)	Fat (g.)	Cholesterol (mg.)	Sodium (mg.)
Gingerbread Cake, w/veg. shortening (1 slice)							
	1.8	158.5	26.0	1.9	5.3	21.5	118.5
Holiday Cake, ETW recipe (1 slice)							
	5.8	385.7	81.8	11.5	3.1	0.4	197.1
Honey, strained or extracted (1 serving)							
	0.7	60.8	16.5	0.1	0	0	1.0
Honey Spice Cake, from mix, w/caramel icing, eggs (1 slice)							
	1.8	176.0	30.4	2.0	5.4	29.0	122.5
Ice Cream, regular, 10% fat (1 serving)							
	2.3	134.3	15.9	2.4	7.2	29.9	58.1
Ice Cream, regular, 12% fat (1 serving)							
	2.3	137.7	13.7	2.7	8.3	30.6	26.6
Ice Cream, rich, 16% fat (1 serving)							
	2.6	174.7	16.0	2.1	11.8	43.7	54.1
Ice Milk, vanilla (1 serving)							
	2.4	94.6	14.9	2.6	2.9	9.5	53.9
Lemon Chiffon Pie, w/lard, no salt in filling (1 slice)							
	3.9	344.3	48.2	7.7	13.9	195.8	287.1
Lemon Chiffon Pie, w/veg. shortening, no salt in filling (1 slice)							
	3.9	344.3	48.2	7.7	13.9	185.9	287.1
Lemon Meringue Pie, w/lard (1 slice)							
	4.9	354.2	52.4	5.1	14.2	138.9	391.7
Lemon Meringue Pie, w/veg. shortening (1 slice)							
	4.9	354.2	52.4	5.1	14.2	129.2	391.7
Maple Syrup (3½ ounces)							
	3.5	249.8	64.4	0	0	0	9.9
Marble Cake, w/boiled white icing, from mix, w/eggs (1 slice)							
	1.8	165.5	31.0	2.2	4.3	25.5	129.5
Merv's Favorite Chocolate-Covered Cherry Cake, ETS recipe (1 slice)							
	3.4	244.2	39.5	4.0	8.7	0	13.3
Mince Pie, w/lard (1 slice)							
	5.6	433.6	65.9	4.0	18.4	17.6	716.8
Mince Pie, w/veg. shortening (1 slice)							
	5.6	433.6	65.9	4.0	18.4	1.6	716.8
Molasses, cane, light (1 serving)							
	0.7	50.4	13.0	0	0	0	3.0
Noodle Pudding, ETW recipe (1 serving)							
	4.0	207.2	46.3	6.0	0.9	0.6	40.5
Peach Pie, w/lard, no salt in filling (1 slice)							
	5.6	408.0	61.1	4.0	17.1	17.6	428.8
Peach Pie, w/veg. shortening, no salt in filling (1 slice)							
	5.6	408.0	61.1	4.0	17.1	0	428.8
Pecan Pie, w/lard, no salt in filling (1 slice)							
	3.5	418.0	51.3	5.1	22.9	70.0	221.0
Pecan Pie, w/veg. shortening, no salt in filling (1 slice)							
	3.5	418.0	51.3	5.1	22.9	63.0	221.0
Pie Crust, from mix, w/water, baked (3½ ounces)							
	3.5	460.4	43.7	6.4	28.9	0	806.7

	Weight (oz.)	Calories	Carbo-hydrates (g.)	Protein (g.)	Fat (g.)	Cholesterol (mg.)	Sodium (mg.)
Pie Crust, w/lard, baked (3½ ounces)							
	3.5	496.1	43.5	6.1	33.1	30.8	606.3
Pie Crust, w/veg. shortening, baked (3½ ounces)							
	3.5	496.1	43.5	6.1	33.1	0	606.3
Pineapple Chiffon Pie, w/lard, no salt in filling (1 slice)							
	3.9	316.8	43.0	7.3	13.3	174.9	281.6
Pineapple Chiffon Pie, w/veg. shortening, no salt in filling (1 slice)							
	3.9	316.8	43.0	7.3	13.3	167.2	281.6
Pineapple Custard Pie, w/lard, no salt in filling (1 slice)							
	5.3	330.0	48.1	6.0	13.0	91.5	279.0
Pineapple Custard Pie, w/veg. shortening, no salt in filling (1 slice)							
	5.3	330.0	48.1	6.0	13.0	82.5	279.0
Pineapple Pie, w/lard, no salt in filling (1 slice)							
	5.6	404.8	61.0	3.5	17.1	17.6	433.6
Pineapple Pie, w/veg. shortening, no salt in filling (1 serving)							
	5.6	404.8	61.0	3.5	17.1	0	433.6
Pineapple Pumpkin Upside-Down Cake, ETS recipe (1 slice)							
	3.7	191.0	46.2	2.4	0.4	0	79.0
Plain Cake, no icing, w/butter (1 slice)							
	1.8	175.0	27.6	2.3	6.3	46.5	210.0
Plain Cake, no icing, w/veg. shortening (1 slice)							
	1.8	182.0	27.9	2.2	6.9	32.5	150.0
Plain Cake, w/chocolate icing, butter (1 slice)							
	1.8	179.0	29.4	2.1	6.5	35.0	156.5
Plain Cake, w/chocolate icing, veg. shortening (1 slice)							
	1.8	184.0	29.7	2.1	6.9	25.0	114.5
Pound Cake, w/butter (1 slice)							
	1.1	131.1	14.5	1.7	7.5	60.9	109.8
Pound Cake, w/veg. shortening (1 slice)							
	1.1	144.6	14.5	1.7	9.0	40.5	30.6
Prune Whip (1 serving)							
	2.8	124.8	29.5	3.5	0.2	0	131.2
Pumpkin Brown Rice Pudding, ETS recipe (1 serving)							
	6.5	178.7	36.6	7.4	0.7	1.7	76.7
Pumpkin Pie, w/lard, no salt in filling (1 slice)							
	5.3	316.5	36.7	6.0	16.8	97.5	321.0
Pumpkin Pie, w/veg. shortening, no salt in filling (1 slice)							
	5.3	316.5	36.7	6.0	16.8	91.5	321.0
Raisin Pie, w/lard (1 slice)							
	4.2	324.0	51.6	3.1	12.8	12.0	342.0
Raisin Pie, w/veg. shortening (1 serving)							
	4.2	324.0	51.6	3.1	12.8	0	342.0
Raspberry Preserves Bars, ETS recipe (1 average)							
	1.7	162.1	21.2	4.0	7.6	0	7.9
Rennin Chocolate Dessert, from mix, w/milk (1 serving)							
	4.6	129.5	17.9	4.3	4.8	15.3	66.0
Rennin Dessert, home-prepared w/tablet (1 serving)							
	4.5	113.0	14.7	3.9	4.4	15.2	104.1

	Weight (oz.)	Calories	Carbo-hydrates (g.)	Protein (g.)	Fat (g.)	Cholesterol (mg.)	Sodium (mg.)
Rennin Dessert, vanilla, caramel, or fruit-flavored (1 serving)							
	4.5	120.7	16.3	4.1	4.6	16.5	58.4
Rhubarb Pie, w/lard, no salt in filling (1 slice)							
	5.6	404.8	61.1	4.0	17.1	17.6	432.0
Rhubarb Pie, w/veg. shortening, no salt in filling (1 serving)							
	5.6	404.8	61.1	4.0	17.1	0	432.0
Rice Pudding, w/raisins (1 serving)							
	3.4	141.1	25.8	3.5	3.0	10.6	68.6
Sherbet, orange-flavored (1 serving)							
	3.4	134.6	29.2	1.1	1.9	6.7	44.0
Sponge Cake (1 slice)							
	1.8	148.5	27.0	3.8	2.8	123.0	83.5
Strawberry Pie, w/lard, no salt in filling (1 slice)							
	3.5	198.0	30.9	1.9	7.9	8.0	194.0
Strawberry Pie, w/veg. shortening, no salt in filling (1 slice)							
	3.5	100.0	15.6	1.0	4.0	0	98.0
Sweet Potato Pie, w/lard, no salt in filling (1 slice)							
	5.6	340.8	37.9	7.2	18.1	96.0	348.8
Sweet Potato Pie, w/veg. shortening, no salt in filling (1 slice)							
	5.6	340.8	37.9	7.2	18.1	86.4	348.8
Tapioca Cream Pudding (1 serving)							
	4.6	174.5	22.3	6.5	6.6	126.3	203.1
Tapioca Dessert, apple (1 serving)							
	4.3	142.8	35.9	0.2	0.1	0	62.2
Vanilla Pudding, home recipe, starch base (1 serving)							
	4.3	135.4	19.4	4.3	4.8	17.1	79.3
White Cake, no icing, w/butter (1 slice)							
	1.8	174.5	26.5	2.3	7.2	20.0	240.5
White Cake, no icing, w/veg. shortening (1 slice)							
	1.8	187.5	27.0	2.3	8.0	1.5	161.5
White Cake, w/chocolate icing, from mix, w/eggs (1 slice)							
	1.8	175.5	31.4	1.9	5.3	1.0	113.5
Yellow Cake, no icing, w/butter (1 slice)							
	1.8	172.5	28.8	2.3	5.8	40.0	184.0
Yellow Cake, no icing, w/veg. shortening (1 slice)							
	1.8	181.5	29.1	2.2	6.3	27.0	129.0
Yellow Cake, w/chocolate icing, butter (1 slice)							
	1.8	176.0	29.9	2.1	6.1	32.0	145.0
Yellow Cake, w/chocolate icing, veg. shortening (1 slice)							
	1.8	182.5	30.2	2.1	6.5	22.0	104.00

EGGS

	Weight (oz.)	Calories	Carbo-hydrates (g.)	Protein (g.)	Fat (g.)	Cholesterol (mg.)	Sodium (mg.)
Cheddar Scramble, ETS recipe (1 serving)							
	4.5	98.4	4.0	12.7	3.2	10.8	344.8
Duck Egg, whole, fresh, raw (1 average)							
	2.6	136.9	1.0	9.5	10.2	654.2	108.0
Egg, fried (1 average)							
	1.8	90.0	0.5	5.8	6.9	267.0	156.5

	Weight (oz.)	Calories	Carbo-hydrates (g.)	Protein (g.)	Fat (g.)	Cholesterol (mg.)	Sodium (mg.)
Egg, hard-cooked (1 average)	1.7	75.8	0.6	5.8	5.3	263.0	66.4
Egg, omelet (1 average)	2.2	91.8	1.3	5.8	6.9	240.6	150.4
Egg, poached (1 average)	1.7	75.4	0.6	5.8	5.3	261.6	140.5
Egg, scrambled (1 average)	2.6	111.0	1.6	7.0	8.3	291.0	181.9
Egg, whole, dried (1 serving)	0.2	41.6	0.3	3.2	2.9	134.3	36.5
Egg, whole, dried, stabilized, glucose-reduced (1 serving)	0.2	43.1	0.2	3.4	3.1	141.2	38.4
Egg, whole, raw (1 average)	1.7	76.1	0.6	5.8	5.3	264.1	66.7
Egg White, flakes, dried (3½ ounces)	3.5	348.3	4.2	76.3	0	0	1147.0
Egg White, powder, dried (3½ ounces)	3.5	373.1	4.5	81.8	0	0	1228.8
Egg White, raw (1 average)	1.1	15.2	0.4	3.1	0	0	47.2
Egg Yolk, dried (3½ ounces)	3.5	681.7	0.4	30.3	60.8	2905.3	89.9
Egg Yolk, fresh, raw (1 serving)	0.6	54.9	0.1	2.5	4.9	221.2	10.7
Goose Egg, whole, fresh, raw (1 average)	3.2	166.5	1.3	12.5	12.0	766.8	124.1
Haas "Scrambled Eggs and Bacon," ETW recipe (1 serving)	4.5	239.3	33.9	16.4	4.4	4.6	824.6
Mushroom Onion Scramble, ETS recipe (1 serving)	5.0	97.6	5.4	13.7	2.1	5.9	322.9
Nova Scramble, ETS recipe (1 serving)	3.5	64.4	3.1	8.9	1.6	6.0	970.9
Turkey Egg, whole, fresh, raw (1 average)	2.8	136.8	0.9	11.0	9.5	746.4	121.0
FAST FOODS							
Apple Pie, McDonald's (1 serving)	3.2	295.0	30.5	2.2	18.3	15.0	408.0
Bean Burrito, Taco Bell (1 serving)	5.9	343.0	48.0	11.0	12.0	25.1	272.0
Bean Burrito, w/o cheese, Taco Bell (1 serving)	4.1	257.3	47.7	5.7	5.0	2.8	140.1
Beef Burrito, Taco Bell (1 serving)	6.5	466.0	37.0	30.0	21.0	110.0	327.0
Beef Taco, Taco Bell (1 serving)	2.9	186.0	14.0	15.0	8.0	90.0	175.0
Beefy Tostada, Taco Bell (1 serving)	6.5	291.0	21.0	19.0	15.0	65.0	138.0

	Weight (oz.)	Calories	Carbo-hydrates (g.)	Protein (g.)	Fat (g.)	Cholesterol (mg.)	Sodium (mg.)
Bellbeefer, Taco Bell (1 serving)	4.3	221.0	23.0	15.0	7.0	90.0	231.0
Bellbeefer, w/cheese, Taco Bell (1 serving)	4.8	278.0	23.0	19.0	12.0	104.9	330.0
Big Mac, McDonald's (1 serving)	6.6	541.0	39.0	25.6	31.4	75.0	963.0
Burrito, combination, Taco Bell (1 serving)	6.2	404.0	43.0	21.0	16.0	110.1	300.0
Burrito Supreme, Taco Bell (1 serving)	7.9	457.0	43.0	21.0	22.0	150.1	245.0
Cheeseburger, Burger King (1 serving)	4.6	305.0	29.0	17.0	13.0	41.0	823.0
Cheeseburger, McDonald's (1 serving)	4.0	306.0	30.4	15.6	13.3	41.0	724.0
Cherry Pie, McDonald's (1 serving)	3.2	296.0	32.4	2.2	17.6	15.0	454.0
Chicken Dinner, Original Recipe, Kentucky Fried Chicken (1 serving)	15.0	830.0	56.0	52.0	46.0	285.2	472.0
Chicken Drumstick, Kentucky Fried Chicken (1 serving)	1.9	136.0	2.0	14.0	8.0	73.0	60.0
Chicken Thigh, Kentucky Fried Chicken (1 serving)	3.4	276.0	12.0	20.0	19.0	147.0	88.0
Chicken Wing, Kentucky Fried Chicken (1 serving)	1.6	151.0	4.0	11.0	10.0	70.0	60.0
Chili, Wendy's (1 serving)	8.8	250.0	23.0	22.0	7.0	70.0	1190.0
Egg McMuffin, McDonald's (1 serving)	4.7	352.0	26.0	18.0	20.0	192.1	911.0
Eggs, scrambled, McDonald's (1 serving)	2.7	161.0	1.9	11.6	11.9	301.0	206.0
Enchirito, Taco Bell (1 serving)	7.3	454.0	42.0	25.0	21.0	109.9	338.0
English Muffin, buttered, McDonald's (1 serving)	2.2	186.0	28.0	5.6	5.6	10.0	446.0
Filet o' Fish, McDonald's (1 serving)	4.6	402.0	34.0	15.0	22.7	43.0	707.0
French Fries, McDonald's (1 serving)	2.4	211.0	25.0	3.1	10.6	10.0	112.0
Hamburger, Burger King (1 serving)	3.2	252.0	29.0	14.0	9.0	26.0	372.0
Hamburger, McDonald's (1 serving)	3.5	257.0	30.1	13.3	9.4	26.0	525.0
Hamburger, single, Wendy's (1 serving)	7.1	440.0	33.0	25.0	25.0	75.0	708.0
Hot Cakes, w/butter and syrup, McDonald's (1 serving)	7.3	472.0	89.0	8.0	9.0	35.0	1071.0
Milk Shake, chocolate, McDonald's (1 serving)	10.2	324.0	51.7	10.7	8.4	28.9	329.0

	Weight (oz.)	Calories	Carbo-hydrates (g.)	Protein (g.)	Fat (g.)	Cholesterol (mg.)	Sodium (mg.)
Milk Shake, strawberry, McDonald's (1 serving)							
	10.3	346.0	57.5	10.3	8.5	29.8	257.0
Milk Shake, vanilla, Burger King (1 serving)							
	11.1	331.0	48.5	13.2	9.5	31.5	306.0
Milk Shake, vanilla, McDonald's (1 serving)							
	10.2	324.0	51.7	10.7	7.8	28.9	250.0
Pintos 'n' Cheese, Taco Bell (1 serving)							
	5.6	168.0	21.0	11.0	5.0	25.1	210.0
Quarter Pounder, McDonald's (1 serving)							
	5.8	418.0	33.0	25.6	20.5	69.0	278.0
Quarter Pounder w/Cheese, McDonald's (1 serving)							
	6.8	518.0	33.0	30.9	28.6	95.9	1206.0
Sausage, pork, McDonald's (1 serving)							
	1.8	191.0	0	8.9	17.2	43.0	487.0
Taco, Taco Bell (1 serving)							
	2.9	186.0	14.0	15.0	8.0	89.6	175.0
Tostada, Taco Bell (1 serving)							
	3.0	179.0	25.0	9.0	6.0	22.0	186.0

FISH/SEAFOOD

	Weight (oz.)	Calories	Carbo-hydrates (g.)	Protein (g.)	Fat (g.)	Cholesterol (mg.)	Sodium (mg.)
Anchovies, pickled, no added oil, not heavily salted (3½ ounces)							
	3.5	174.6	0.3	19.1	10.2	54.6	816.6
Anchovy Paste (3½ ounces)							
	3.5	198.4	4.3	19.8	11.3	70.8	7229.1
Barracuda, Pacific, raw (1 serving)							
	3.5	112.1	0	20.8	2.6	54.6	39.7
Bass, Black Sea, raw (3½ ounces)							
	3.5	92.3	0	19.1	1.2	54.6	67.5
Bluefish, baked or broiled (1 serving)							
	3.5	157.8	0	26.0	5.2	69.5	103.2
Bluefish, raw (3½ ounces)							
	3.5	116.1	0	20.3	3.3	54.6	73.4
Bonito, raw (3½ ounces)							
	3.5	166.7	0	23.8	7.2	54.6	39.7
Broiled Shrimp, ETS recipe (1 serving)							
	6.0	229.7	17.9	30.0	3.6	153.8	390.4
Butterfish, from Gulf waters, raw (1 serving)							
	3.5	94.3	0	16.1	2.9	54.6	53.6
Carp, raw (3½ ounces)							
	3.5	114.1	0	17.9	4.2	54.6	49.6
Catfish, freshwater, raw (1 serving)							
	3.5	102.2	0	17.5	3.1	54.6	59.5
Caviar, sturgeon, granular (1 serving)							
	0.7	52.4	0.7	5.4	3.0	60.0	440.0
Caviar, sturgeon, pressed (1 serving)							
	0.7	63.2	1.0	6.9	3.3	76.8	440.0
Clam Fritters (1 serving)							
	3.5	308.6	30.7	11.3	14.9	128.0	119.1

	Weight (oz.)	Calories	Carbo-hydrates (g.)	Protein (g.)	Fat (g.)	Cholesterol (mg.)	Sodium (mg.)
Clams, canned, drained solids (1 serving)	3.5	97.2	1.9	15.7	2.5	62.5	119.1
Clams, canned, solids and liquid (1 serving)	3.5	51.6	2.8	7.8	0.7	31.8	565.6
Cod, broiled (1 serving)	3.5	168.7	0	28.3	5.3	80.4	109.1
Cod, raw (3½ ounces)	3.5	77.4	0	17.5	0.3	49.6	69.5
Crab, canned (1 serving)	3.5	100.2	1.1	17.3	2.5	100.2	992.2
Crab, steamed (1 serving)	3.5	92.3	0.5	17.2	1.9	99.2	208.4
Fish and Mushroom Marinade, ETW recipe (1 serving)	6.0	270.8	5.4	32.9	6.9	90.7	264.7
Fish Sticks, frozen, cooked (4½ average)	3.5	174.6	6.4	16.5	8.8	46.6	175.6
Flounder, baked (1 serving)	3.5	200.4	0	29.8	8.1	89.3	235.2
Frog Legs, raw (4 large)	3.5	72.4	0	16.3	0.3	49.6	57.5
Grouper, raw (3½ ounces)	3.5	86.3	0	19.2	0.5	54.6	60.5
Haddock, fried (1 serving)	3.5	163.7	5.8	19.4	6.4	63.5	175.6
Haddock, raw (3½ ounces)	3.5	78.4	0	18.2	0.1	59.5	60.5
Haddock, smoked (1 serving)	3.5	102.2	0	23.0	0.4	75.4	6182.6
Halibut, broiled (1 serving)	3.5	169.7	0	25.0	6.9	59.5	133.0
Herring, Bismarck type, pickled (1 serving)	3.5	231.2	0	20.2	15.0	99.2	6182.6
Herring, bloaters, smoked (1 serving)	3.5	194.5	0	19.4	12.3	95.3	6182.6
Herring, canned in tomato sauce, solids and liquid (1 serving)	3.5	174.6	3.7	15.7	10.4	77.4	73.4
Herring, kippered, smoked (1 serving)	3.5	209.4	0	22.0	12.8	108.2	6182.6
Herring, plain, canned, solids and liquid (1 serving)	3.5	206.4	0	19.7	13.5	96.2	73.4
Lobster, steamed (1 serving)	1.0	25.8	0.1	4.8	0.5	23.8	60.1
Lobster Paste, canned (3½ ounces)	3.5	178.6	1.5	20.6	9.3	170.7	138.9
Mackerel, Atlantic, broiled w/butter (1 serving)	3.5	234.2	0	21.6	15.7	100.2	73.4
Mackerel, Atlantic, canned, solids and liquid (1 serving)	3.5	181.6	0	19.2	11.0	93.3	73.4

	Weight (oz.)	Calories	Carbo-hydrates (g.)	Protein (g.)	Fat (g.)	Cholesterol (mg.)	Sodium (mg.)
Mackerel, Pacific, canned, solids and liquid (1 serving)	3.5	178.6	0	20.9	9.9	93.3	73.4
Mackerel, Pacific, raw (3½ ounces)	3.5	157.8	0	21.7	7.2	94.3	73.4
Mussels, Pacific, canned, drained solids (1 serving)	3.5	113.1	1.5	18.1	3.3	44.7	286.8
Ocean Perch, Atlantic, fried (1 serving)	3.5	225.2	6.7	18.9	13.2	57.5	151.8
Ocean Perch, Atlantic, raw (3½ ounces)	3.5	87.3	0	17.9	1.2	54.6	78.4
Oysters, canned, solids and liquid (1 serving)	3.5	75.4	4.9	8.4	2.2	44.7	377.0
Oysters, Eastern, meat only, raw (3½ ounces)	3.5	65.5	3.4	8.3	1.8	49.6	72.4
Oysters, Pacific and Western, Olympia, meat only, raw (3½ ounces)	3.5	90.3	6.4	10.5	2.2	49.6	72.4
Perch, white, raw (3½ ounces)	3.5	117.1	0	19.2	4.0	54.6	49.6
Pike, blue, raw (3½ ounces)	3.5	89.3	0	19.0	0.9	54.6	50.6
Poached Salmon, ETS recipe (1 serving)	7.5	247.1	8.9	27.7	7.7	46.6	189.8
Roe, from salmon, sturgeon, or turbot, raw (3½ ounces)	3.5	205.4	1.4	25.0	10.3	357.2	72.4
Salmon, Atlantic, canned, solids and liquid (3½ ounces)	3.5	201.4	0	21.5	12.1	36.7	73.4
Salmon, Atlantic, raw (3½ ounces)	3.5	215.3	0	22.3	13.3	38.7	73.4
Salmon, broiled or baked (1 serving)	3.5	180.6	0	26.8	7.3	46.6	115.1
Salmon, pink, canned, solids and liquid, w/o salt (1 serving)	3.5	139.9	0	20.3	5.9	34.7	63.5
Salmon, pink, canned, solids and liquid, w/salt (1 serving)	3.5	139.9	0	20.3	5.9	34.7	384.0
Salmon, smoked (3½ ounces)	3.5	174.6	0	21.4	9.2	37.7	6182.6
Sardines, Atlantic, canned in oil, drained solids (3½ ounces)	3.5	201.4	0	23.8	11.0	138.9	816.6
Sardines, Pacific, canned in mustard, solid and liquid (3½ ounces)	3.5	194.5	1.7	18.7	11.9	109.1	754.1
Sardines, Pacific, canned in oil, drained solids (3½ ounces)	3.5	201.4	0	23.8	11.0	119.1	816.6
Scallops, frozen, fried (1 serving)	3.5	192.5	10.4	17.9	8.3	40.7	119.1
Scallops, steamed (3½ ounces)	3.5	112.0	4.5	23.2	1.4	35.0	262.0
Shad, American, baked (1 serving)	3.5	199.4	0	23.0	11.2	68.5	78.4

	Weight (oz.)	Calories	Carbo-hydrates (g.)	Protein (g.)	Fat (g.)	Cholesterol (mg.)	Sodium (mg.)
Shrimp, canned, wet pack, drained solids (3½ ounces)	3.5	115.1	0.7	24.0	1.1	148.8	138.9
Shrimp, canned, wet pack, solids and liquid (3½ ounces)	3.5	79.4	0.8	16.1	0.8	133.0	138.9
Shrimp, fried (1 serving)	3.5	223.3	9.9	20.1	10.7	148.8	184.6
Swordfish, broiled (1 serving)	3.5	172.6	0	27.8	6.0	79.4	133.0
Trout, brook, raw (3½ ounces)	3.5	100.2	0	19.1	2.1	48.6	46.6
Tuna, canned in water, solids and liquid, w/o salt (1 serving)	3.5	126.0	0	27.8	0.8	62.5	40.7
Tuna, canned in water, solids and liquid, w/salt (1 serving)	3.5	126.0	0	27.8	0.8	62.5	868.2
Turbot, raw (3½ ounces)	3.5	81.4	0	17.3	0.9	54.6	60.5
Whitefish, smoked (1 serving)	3.5	153.8	0	20.7	7.2	60.5	6182.6

FLOURS/FLOUR MIXES/DOUGH

	Weight (oz.)	Calories	Carbo-hydrates (g.)	Protein (g.)	Fat (g.)	Cholesterol (mg.)	Sodium (mg.)
Buckwheat Flour, light (3½ ounces)	3.5	344.3	78.9	6.4	1.2	0	2.0
Cornmeal, unrefined (3½ ounces)	3.5	359.2	73.9	8.9	3.4	0	1.0
Cornmeal, white, degermed, cooked w/o salt (1 serving)	8.5	120.0	25.7	2.6	0.5	0	0
Lima Bean Flour (3½ ounces)	3.5	340.3	62.5	21.3	1.4	0	4.0
Muffin Mix, corn, w/nonfat dry milk (3½ ounces)	3.5	405.8	71.0	6.2	10.6	6.0	804.7
Pancake Mix, buckwheat, dry form (3½ ounces)	3.5	325.5	69.8	10.4	1.9	0	1323.6
Roll Dough, frozen, unraised (3½ ounces)	3.5	265.9	47.0	7.4	5.0	5.0	478.3
Rye Flour, medium (3½ ounces)	3.5	347.3	74.2	11.3	1.7	0	1.0
Soybean Flour, defatted (3½ ounces)	3.5	323.5	37.8	46.6	0.9	0	1.0
Soybean Flour, high-fat (3½ ounces)	3.5	377.0	33.0	40.9	12.0	0	1.0
Waffle Mix, dry form (3½ ounces)	3.5	454.4	64.9	6.4	19.1	0	1019.0
Wheat Flour, all-purpose (3½ ounces)	3.5	361.2	75.5	10.4	1.0	0	2.0
Wheat Flour, bread type (3½ ounces)	3.5	362.2	74.1	11.7	1.1	0	2.0

	Weight (oz.)	Calories	Carbo-hydrates (g.)	Protein (g.)	Fat (g.)	Cholesterol (mg.)	Sodium (mg.)
Wheat Flour, cake or pastry type (3½ ounces)							
	3.5	361.2	78.8	7.4	0.8	0	2.0
Wheat Flour, gluten, 45% gluten, 55% patent (3½ ounces)							
	3.5	375.1	46.8	41.1	1.9	0	2.0
Wheat Flour, self-rising, w/anhydrous monocal phosphate (3½ ounces)							
	3.5	349.3	73.6	9.2	1.0	0	1070.6
Wheat Flour, self-rising, w/sodium acid pyrophosphate (3½ ounces)							
	3.5	349.3	73.6	9.2	1.0	0	1349.4
Wheat Flour, whole wheat (3½ ounces)							
	3.5	330.4	70.4	13.2	2.0	0	3.0

FRUIT

	Weight (oz.)	Calories	Carbo-hydrates (g.)	Protein (g.)	Fat (g.)	Cholesterol (mg.)	Sodium (mg.)
Acerola, raw (3½ ounces)							
	3.5	31.8	7.6	0.4	0.3	0	6.9
Amaranth, raw (3½ ounces)							
	3.5	35.7	6.4	3.5	0.5	0	70.4
Apple, dried, cooked w/o sugar (3½ ounces)							
	3.5	56.6	15.2	0.2	0.1	0	19.8
Apple, dried, sulfured (3½ ounces)							
	3.5	241.1	65.4	0.9	0.3	0	86.3
Apple, raw, w/o skin (1 average)							
	5.3	85.5	22.2	0.1	0.4	0	1.7
Apple, raw, w/skin (1 average)							
	5.3	88.5	22.9	0.3	0.6	0	1.7
Applesauce, canned, w/o sugar (1 serving)							
	4.3	50.0	13.2	0.2	0.2	0	2.5
Applesauce, ETS recipe (1 serving)							
	7.5	140.9	35.4	0.7	0.6	0	2.9
Apricot, canned, solids and liquid, juice pack (1 serving)							
	9.1	123.8	31.7	1.5	0	0	10.3
Apricot, dried (3½ ounces)							
	3.5	236.2	61.3	3.6	0.5	0	9.9
Apricot, raw (3½ ounces)							
	3.5	47.6	11.0	1.4	0.4	0	0.9
Apricot Nectar, canned, 40% fruit (1 serving)							
	8.9	143.0	36.6	0.8	0.3	0	7.5
Avocado, raw, pitted (1 serving)							
	5.3	241.5	11.1	3.0	22.9	0	15.0
Banana, common, raw (1 average)							
	5.3	138.0	35.1	1.5	0.8	0	2.0
Banana Puree (3½ ounces)							
	3.5	84.0	21.8	1.1	0.2	0	1.3
Blackberries, raw (3½ ounces)							
	3.5	51.6	12.7	0.7	0.4	0	0.7
Blueberries, frozen, w/o sugar (3½ ounces)							
	3.5	50.6	12.1	0.4	0.6	0	0.9

	Weight (oz.)	Calories	Carbo-hydrates (g.)	Protein (g.)	Fat (g.)	Cholesterol (mg.)	Sodium (mg.)
Blueberries, raw (3½ ounces)	3.5	55.6	14.0	0.7	0.4	0	6.0
Boysenberries, raw (3½ ounces)	3.5	51.6	12.7	0.7	0.4	0	0.8
Cantaloupe, raw (¼ average)	3.5	34.7	8.3	0.9	0.3	0	8.9
Casaba Melon, raw (1 slice)	3.5	26.0	6.2	0.9	0.1	0	12.0
Cherries, maraschino, bottled, solids and liquid (3½ ounces)	3.5	115.1	29.2	0.2	0.2	0	1.0
Cherries, sour, red, raw (3½ ounces)	3.5	49.6	12.1	1.0	0.3	0	3.0
Cherries, sweet, canned, water pack, solids and liquid (3½ ounces)	3.5	45.6	11.7	0.8	0.1	0	1.0
Cherries, sweet, raw (3½ ounces)	3.5	71.4	16.5	1.2	1.0	0	1.5
Crabapple, raw (3½ ounces)	3.5	75.4	19.7	0.4	0.3	0	1.0
Cranberries, raw (3½ ounces)	3.5	48.6	12.6	0.4	0.2	0	1.0
Currants, black, European, raw (3½ ounces)	3.5	62.5	15.3	1.4	0.4	0	2.0
Dates, domestic, natural, dry (3½ ounces)	3.5	272.9	72.9	2.0	0.4	0	3.0
Elderberries, raw (3½ ounces)	3.5	72.4	18.3	0.7	0.5	0	0
Figs, dried, uncooked (3½ ounces)	3.5	253.0	64.9	3.1	1.2	0	10.9
Fruit Cocktail, canned, water pack, solids and liquid (1 serving)	3.9	35.6	9.4	0.4	0.1	0	4.4
Gooseberries, raw (3½ ounces)	3.5	43.7	10.1	0.9	0.6	0	1.0
Grapefruit, canned segments, water pack, solids and liquid (1 serving)	3.5	36.0	9.1	0.6	0.1	0	2.0
Grapefruit, raw (½ average)	3.5	32.0	8.1	0.6	0.1	0	1.0
Grapes, American type, slip skin, raw (33 average)	5.3	94.5	25.6	0.9	0.6	0	3.0
Grapes, European type, adherent skin, raw (36 average)	5.6	113.6	28.5	1.1	1.0	0	3.2
Grapes, seedless, canned, water pack, solids and liquid (3½ ounces)	3.5	39.7	10.2	0.5	0.1	0	6.0
Guava, common, whole, raw (1 average)	3.5	51.0	11.9	0.8	0.6	0	3.0
Honeydew Melon, raw (¼ average)	5.3	52.5	13.8	0.8	0.1	0	15.0

	Weight (oz.)	Calories	Carbo- hydrates (g.)	Protein (g.)	Fat (g.)	Cholesterol (mg.)	Sodium (mg.)
Kumquat, raw (5 average)							
	3.5	63.0	16.4	0.9	0.1	0	6.0
Lemon, raw, peeled (1 average)							
	3.5	29.0	9.3	1.1	0.3	0	2.0
Longan, raw (3½ ounces)							
	3.5	59.5	15.0	1.3	0.1	0	0
Loquat, raw (1 serving)							
	3.5	47.0	12.1	0.4	0.2	0	1.0
Lychee, raw (3½ ounces)							
	3.5	65.5	16.4	0.8	0.4	0	1.0
Mango, raw (½ average)							
	3.5	65.0	17.0	0.5	0.3	0	2.0
Nectarine, raw (2 average)							
	3.5	49.0	11.8	0.9	0.5	0	0
Olives, Greek, salt-cured (3½ ounces)							
	3.5	332.2	8.5	1.9	35.2	0	3267.2
Olives, green (3½ ounces)							
	3.5	114.5	1.5	1.5	12.2	0	2381.4
Orange, California Navel, winter, peeled, raw (1 small)							
	5.3	69.0	17.4	1.5	0.1	0	1.5
Orange, California Valencia, summer, peeled, raw (1 average)							
	5.6	78.4	19.0	1.6	0.5	0	0
Orange, Florida, all commercial varieties, peeled, raw (1 average)							
	7.1	92.0	23.0	1.4	0.4	0	0
Orange Rind, grated (3½ ounces)							
	3.5	79.4	15.9	1.6	0.4	0	4.0
Papaya, dried (3½ ounces)							
	3.5	260.0	67.8	3.1	0.7	0	15.9
Papaya, raw (⅓ average)							
	3.5	39.0	9.8	0.6	0.1	0	3.0
Peach, canned, juice pack, solids and liquid (1 serving)							
	3.5	44.0	11.6	0.6	0	0	4.0
Peach, dried, sulfured, uncooked (3½ ounces)							
	3.5	237.1	60.8	3.6	0.8	0	6.9
Peach, raw (1 average)							
	3.5	43.0	11.1	0.7	0.1	0	0.9
Pear, canned, juice pack, solids and liquid (1 small)							
	3.5	50.0	12.9	0.3	0.1	0	4.0
Pear, raw, w/skin (1 average)							
	7.1	118.0	30.2	0.8	0.8	0	0
Persimmon, native, raw (1 average)							
	3.5	127.0	33.5	0.8	0.4	0	1.0
Pineapple, canned, juice pack, solids and liquid (1 slice)							
	4.7	79.9	20.9	0.5	0.1	0	1.3
Pineapple, dried (3½ ounces)							
	3.5	260.0	67.8	3.1	0.7	0	15.9
Pineapple, raw (1 slice)							
	3.5	49.0	12.4	0.4	0.4	0	1.0
Plantain, raw (1 small)							
	3.5	122.0	31.9	1.3	0.4	0	4.0

	Weight (oz.)	Calories	Carbo-hydrates (g.)	Protein (g.)	Fat (g.)	Cholesterol (mg.)	Sodium (mg.)
Plum, Damson, raw (2 average)	3.5	66.0	17.8	0.5	0	0	2.0
Plum, purple, canned, water pack, solids and liquid (2 average)	3.5	41.0	11.0	0.4	0	0	1.0
Pomegranate, raw, pulp (1 average)	3.5	68.0	17.2	0.9	0.3	0	3.0
Prune, dried, cooked fruit and liquid, w/o sugar (5 average)	3.9	137.8	36.6	1.2	0.2	0	2.2
Prune, dried, uncooked (1 large)	0.4	25.5	6.7	0.2	0	0	0.8
Quince, raw (1 serving)	3.5	57.0	15.3	0.4	0.1	0	4.0
Raisins, seedless, natural, unbleached, uncooked (3½ ounces)	3.5	297.7	78.5	3.2	0.5	0	11.9
Raspberries, red, raw (3½ ounces)	3.5	72.6	15.5	1.5	1.4	0	0.7
Sapodillo, raw, pulp (1 serving)	3.5	83.0	20.0	0.4	1.1	0	12.0
Sapote, raw (1 serving)	3.5	134.0	33.8	2.1	0.6	0	10.0
Strawberries, raw (3½ ounces)	3.5	29.8	6.9	0.6	0.4	0	1.0
Strawberries, sliced, frozen, sweetened (1 serving)	4.4	120.0	32.4	0.6	0.1	0	3.7
Tangerine, fancy variety, raw (2 small)	3.5	44.0	11.2	0.6	0.2	0	1.0
Watermelon, raw (1 slice)	21.2	192.0	43.2	3.6	2.4	0	12.0

INFANT FOOD

	Weight (oz.)	Calories	Carbo-hydrates (g.)	Protein (g.)	Fat (g.)	Cholesterol (mg.)	Sodium (mg.)
Apples and Apricots, canned, strained, Jr. (3½ ounces)	3.5	44.7	11.5	0.2	0.2	0	3.0
Applesauce, canned, strained, Jr. (3½ ounces)	3.5	40.7	10.8	0.2	0.2	0	2.0
Bananas with Tapioca, canned, strained, Jr. (3½ ounces)	3.5	56.6	15.2	0.4	0.1	0	8.9
Beans, green, canned, strained, Jr. (3½ ounces)	3.5	24.8	5.9	1.3	0.1	0	2.0
Beef, canned, strained, Jr. (3½ ounces)	3.5	106.2	0	13.5	5.4	93.3	80.4
Beef, w/beef heart, canned, strained, Jr. (3½ ounces)	3.5	93.3	0	12.6	4.4	271.9	62.5
Beets, canned, strained, Jr. (3½ ounces)	3.5	33.7	7.6	1.3	0.1	0	82.4
Carrots, canned, strained, Jr. (3½ ounces)	3.5	26.8	6.0	0.8	0.1	0	36.7
Cereal, mixed grain, cooked, dry, Jr. (3½ ounces)	3.5	369.1	70.5	13.0	4.0	0	466.3
Cereal, oatmeal, cooked, dry, Jr. (3½ ounces)	3.5	394.9	68.7	13.5	7.7	0	433.6

	Weight (oz.)	Calories	Carbo-hydrates (g.)	Protein (g.)	Fat (g.)	Cholesterol (mg.)	Sodium (mg.)
Cereal, rice, cooked, dry, Jr. (3½ ounces)							
	3.5	379.0	75.8	6.8	4.5	0	525.9
Chicken, canned, strained, Jr. (3½ ounces)							
	3.5	129.0	0.1	13.6	7.8	86.3	46.6
Chocolate Pudding, strained, Jr. (3½ ounces)							
	3.5	83.3	16.0	1.9	1.7	88.3	22.8
Dinner, beef and egg noodle, canned, strained, Jr. (3½ ounces)							
	3.5	52.6	6.9	2.3	1.7	10.9	28.8
Dinner, chicken and noodle, strained, Jr. (3½ ounces)							
	3.5	51.6	7.4	2.1	1.5	7.9	15.9
Dinner, high meat, beef and vegetables, strained, Jr. (3½ ounces)							
	3.5	74.4	4.2	5.7	4.2	27.8	35.7
Dinner, high meat, chicken and vegetables, strained, Jr. (3½ ounces)							
	3.5	77.4	5.9	6.2	3.6	27.8	26.8
Dinner, high meat, turkey and vegetables, strained, Jr. (3½ ounces)							
	3.5	86.3	6.0	5.6	4.8	24.8	29.8
Dinner, high meat, veal and vegetables, strained, Jr. (3½ ounces)							
	3.5	68.5	6.1	5.9	2.7	26.8	23.8
Dinner, macaroni, tomatoes, beef, strained, Jr. (3½ ounces)							
	3.5	54.6	8.7	2.2	1.1	9.9	16.9
Dinner, split peas, vegetables, ham or bacon, Jr. (3½ ounces)							
	3.5	70.4	11.2	3.3	1.3	10.9	13.9
Dinner, vegetables and beef, strained, Jr. (3½ ounces)							
	3.5	52.6	6.9	2.0	2.0	9.9	20.8
Dinner, vegetables and chicken, strained, Jr. (3½ ounces)							
	3.5	42.7	6.5	1.9	1.1	7.9	10.9
Dinner, vegetables and ham, strained, Jr. (3½ ounces)							
	3.5.	47.6	6.8	1.8	1.7	10.9	11.9
Dinner, vegetables and lamb, strained, Jr. (3½ ounces)							
	3.5	51.6	6.8	2.0	2.0	7.9	19.8
Dinner, vegetables and liver, strained, Jr. (3½ ounces)							
	3.5	38.7	6.8	2.2	0.4	11.9	17.9
Dinner, vegetables and turkey, strained, Jr. (3½ ounces)							
	3.5	41.7	6.5	1.7	1.2	7.9	12.9
Dinner, vegetables, noodles, chicken, strained, Jr. (3½ ounces)							
	3.5	62.5	7.8	2.0	2.5	7.9	19.8
Egg Yolks, canned, strained, Jr. (3½ ounces)							
	3.5	201.4	1.0	9.9	17.2	779.9	38.7
Lamb, canned, strained, Jr. (3½ ounces)							
	3.5	102.2	0.1	14.0	4.7	97.2	61.5
Liver, canned, strained, Jr. (3½ ounces)							
	3.5	100.2	1.4	14.2	3.8	181.6	73.4
Liver and Bacon, canned, strained, Jr. (3½ ounces)							
	3.5	122.0	1.3	13.6	6.5	261.9	299.7
Peaches, canned, w/sugar, strained, Jr. (3½ ounces)							
	3.5	70.4	18.8	0.5	0.2	0	6.0
Pears, canned, strained, Jr. (3½ ounces)							
	3.5	40.7	10.7	0.3	0.2	0	2.0

	Weight (oz.)	Calories	Carbo- hydrates (g.)	Protein (g.)	Fat (g.)	Cholesterol (mg.)	Sodium (mg.)
Pears and Pineapple, canned, strained, Jr. (3½ ounces)	3.5	40.7	10.8	0.3	0.1	0	4.0
Plums with Tapioca, canned, strained, Jr. (3½ ounces)	3.5	70.4	19.5	0.1	0	0	6.0
Pork, canned, strained, Jr. (3½ ounces)	3.5	123.0	0	13.9	7.0	88.3	41.7
Prunes with Tapioca, canned, strained, Jr. (3½ ounces)	3.5	69.5	18.4	0.6	0.1	0	5.0
Spinach, creamed, canned, strained, Jr. (3½ ounces)	3.5	36.7	5.7	2.5	1.3	0	48.6
Squash, canned, strained, Jr. (3½ ounces)	3.5	23.8	5.6	0.8	0.2	0	2.0
Sweet Potatoes, canned, strained, Jr. (3½ ounces)	3.5	56.6	13.1	1.1	0.1	0	19.8
Teething Biscuit, Jr. (3½ ounces)	3.5	389.0	75.8	10.6	4.2	0	359.2
Tomato Soup, canned, strained, Jr. (3½ ounces)	3.5	53.6	13.4	1.9	0.1	0	291.7
Vanilla Pudding, strained, Jr. (3½ ounces)	3.5	84.3	16.0	1.6	2.0	88.3	27.8
Veal, canned, strained, Jr. (3½ ounces)	3.5	100.2	0	13.4	4.8	100.2	63.5
Vegetables, mixed, canned, strained, Jr. (3½ ounces)	3.5	40.7	7.9	1.2	0.5	0	12.9

JUICES (FRUIT/VEGETABLE)

	Weight (oz.)	Calories	Carbo- hydrates (g.)	Protein (g.)	Fat (g.)	Cholesterol (mg.)	Sodium (mg.)
Acerola Juice, raw (1 cup)	8.7	52.1	11.9	1.0	0.7	0	7.4
Apple Juice, unsweetened (1 cup)	8.7	116.6	29.0	0.2	0.2	0	7.4
Apple Juice Concentrate, undiluted, unsweetened (1 cup)	8.8	300.0	70.0	4.3	0.4	0	3.7
Blackberry Juice, canned, w/o sugar (1 cup)	8.6	90.7	19.1	0.7	1.5	0	2.5
Cranberry Juice Cocktail, 33% juice, bottled (1 cup)	8.5	139.2	35.8	0	0.2	0	9.6
Grapefruit Juice, canned, unsweetened (1 cup)	9.0	97.1	23.0	1.3	0.3	0	2.6
Grapefruit Juice, fresh (1 cup)	9.0	99.6	23.5	1.3	0.3	0	2.6
Grapefruit Juice Concentrate, undiluted, w/o sugar (1 cup)	8.8	365.0	86.5	5.0	1.3	0	7.5
Grape Juice, canned or bottled (1 cup)	9.0	155.8	38.3	1.5	0.3	0	7.7
Grape Juice Concentrate, undiluted, w/sugar (1 cup)	8.8	447.5	111.0	1.5	0.7	0	17.5

	Weight (oz.)	Calories	Carbo-hydrates (g.)	Protein (g.)	Fat (g.)	Cholesterol (mg.)	Sodium (mg.)
Lemonade, from concentrate, diluted 4⅓ parts water (1 cup)							
	8.8	110.0	28.5	0.3	0	0	0
Lemon Juice, canned or bottled, unsweetened (1 cup)							
	8.5	50.4	15.6	1.0	0.7	0	50.4
Lemon Juice, frozen, concentrate, unsweetened (1 cup)							
	8.8	290.0	93.5	5.7	2.2	0	12.5
Lemon Juice, fresh (1 cup)							
	8.5	60.0	20.6	1.0	0	0	2.4
Limeade from concentrate, diluted 4⅓ parts water (1 cup)							
	8.8	102.3	27.5	0	0	0	0
Limeade Concentrate, frozen, undiluted (1 cup)							
	8.8	467.5	123.7	0.5	0.2	0	0
Lime Juice, canned or bottled, unsweetened (1 cup)							
	8.5	50.4	16.1	0.7	0.5	0	38.4
Lime Juice, fresh (1 cup)							
	8.5	64.8	21.6	1.0	0.2	0	2.4
Orange Juice, fresh (1 cup)							
	9.0	114.9	26.6	1.8	0.5	0	2.6
Orange Juice Concentrate, undiluted, unsweetened (1 cup)							
	8.8	397.5	95.5	6.0	0.5	0	7.5
Pineapple Juice, canned, unsweetened (1 cup)							
	9.0	143.0	35.2	0.8	0.3	0	2.6
Pineapple Juice Concentrate, undiluted, unsweetened (1 cup)							
	8.8	447.5	110.7	3.2	0.2	0	7.5
Prune Juice, canned or bottled (1 cup)							
	8.5	170.4	41.8	1.4	0	0	9.6
Sauerkraut Juice, canned (1 cup)							
	8.8	25.0	5.7	1.7	0	0	1967.5
Tangelo Juice, raw (1 cup)							
	9.0	104.7	24.8	1.3	0.3	0	2.6
Tangerine Juice, fancy variety, raw (1 cup)							
	9.0	109.8	25.8	1.3	0.5	0	2.6
Tomato Juice (1 cup)							
	8.6	46.0	10.4	2.2	0.2	0	486.0
Tomato Juice, canned or bottled, low-sodium (1 cup)							
	8.5	45.6	10.3	1.9	0.2	0	7.2
Tomato Juice, canned or bottled, regular pack (1 cup)							
	8.5	45.6	10.3	2.2	0.2	0	480.5
Tomato Juice Cocktail, canned or bottled (1 cup)							
	8.5	50.5	12.0	1.7	0.2	0	480.5
Vegetable Juice, V-8, no salt added (1 cup)							
	8.6	53.3	12.0	1.3	0	0	66.7
Vegetable Juice Cocktail, canned (1 cup)							
	8.5	40.8	8.6	2.2	0.2	0	480.5

MEATS

	Weight	Calories	Carbo	Protein	Fat	Cholesterol	Sodium
Bacon, Canadian, broiled or fried, drained (1 serving)							
	3.5	271.9	0.3	26.8	17.4	82.4	2535.2
Bacon, cured, broiled or fried, drained (1 serving)							
	3.5	594.0	3.2	26.3	52.0	89.0	1021.0

	Weight (oz.)	Calories	Carbo-hydrates (g.)	Protein (g.)	Fat (g.)	Cholesterol (mg.)	Sodium (mg.)
Beef Chuck, lean, choice grade, braised (1 serving)							
	3.5	212.3	0	29.8	9.4	90.3	52.1
Beef Club Steak, lean, choice grade, broiled (1 serving)							
	3.5	242.1	0	29.4	12.9	90.3	71.9
Beef Double-Bone Sirloin, lean, choice grade, broiled (1 serving)							
	3.5	214.3	0	30.4	9.4	90.3	74.4
Beef Flank Steak, total edible, lean, choice, braised (1 serving)							
	3.5	194.5	0	30.3	7.2	93.3	53.0
Beef Heart, lean, braised (1 serving)							
	3.5	186.5	0.7	31.1	5.7	271.9	103.2
Beef Liver, fried (1 serving)							
	3.5	227.2	5.3	26.2	10.5	434.6	182.6
Beef Porterhouse, lean, choice grade, broiled (1 serving)							
	3.5	222.3	0	30.0	10.4	90.3	73.4
Beef Rump, lean, choice grade, roasted (1 serving)							
	3.5	206.4	0	28.9	9.2	90.3	70.7
Beef Sirloin Steak, lean, choice grade, broiled (1 serving)							
	3.5	205.4	0	31.9	7.6	90.3	78.3
Beef T-Bone, lean, choice grade, broiled (1 serving)							
	3.5	221.3	0	30.2	10.2	90.3	73.9
Beef Tongue, medium fat, braised (1 serving)							
	3.5	242.1	0.4	21.3	16.6	93.3	60.5
Bologna, all meat, w/beef, pork (1 serving)							
	3.5	313.5	2.8	11.6	28.1	54.6	1011.1
Brains, all kinds, raw (1 serving)							
	3.5	124.0	0.8	10.3	8.5	1984.5	124.0
Calf Liver, fried (1 serving)							
	3.5	259.0	4.0	29.3	13.1	434.6	117.1
Calf Sweetbread, braised (1 serving)							
	3.5	166.7	0	32.3	3.2	462.4	115.1
Corned Beef, medium fat, cooked (1 serving)							
	3.5	290.7	0	15.7	24.8	67.5	1289.9
Dried Chipped Beef, cooked, creamed (1 serving)							
	3.5	152.8	7.0	8.1	10.2	39.7	710.4
Frankfurter, cooked (1 serving)							
	3.5	301.6	1.6	12.3	27.0	61.5	1091.5
Ground Beef, lean, 21% fat, cooked medium rare (1 serving)							
	3.5	283.8	0	24.0	20.1	93.3	58.8
Ham, deviled, canned (1 serving)							
	3.5	348.3	0	13.8	32.0	64.5	1224.4
Ham, luncheon meat, sliced, regular, boiled (1 serving)							
	3.5	180.6	3.1	17.5	10.5	56.6	1306.8
Hog Liver, fried (1 serving)							
	3.5	239.1	2.5	29.7	11.4	434.6	110.1
Hog Tongue, braised (1 serving)							
	3.5	251.0	0.5	21.8	17.3	87.3	60.5
Knackwurst, w/pork, beef (1 serving)							
	3.5	305.6	1.8	11.8.	27.6	57.5	1002.2
Lamb Leg, lean, choice grade, roasted (1 serving)							
	3.5	184.6	0	28.5	6.9	99.2	69.8

	Weight (oz.)	Calories	Carbo-hydrates (g.)	Protein (g.)	Fat (g.)	Cholesterol (mg.)	Sodium (mg.)
Lamb Loin, lean, prime grade, broiled (1 serving)							
	3.5	195.5	0	27.8	8.5	99.2	68.1
Lamb Rib, lean, choice grade, broiled (1 serving)							
	3.5	209.4	0	27.0	10.4	99.2	66.1
Liverwurst, pork, fresh (1 serving)							
	3.5	323.5	2.2	14.0	28.3	156.8	853.3
Luncheon Meat, w/pork, beef, chopped together (1 serving)							
	3.5	350.3	2.3	12.5	31.9	54.6	1283.0
Pigs' Feet, pickled (1 serving)							
	3.5	197.5	0	16.6	14.7	88.3	69.5
Pork, Boston butt, lean, medium-fat, roasted (1 serving)							
	3.5	242.1	0	26.8	14.2	87.3	65.7
Pork, ham, lean, light cure, medium-fat, roasted (1 serving)							
	3.5	185.5	0	25.1	8.7	87.3	898.7
Pork, lean cuts, medium-fat, roasted (1 serving)							
	3.5	234.2	0	27.8	12.8	87.3	68.1
Pork Loin, lean, retail, medium-fat, broiled (1 serving)							
	3.5	267.9	0	30.4	15.3	87.3	74.4
Pork Sausage, links or bulk, cooked (1 serving)							
	3.5	366.1	1.0	19.4	31.0	82.4	1283.9
Pork Spareribs, total edible, medium-fat, braised (1 serving)							
	3.5	436.6	0	20.6	38.6	88.3	36.1
Salami, w/pork, beef, cooked (1 serving)							
	3.5	248.1	2.3	13.8	19.9	64.5	1056.7
Sausage, brown-and-serve, browned (1 serving)							
	3.5	392.9	2.7	13.7	36.0	70.4	798.7
Veal Loin, total edible, medium-fat, broiled (1 serving)							
	3.5	232.2	0	26.2	13.3	100.2	64.2
Veal Scallopini, ETW recipe (1 serving)							
	12.5	477.0	33.4	43.3	14.1	107.7	744.3
Venison, lean, raw (1 serving)							
	3.5	125.0	0	20.8	4.0	64.5	89.3
Vienna Sausage, w/beef, pork, canned (1 serving)							
	3.5	267.9	2.0	10.2	25.0	51.6	945.6
MILK/MILK MIXES							
Buttermilk, cultured, from skim milk (1 cup)							
	3.4	38.4	4.6	3.2	0.9	3.8	100.7
Condensed Milk, sweetened, canned (1 cup)							
	10.5	963.0	163.2	23.7	26.1	101.2	381.0
Dry Milk, whole (1 cup)							
	3.5	496.0	38.4	26.3	26.7	96.2	371.3
Evaporated Milk, whole, unsweetened (1 cup)							
	8.9	338.0	25.3	17.2	19.1	74.2	266.0
Evaporated Skim Milk, unsweetened (1 cup)							
	9.0	198.0	28.9	19.3	0.5	10.0	294.0
Goat Milk, fluid (1 cup)							
	8.6	168.4	10.7	8.8	10.0	26.8	121.5

THE FOOD COMPOSITION TABLES • 267

	Weight (oz.)	Calories	Carbo-hydrates (g.)	Protein (g.)	Fat (g.)	Cholesterol (mg.)	Sodium (mg.)
Human Milk, U.S. samples (1 cup)	8.5	168.0	16.6	2.4	10.6	33.6	40.6
Malted Milk, beverage (1 cup)	9.4	236.1	26.5	10.9	10.1	37.3	215.6
Malted Milk, dry powder (1 cup)	8.8	1027.5	181.3	32.7	21.3	49.9	1141.7
Milk, whole, 3.5% fat (1 cup)	8.6	148.9	11.5	8.1	8.1	34.2	119.6
Nonfat Dry Milk, skim solids, instant (1 cup)	2.1	214.8	31.3	21.1	0.4	10.7	329.2
Nonfat Dry Milk, skim solids, regular (1 cup)	2.5	253.5	36.4	25.4	0.6	14.2	374.9
Reindeer Milk (1 cup)	8.6	571.0	10.0	26.4	47.8	34.2	383.1
Skim Milk (1 cup)	8.6	85.4	12.0	8.3	0.5	4.9	125.7
Skim Milk, 2% nonfat milk solids (1 cup)	8.6	136.7	13.4	9.5	4.9	19.5	143.5
Soybean Milk, fluid (1 cup)	9.3	86.8	5.8	8.9	3.9	0	0
Soybean Milk, powder, dry form (3½ ounces)	3.5	425.7	27.8	41.5	20.1	0	1.0
Yogurt, plain, from partially skimmed milk (1 cup)	8.0	113.5	11.8	7.7	3.9	18.2	115.8
Yogurt, plain, from whole milk (1 cup)	8.0	138.5	10.7	7.9	7.5	29.5	105.3

MISCELLANEOUS

	Weight	Calories	Carbo	Protein	Fat	Cholesterol	Sodium
Almond Flavoring (3½ ounces)	3.5	297.7	29.8	0	0	0	0
Arrowroot Powder (3½ ounces)	3.5	359.7	86.8	0	0	0	49.6
Bacon Chips, imitation (1 serving)	0.3	38.0	2.7	3.2	1.6	0	473.0
Baking Powder, home use, low-sodium (3½ ounces)	3.5	82.4	19.9	0.1	0	0	6.0
Baking Powder, home use, tartrate (3½ ounces)	3.5	77.1	18.7	0.1	0	0	7214.1
Baking Powder, w/calcium carbonate (3½ ounces)	3.5	77.4	18.8	0.1	0	0	11527.8
Baking Soda (3½ ounces)	3.5	0	0	0	0	0	27154.1
Banana Flavoring (1 serving)	0.2	15.0	1.5	0	0	0	0
Butter Buds, mixed w/water (1 serving)	1.0	12.0	3.0	0	0	0.7	250.0
Butter Buds, packaged, dry (1 serving)	0.5	48.0	12.0	0	0	2.8	1000.0

	Weight (oz.)	Calories	Carbo-hydrates (g.)	Protein (g.)	Fat (g.)	Cholesterol (mg.)	Sodium (mg.)
Carob Powder (3½ ounces)							
	3.5	385.0	91.0	3.5	0	0	10.5
Cornstarch (3½ ounces)							
	3.5	359.2	86.9	0.3	0	0	0
Dextrose, anhydrous (3½ ounces)							
	3.5	363.2	98.7	0	0	0	0
Equal Sweetener (3½ ounces)							
	3.5	396.9	0	9.9	0	0	0
Fructose, granulated (3½ ounces)							
	3.5	396.9	99.2	0	0	0	0
Fructose, liquid (3½ ounces)							
	3.5	396.9	99.2	0	0	0	0
Gelatin, dry (1 serving)							
	0.2	23.5	0	6.0	0+	0	6.3
Malt, dry (1 serving)							
	1.0	103.1	21.7	3.7	0.5	0	22.4
Malt, extract, dried (1 serving)							
	0.4	36.7	8.9	0.6	0	0	8.0
Meat Tenderizer, Adolph's (1 serving)							
	0.2	2.0	0.5	0	0	0	1745.0
PAM (1 serving)							
	0+	7.0	0	0	0.8	0	0
Rice Syrup (3½ ounces)							
	3.5	396.9	99.2	0	0	0	0
Soybean Protein (3½ ounces)							
	3.5	319.5	15.0	74.3	0.1	0	208.4
Sugar, brown (3½ ounces)							
	3.5	370.1	95.7	0	0	0	29.8
Sugar, granulated (3½ ounces)							
	3.5	382.0	98.7	0	0	0	1.0
Sugar, powdered (3½ ounces)							
	3.5	382.0	98.7	0	0	0	1.0
TwinSport QuickFix (1 serving)							
	0.3	23.0	6.0	0	0	0	0
TwinSport Weight Control Powder (1 serving)							
	1.0	90.0	18.0	5.0	0.5	3.0	75.0
TwinSport Weight Gain Powder (1 serving)							
	1.5	249.0	28.0	7.4	5.0	4.0	111.0
Vanilla Flavoring (3½ ounces)							
	3.5	297.7	29.8	0	0	0	0
Vegex, vegetable bouillon cube (1 average)							
	0.1	8.0	1.0	1.0	0	0	900.0
Vinegar, cider (1 serving)							
	0.5	2.1	0.9	0	0	0	0.1
Vinegar, distilled (3½ ounces)							
	3.5	13.2	5.3	0	0	0	0
Vinegar, red wine (1 serving)							
	0.5	1.8	0.7	0	0	0	0.1

	Weight (oz.)	Calories	Carbo-hydrates (g.)	Protein (g.)	Fat (g.)	Cholesterol (mg.)	Sodium (mg.)
Whey, sweet, dried (3½ ounces)	3.5	350.3	73.9	12.8	1.1	6.0	10.7
Whey, sweet, fluid (3½ ounces)	3.5	26.8	5.1	0.9	0.4	2.0	53.1
Yeast, bakers', compressed (3½ ounces)	3.5	85.3	10.9	12.0	0.4	0	15.9
Yeast, brewers', debittered (1 serving)	0.3	22.6	3.1	3.1	0.1	0	9.7
Yeast, torula (1 serving)	0.3	22.2	3.0	3.1	0.1	0	1.2

NUTS/SEEDS

	Weight (oz.)	Calories	Carbo-hydrates (g.)	Protein (g.)	Fat (g.)	Cholesterol (mg.)	Sodium (mg.)
Almonds, raw (3½ ounces)	3.5	593.2	19.4	18.4	53.8	0	4.2
Almonds, roasted, w/salt (3½ ounces)	3.5	622.1	19.3	18.5	57.3	0	196.5
Brazil Nuts, raw (3½ ounces)	3.5	649.2	10.8	14.2	66.4	0	0.7
Cashews, roasted, w/o salt (3½ ounces)	3.5	556.6	29.1	17.1	45.3	·0	14.9
Cashews, roasted, w/salt (3½ ounces)	3.5	556.6	29.1	17.1	45.3	0	198.4
Chestnuts, dried (3½ ounces)	3.5	374.1	78.0	6.6	4.1	0	11.9
Chestnuts, fresh (3½ ounces)	3.5	192.5	41.8	2.9	1.5	0	6.0
Coconut Meat, dry, shredded, unsweetened (3½ ounces)	3.5	656.9	22.8	7.1	64.4	0	19.8
Coconut Meat, fresh (3½ ounces)	3.5	343.3	9.3	3.5	35.0	0	22.8
Filberts (3½ ounces)	3.5	629.1	16.6	12.5	61.9	0	2.0
Hickory Nuts (3½ ounces)	3.5	667.8	12.7	13.1	68.2	0	1.0
Macadamia Nuts (3½ ounces)	3.5	685.6	15.8	7.7	71.0	0	1.0
Peanut Butter, w/added fat, salt (3½ ounces)	3.5	576.5	17.1	27.6	49.0	0	602.3
Peanuts, roasted, w/skins, salted (3½ ounces)	3.5	577.5	20.4	26.0	48.3	0	414.8
Pecans, halves, raw (3½ ounces)	3.5	681.7	14.5	9.1	70.6	0	0
Pine Nuts (3½ ounces)	3.5	628.4	16.5	15.2	60.9	0	19.8
Pistachio Nuts, w/o added salt (3½ ounces)	3.5	589.4	18.9	19.2	53.3	0	1.0

	Weight (oz.)	Calories	Carbo-hydrates (g.)	Protein (g.)	Fat (g.)	Cholesterol (mg.)	Sodium (mg.)
Pumpkin Seed, kernels, dry (3½ ounces)							
	3.5	548.7	14.9	28.8	46.3	0	0
Sesame Seeds, decorticated, dry (3½ ounces)							
	3.5	583.5	9.3	26.2	54.3	0	39.0
Squash Seeds, kernels, dry (3½ ounces)							
	3.5	548.7	14.9	28.8	46.3	0	0
Sunflower Seeds, kernels, dry (3½ ounces)							
	3.5	555.7	19.7	23.8	46.9	0	29.8
Walnuts, black, chopped, raw (3½ ounces)							
	3.5	623.1	14.7	20.3	58.8	0	3.2
Walnuts, English, halves, raw (3½ ounces)							
	3.5	645.9	15.7	14.7	63.5	0	2.0

OILS/FATS

	Weight (oz.)	Calories	Carbo-hydrates (g.)	Protein (g.)	Fat (g.)	Cholesterol (mg.)	Sodium (mg.)
Butter, salted (1 tablespoon)							
	0.5	107.6	0+	0.1	12.2	32.9	124.0
Butter, unsalted (1 tablespoon)							
	0.5	107.6	0+	0.1	12.2	32.9	1.7
Lard (1 tablespoon)							
	0.5	117.0	0	0	13.0	12.0	0+
Margarine, regular, w/o salt (1 tablespoon)							
	0.5	107.1	0.1	0.1	12.0	0	0.3
Margarine, regular, w/salt (1 tablespoon)							
	0.5	107.9	0.1	0.1	12.1	0	141.5
Margarine, soft, w/o salt (1 tablespoon)							
	0.4	85.9	0.1	0.1	9.6	0	3.3
Margarine, soft, w/salt (1 tablespoon)							
	0.4	85.9	0.1	0.1	9.6	0	129.4
Olive Oil (1 tablespoon)							
	0.5	123.8	0	0	14.0	0	0
Peanut Oil (1 tablespoon)							
	0.5	123.8	0	0	14.0	0	0+
Safflower Oil (1 tablespoon)							
	0.5	123.8	0	0	14.0	0	0
Sesame Oil (1 tablespoon)							
	0.5	123.8	0	0	14.0	0	0
Soybean Oil (1 tablespoon)							
	0.5	123.8	0	0	14.0	0	0
Vegetable Shortening, cooking (1 tablespoon)							
	0.5	123.8	0	0	14.0	0	0

PANCAKES/WAFFLES/CREPES

	Weight (oz.)	Calories	Carbo-hydrates (g.)	Protein (g.)	Fat (g.)	Cholesterol (mg.)	Sodium (mg.)
Buckwheat Pancakes, ETW recipe (6 average)							
	7.0	244.1	41.9	15.6	2.0	2.4	824.2
Cinnamon French Toast, ETS recipe (2 slices)							
	3.5	150.2	26.4	9.4	1.5	2.6	310.8
Corn Cakes, ETS recipe (2 average)							
	8.6	264.8	57.1	10.0	1.5	1.7	68.6

	Weight (oz.)	Calories	Carbo-hydrates (g.)	Protein (g.)	Fat (g.)	Cholesterol (mg.)	Sodium (mg.)
Hawaiian Pancakes, ETS recipe (2 large)							
	6.6	242.4	42.3	5.2	6.6	0.8	39.9
Need-No-Syrup Banana Pancakes, ETS recipe (2 average)							
	8.2	259.2	59.4	7.2	1.5	0.8	39.5
Pancakes, buckwheat, w/egg, milk (3 average)							
	4.8	270.0	32.1	9.2	12.3	89.1	626.4
Pancakes, from mix, w/egg, milk (3 average)							
	4.8	303.8	43.7	9.7	9.9	99.9	761.4
Potato Pancakes, ETS recipe (1 average)							
	6.0	124.8	24.0	6.0	0.7	1.3	130.3
Waffles, from mix, w/egg, milk (1 average)							
	2.6	206.3	27.1	6.6	7.9	45.0	514.5
Waffles, from mix, w/water (1 average)							
	2.6	228.8	30.1	3.6	10.5	0	420.0
Waffles, frozen (1 average)							
	1.3	93.6	15.5	2.6	2.3	22.2	238.3

PASTA

	Weight (oz.)	Calories	Carbo-hydrates (g.)	Protein (g.)	Fat (g.)	Cholesterol (mg.)	Sodium (mg.)
Macaroni, cooked firm (1 serving)							
	4.9	207.3	42.2	7.0	0.7	0	1.4
Macaroni, cooked tender (1 serving)							
	4.9	155.5	32.2	4.8	0.6	0	1.4
Macaroni, dry form (1 serving)							
	1.8	184.5	37.6	6.2	0.6	0	1.0
Macaroni, whole wheat, dry (1 serving)							
	3.9	405.9	82.7	13.8	1.3	0	2.2
Macaroni and Cheese Lombardo, ETW recipe (1 serving)							
	5.2	234.3	29.3	19.9	3.8	26.0	396.7
Noodles, chow mein, canned (1 serving)							
	1.8	244.5	29.0	6.6	11.8	6.0	500.0
Noodles, egg, cooked (1 serving)							
	5.6	200.0	37.3	6.6	2.4	49.6	3.2
Noodles, egg, dry (1 serving)							
	2.6	283.4	52.6	9.3	3.4	68.7	3.7
Noodles, "No Yolk" thin, cooked (3½ ounces)							
	3.5	52.5	10.0	2.0	0.5	0	0.5
Noodles, "No Yolk" thin, dry (3½ ounces)							
	3.5	367.5	70.0	14.0	3.5	0	3.5
Noodles, spinach, w/o egg, dry (3½ ounces)							
	3.5	367.5	70.0	14.0	3.5	0	3.5
Noodles Romanoff, ETS recipe (1 serving)							
	12.0	263.0	37.1	19.4	3.6	10.1	931.0
Pasta and Garlic Sauce, ETW recipe (1 serving)							
	8.2	311.8	49.4	22.8	1.9	6.2	553.0
Pasta e Fagioli, ETS recipe (1 serving)							
	15.0	353.4	62.4	21.0	3.1	3.9	354.3
Spaghetti, cooked firm, 8–10 minutes (1 serving)							
	5.2	217.6	44.3	7.4	0.7	0	1.5

	Weight (oz.)	Calories	Carbo-hydrates (g.)	Protein (g.)	Fat (g.)	Cholesterol (mg.)	Sodium (mg.)
Spaghetti, cooked tender, 14–20 minutes (1 serving)	5.3	166.5	34.5	5.1	0.6	0	1.5
Spaghetti, dry form (1 serving)	1.3	140.4	28.6	4.8	0.5	0	0.8
Stuffed Shells, ETS recipe (1 serving)	13.7	461.5	72.4	30.0	5.6	15.4	1658.1
Tini Linguini, ETW recipe (1 serving)	8.2	380.3	47.2	31.6	6.3	45.8	746.0
Veal Lasagna, ETS recipe (1 serving)	10.5	330.1	38.7	27.2	7.1	41.9	1229.8
PICKLES/RELISHES							
Pickle Relish, sour (1 tablespoon)	0.5	2.9	0.4	0.1	0.1	0	203.0
Pickle Relish, sweet (1 tablespoon)	0.5	20.7	5.1	0.1	0.1	0	106.8
Pickles, bread-and-butter, fresh (1 tablespoon)	0.4	9.1	2.2	0.1	0+	0	84.1
Pickles, dill (1 tablespoon)	0.4	1.4	0.3	0.1	0+	0	178.5
Pickles, sour (1 tablespoon)	0.4	1.3	0.3	0.1	0+	0	169.1
Pickles, sweet (1 tablespoon)	0.4	18.3	4.6	0.1	0+	0	89.0
PIZZA							
Pizza, w/cheese (1 slice)	3.5	245.0	36.3	9.2	6.8	18.0	633.0
Pizza, w/sausage, cheese (1 slice)	3.5	282.0	27.4	12.9	13.3	29.0	668.0
Pizza, w/sausage, w/o cheese (1 slice)	3.5	234.0	29.6	7.8	9.3	19.0	729.0
POULTRY							
Capon, flesh and skin, raw (1 serving)	3.5	232.2	0	18.7	17.0	74.4	44.7
Chicken, all classes, dark meat, w/o skin, roasted (1 serving)	3.5	174.6	0	27.8	6.3	85.9	85.3
Chicken, all classes, light meat, roasted (1 serving)	3.5	164.7	0	31.4	3.4	85.9	63.5
Chicken, broiler, flesh only, broiled (1 serving)	3.5	134.9	0	23.6	3.8	86.3	65.5
Chicken, fryer, breast, w/skin, fried (1 serving)	3.5	220.3	1.6	31.6	8.8	88.3	75.4
Chicken, fryer, flesh only, fried (1 serving)	3.5	217.3	1.7	30.4	9.0	93.3	90.3

	Weight (oz.)	Calories	Carbo-hydrates (g.)	Protein (g.)	Fat (g.)	Cholesterol (mg.)	Sodium (mg.)
Chicken, light meat, w/o skin, raw (3½ ounces)	3.5	117.0	0	23.4	1.9	78.0	50.0
Chicken, roaster, flesh and skin, roasted (1 serving)	3.5	221.3	0	23.8	13.3	75.4	72.4
Chicken, roaster, flesh only, roasted (1 serving)	3.5	165.7	0	24.8	6.5	74.4	74.4
Chicken, roaster, giblets only, raw (1 serving)	3.5	126.0	1.1	18.0	5.0	234.2	76.4
Chicken Gizzard, simmered (1 serving)	3.5	151.8	1.1	26.9	3.7	192.5	66.5
Chicken Heart, simmered (1 serving)	3.5	183.6	0.1	26.2	7.8	240.1	47.6
Chicken Liver, simmered (1 serving)	3.5	155.8	0.9	24.2	5.4	626.1	50.6
Chicken Tetrazzini, ETS recipe (1 serving)	6.4	208.5	26.6	18.9	1.9	45.9	117.8
Cornish Hen, flesh, w/o skin, roasted (3½ ounces)	3.5	183.0	0	29.5	6.3	71.0	77.0
Cornish Hens, ETS recipe (1 serving)	11.5	487.6	44.2	45.5	14.4	101.4	242.5
Duck, domesticated, flesh only, raw (1 serving)	3.5	131.0	0	18.2	5.9	76.4	73.4
Duck, domesticated, total edible, raw (1 serving)	3.5	323.5	0	15.9	28.4	97.2	73.4
Duck, wild, flesh only, raw (1 serving)	3.5	136.9	0	21.1	5.2	80.4	73.4
Duck, wild, total edible, raw (1 serving)	3.5	231.2	0	20.9	15.7	97.2	73.4
Goose, domesticated, flesh and skin, roasted (1 serving)	3.5	302.6	0	25.0	21.7	90.3	69.5
Goose, domesticated, flesh only, roasted (1 serving)	3.5	236.2	0	28.8	12.6	95.3	75.4
Pâté de Foie Gras, canned (1 serving)	0.5	69.3	0.7	1.7	6.6	22.5	104.6
Pheasant, flesh and skin, raw (1 serving)	3.5	179.6	0	22.5	9.2	70.4	39.7
Pheasant, flesh only, raw (1 serving)	3.5	132.0	0	23.4	3.6	65.5	36.7
Sweet and Sour Chicken, ETW recipe (1 serving)	14.0	491.1	76.6	37.5	4.3	98.2	405.4
Turkey, flesh and skin, roasted (1 serving)	3.5	206.4	0	27.9	9.6	81.4	67.5
Turkey, flesh only, roasted (1 serving)	3.5	168.7	0	29.1	5.0	75.4	69.5
Turkey Gizzard, simmered (1 serving)	3.5	175.6	2.1	26.6	6.1	224.2	54.6

	Weight (oz.)	Calories	Carbo- hydrates (g.)	Protein (g.)	Fat (g.)	Cholesterol (mg.)	Sodium (mg.)
Turkey Liver, simmered (1 serving)	3.5	167.7	3.4	23.8	5.9	621.1	63.5

PRESERVES/JAMS/JELLIES

	Weight (oz.)	Calories	Carbo- hydrates (g.)	Protein (g.)	Fat (g.)	Cholesterol (mg.)	Sodium (mg.)
Apple Butter (1 tablespoon)	0.7	37.2	9.4	0.1	0.2	0	0.4
Grape Jam (1 tablespoon)	0.7	54.4	14.0	0.1	0+	0	2.4
Guava Jelly (1 tablespoon)	0.7	54.6	14.1	0+	0+	0	3.4
Orange Marmalade (1 tablespoon)	0.7	54.4	14.1	0.1	0+	0	2.5
Raspberry Preserves (1 tablespoon)	0.7	54.4	14.0	0.1	0+	0	2.4
Red Cherry Preserves (1 tablespoon)	0.7	54.4	14.0	0.1	0+	0	2.4
Strawberry Preserves (1 tablespoon)	0.7	54.4	14.0	0.1	0+	0	2.4

SALADS

	Weight (oz.)	Calories	Carbo- hydrates (g.)	Protein (g.)	Fat (g.)	Cholesterol (mg.)	Sodium (mg.)
Apple Raisin Salad, ETS recipe (1 serving)	5.1	224.8	33.2	6.1	9.8	0.7	50.7
Bean and Vegetable Salad, ETW recipe (1 serving)	11.8	274.8	55.2	14.6	1.6	0	157.2
Bean Salad, ETS recipe (1 serving)	7.0	210.1	40.3	10.7	1.9	0	274.2
Broccoli and Onion Salad, ETW recipe (1 serving)	5.3	46.3	9.2	4.3	0.4	0	100.7
Carrot Salad Waldorf, ETS recipe (1 serving)	11.1	250.0	50.8	5.0	5.1	1.7	108.2
Cauliflower Broccoli Salad, ETS recipe (1 serving)	5.4	51.8	7.2	6.3	0.6	1.4	130.7
Chicken Salad, ETW recipe (1 serving)	6.4	181.0	9.3	27.8	3.3	66.4	227.0
Chicken Salad Supreme, ETS recipe (1 serving)	9.9	251.5	25.5	19.3	9.3	44.9	129.5
Chickpea Pasta Salad, ETS recipe (1 serving)	8.1	197.0	33.3	11.7	3.0	3.0	414.0
Coleslaw, w/commercial French dressing (1 serving)	4.2	114.0	9.1	1.4	8.8	13.2	321.6
Coleslaw, w/mayonnaise (1 serving)	4.2	172.8	5.8	1.6	16.8	10.8	144.0
Coleslaw, w/mayonnaise-type salad dressing (1 serving)	4.2	118.8	8.5	1.4	9.5	10.8	148.8
Corn Salad, ETS recipe (1 serving)	7.3	138.5	31.2	5.6	1.3	0.5	75.3
Cucumber Salad, ETW recipe (1 serving)	3.5	13.4	3.5	0.4	0+	0	21.0

	Weight (oz.)	Calories	Carbo- hydrates (g.)	Protein (g.)	Fat (g.)	Cholesterol (mg.)	Sodium (mg.)
Grape and Chicken Salad, ETS recipe (1 serving)							
	8.4	249.8	27.7	27.3	3.3	65.4	112.4
Lobster Salad, ETS recipe (1 serving)							
	6.7	109.0	5.1	17.7	1.9	50.4	409.7
Oriental Salad, ETS recipe (1 serving)							
	8.7	234.5	10.7	23.0	11.9	48.3	282.8
Potato Salad, w/cooked salad dressing, butter (1 serving)							
	8.8	247.5	40.7	6.7	7.0	65.0	1320.0
Potato Salad, w/cooked salad dressing, margarine (1 serving)							
	8.8	247.5	40.7	6.7	7.0	0	1320.0
Potato Salad, w/hard-cooked eggs, mayonnaise dressing (1 serving)							
	8.8	362.5	33.5	7.5	23.0	162.5	1200.0
Red Cabbage and Apple Slaw, ETS recipe (1 serving)							
	7.8	125.3	31.1	2.4	0.6	0	80.5
Red Potato Salad, ETS recipe (1 serving)							
	9.1	145.8	28.4	6.9	1.0	3.2	211.4
Salad, w/lettuce, tomato (1 large)							
	6.0	40.0	8.2	2.2	0.5	0	9.0
Shrimp Salad, ETS recipe (1 serving)							
	7.5	274.3	34.0	28.9	1.8	115.7	319.9
Spinach Salad, ETS recipe (1 serving)							
	5.7	140.2	7.5	10.9	8.0	5.8	308.7
Sweet Slaw, ETS recipe (1 serving)							
	4.3	145.1	18.4	5.3	6.6	2.2	97.0
Tuna Bean Salad, ETS recipe (1 serving)							
	7.7	196.7	24.9	18.3	2.3	22.3	305.5
Vegetable Potato Salad, ETS recipe (1 serving)							
	11.6	192.8	36.5	11.6	1.0	2.3	455.5
Waldorf Salad Deluxe, ETW recipe (1 serving)							
	10.3	257.7	59.9	6.4	1.9	4.9	172.0

SAUCES/SPREADS/CREAMS

	Weight (oz.)	Calories	Carbo- hydrates (g.)	Protein (g.)	Fat (g.)	Cholesterol (mg.)	Sodium (mg.)
Apple Butter, ETW recipe (1 tablespoon)							
	0.6	8.8	2.3	0+	0+	0	0.3
Apple Cranberry Sauce, ETS recipe (1 tablespoon)							
	0.6	10.0	2.1	0.1	0+	0	0.2
Barbecue Sauce (1 tablespoon)							
	0.5	11.3	1.9	0.3	0.3	0	122.3
Catsup, bottled, w/o salt (1 tablespoon)							
	0.5	15.9	3.8	0.3	0.1	0	3.0
Catsup, bottled, w/salt (1 tablespoon)							
	0.5	15.9	3.8	0.3	0.1	0	156.3
Chili Sauce, hot, green, canned (1 tablespoon)							
	0.6	3.4	0.9	0.1	0+	0	4.3
Cream, Half and Half (1 tablespoon)							
	0.5	19.5	0.6	0.5	1.7	5.6	6.1
Cream, heavy whipping (1 tablespoon)							
	0.5	51.8	0.4	0.3	5.6	20.6	5.6

	Weight (oz.)	Calories	Carbo-hydrates (g.)	Protein (g.)	Fat (g.)	Cholesterol (mg.)	Sodium (mg.)
Cream, light, coffee or table (1 tablespoon)	0.5	29.3	0.6	0.4	2.9	9.9	5.9
Cream, light whipping (1 tablespoon)	0.5	43.8	0.5	0.3	4.6	16.7	5.1
Cream, substitute, w/skim milk, lactose (1 tablespoon)	0.5	76.2	9.2	1.3	4.0	0	86.3
Dill Sauce Deluxe, ETW recipe (1 tablespoon)	0.6	12.9	0.8	1.7	0.3	1.0	59.7
Eggplant Sauce, ETS recipe (3½ ounces)	3.5	52.3	8.5	1.7	1.6	0	349.9
Fruit Spread, ETS recipe (1 tablespoon)	0.6	28.2	3.3	1.7	1.1	0.6	46.6
Haas Mayonnaise Spread, ETW recipe (1 tablespoon)	0.7	14.2	0.6	2.4	0.2	0.9	88.1
Haas Peanut Butter, ETW recipe (1 tablespoon)	0.9	45.9	8.1	2.4	0.9	0	0.5
Horseradish Sauce, prepared (1 tablespoon)	0.5	5.7	1.4	0.2	0+	0	14.4
Hot Sauce (1 tablespoon)	0.5	2.4	0.3	0.3	0	0	66.0
Marinara Sauce, ETW recipe (3½ ounces)	3.5	25.5	5.1	1.2	0.3	0	175.6
Mayonnaise, w/soybean oil, salt (1 tablespoon)	0.5	100.4	0.4	0.2	11.1	8.3	79.6
Mustard, brown, prepared (1 tablespoon)	0.5	13.7	0.8	0.9	0.9	0	196.0
Mustard, yellow, prepared (1 tablespoon)	0.5	11.3	1.0	0.7	0.7	0	187.8
Pesto, ETS recipe (1 tablespoon)	0.5	19.3	1.4	0.7	1.4	0.5	74.0
Pimiento Cheese Spread, past. process (3½ ounces)	3.5	372.1	1.7	21.9	31.0	93.3	1416.4
Quick Tomato Sauce, ETS recipe (1 tablespoon)	0.9	14.3	3.0	0.5	0.1	0.2	125.2
Tabasco Sauce (1 tablespoon)	0.5	2.4	0.3	0.3	0	0	66.0
Tamari (1 tablespoon)	0.5	9.6	1.2	1.3	0	0	857.9
Tamari, diluted ½ part water (1 tablespoon)	0.5	4.8	0.6	0.7	0	0	428.9
Tartar Sauce, low-cal (1 tablespoon)	0.7	44.8	1.3	0.1	4.5	10.2	141.4
Tartar Sauce, regular (1 tablespoon)	0.5	74.3	0.6	0.2	8.1	7.1	99.0
Tuna Haas, ETW recipe (3½ ounces)	3.5	72.4	2.7	13.4	0.7	22.0	171.3
White Sauce, medium (1 tablespoon)	0.6	25.9	1.4	0.6	2.0	6.6	60.6
Worcestershire Sauce (1 tablespoon)	0.5	12.0	2.7	0.3	0	0	147.0

	Weight (oz.)	Calories	Carbo-hydrates (g.)	Protein (g.)	Fat (g.)	Cholesterol (mg.)	Sodium (mg.)

SOUP/STEWS

	Weight (oz.)	Calories	Carbo-hydrates (g.)	Protein (g.)	Fat (g.)	Cholesterol (mg.)	Sodium (mg.)
Bean Soup, canned, w/equal volume of water (1 cup)	8.5	169.0	21.7	7.2	4.8	0	831.0
Bean with Pork Soup, canned, w/equal volume of water (1 cup)	8.8	170.0	22.5	7.7	6.0	2.5	940.0
Beef and Vegetable Stew, canned (1 cup)	8.3	185.9	16.7	13.6	7.3	32.9	967.1
Beef Noodle Soup, canned, w/equal volume of water (1 cup)	8.6	83.3	9.1	4.9	3.2	4.9	955.5
Black Bean Soup, ETS recipe (1 cup)	8.3	236.3	43.0	15.4	1.0	0	164.9
Black-Eyed Pea Soup, ETW recipe (1 cup)	8.0	175.8	34.2	9.7	0.7	0	163.1
Chicken Broth, defatted (1 cup)	8.8	27.0	1.0	4.9	0	0	795.0
Chicken Consommé, canned, w/equal volume of water (1 cup)	8.8	40.0	1.0	5.0	1.5	7.5	795.0
Chicken Noodle Soup, canned, w/equal volume of water (1 cup)	8.5	74.4	9.4	4.1	2.4	7.2	1101.6
Chicken Vegetable Soup, canned, w/equal volume of water (1 cup)	8.6	76.0	8.8	3.7	2.9	9.8	960.4
Chicken with Rice Soup, canned, w/equal volume of water (1 cup)	8.5	60.0	7.2	3.6	1.9	7.2	811.2
Chili, ETS recipe (1 cup)	10.4	343.2	34.7	28.2	10.5	68.7	576.6
Chili Bean and Rice Soup, ETW recipe (1 cup)	10.5	213.5	41.6	10.9	1.1	0	347.0
Chili con Carne, canned, w/beans (1 cup)	8.1	306.0	28.1	17.3	14.0	39.1	1221.5
Chili con Carne, canned, w/o beans (1 cup)	8.1	460.1	13.3	23.7	34.0	59.8	1221.5
Chunky Chicken Noodle Soup, ETS recipe (1 cup)	10.8	266.2	28.2	29.9	2.8	59.4	1171.0
Corn Chowder, ETS recipe (1 cup)	8.0	153.5	33.2	6.0	1.2	1.5	41.8
Cream of Asparagus Soup, canned, w/equal volume of milk (1 cup)	8.5	156.0	15.8	6.2	7.9	21.6	1008.0
Cream of Celery Soup, canned, w/equal volume of milk (1 cup)	8.5	158.4	14.2	5.5	9.4	31.2	976.8
Cream of Chicken Soup, canned, w/equal volume of milk (1 cup)	8.5	184.8	14.4	7.2	11.0	26.4	1012.8
Cream of Mushroom Soup, canned, w/equal volume of milk (1 cup)	8.5	196.8	14.6	5.8	13.2	19.2	1041.6
Cream of Potato Soup, canned w/equal volume of milk (1 cup)	8.5	182.4	18.0	7.7	9.4	31.2	1238.4
Green Pea Soup, canned, w/equal volume of milk (1 cup)	8.5	225.6	30.5	12.0	6.7	16.8	988.8
Hearty Vegetable Soup, ETS recipe (1 cup)	8.7	314.1	63.6	16.4	1.7	0	373.4

	Weight (oz.)	Calories	Carbo-hydrates (g.)	Protein (g.)	Fat (g.)	Cholesterol (mg.)	Sodium (mg.)
Howard's Onion Soup, ETW recipe (1 cup)	9.2	147.9	25.9	6.8	1.8	3.0	389.6
Kidney Bean Soup, ETW recipe (1 cup)	10.2	110.6	21.3	6.1	0.5	0	399.4
Lentil Barley Soup, ETS recipe (1 cup)	12.5	240.9	43.8	15.9	0.7	0	1214.0
Lentil Soup (1 cup)	8.5	169.0	21.7	7.2	4.8	0	831.0
Manhattan Clam Chowder, w/tomatoes, canned, w/equal water (1 cup)	8.6	78.4	12.3	4.2	2.2	2.5	1815.5
Minestrone Soup, canned, w/equal volume of water (1 cup)	8.6	83.3	11.5	4.4	2.5	2.5	926.1
Navy Bean Soup, ETS recipe (1 cup)	13.1	170.8	32.0	10.5	0.8	0	158.8
New England Clam Chowder, frozen, w/equal volume of water (1 cup)	8.5	129.6	10.6	4.3	7.7	24.0	1044.0
Onion Soup, canned, w/equal volume of water (1 cup)	8.5	57.6	8.2	3.8	1.7	12.0	1048.8
Onion Soup, dehydrated, dry form (1 serving)	0.4	32.3	5.9	1.3	0.7	0.6	985.3
Onion Soup, Lipton 20% less salt, dry form (1 serving)	1.2	35.0	6.0	1.0	0.5	0	640.0
Oyster Stew, commercial, w/equal volume of milk (1 cup)	8.5	202.4	14.2	10.1	11.8	50.6	881.9
Oyster Stew, commercial, w/equal volume of water (1 cup)	8.5	122.9	8.2	5.5	7.7	26.5	819.3
Potato Soup, ETW recipe (1 cup)	8.0	166.7	33.2	8.6	0.4	2.5	278.9
Ranchero Chili, ETW recipe (1 cup)	8.3	182.9	34.9	10.9	0.9	0	185.1
Split Pea Soup, canned, w/equal volume of water (1 cup)	8.6	183.8	27.2	10.0	4.2	7.4	975.1
Split Pea Soup, ETS recipe (1 cup)	8.7	204.2	38.0	13.6	0.6	0	232.9
Sweet Potato Soup, ETW recipe (1 cup)	8.3	239.7	35.4	4.6	1.9	4.3	320.4
Tomato Rice Soup, ETS recipe (1 cup)	10.3	108.9	20.0	6.4	0.6	0	868.9
Tomato Soup, canned, w/equal volume of water (1 cup)	8.6	85.8	16.7	2.0	2.0	0	874.7
Turkey Noodle Soup, canned w/equal volume of water (1 cup)	8.5	67.2	8.4	3.8	1.9	4.8	801.6
Vegetable Beef Soup, canned, w/equal volume of water (1 cup)	8.6	78.4	10.3	5.6	2.0	4.9	960.4
Vegetarian Vegetable Soup, canned, w/equal volume of water (1 cup)	8.6	73.5	12.3	2.2	2.0	0	835.5

	Weight (oz.)	Calories	Carbo-hydrates (g.)	Protein (g.)	Fat (g.)	Cholesterol (mg.)	Sodium (mg.)
SPICES							
Allspice, ground (1 teaspoon)	0.1	5.0	1.4	0.1	0.2	0	1.0
Basil, ground (1 teaspoon)	0.1	6.0	1.3	0.3	0.1	0	0
Bay Leaf, crumbled (1 teaspoon)	0+	2.0	0.5	0+	0+	0	0
Celery Seed (1 teaspoon)	0.1	8.0	0.8	0.4	0.5	0	3.0
Chervil, dried (1 teaspoon)	0+	1.0	0.3	0.1	0+	0	0
Chili Powder (1 teaspoon)	0.1	8.2	1.4	0.3	0.4	0	26.3
Cinnamon, ground (1 teaspoon)	0.1	6.0	1.8	0.1	0.1	0	1.0
Coriander Seed (1 teaspoon)	0.1	5.0	1.0	0.2	0.3	0	1.0
Cumin Seed (1 teaspoon)	0.1	8.0	0.9	0.4	0.5	0	4.0
Curry Powder (1 teaspoon)	0.1	6.0	1.2	0.3	0.3	0	1.0
Dill Weed, dried (1 teaspoon)	0+	3.0	0.6	0.2	0	0	2.0
Fennel Seed (1 teaspoon)	0.1	7.0	1.0	0.3	0.3	0	2.0
Garlic Clove, raw (1 ounce)	1.0	37.8	8.5	1.9	0	0	9.4
Garlic Powder (1 teaspoon)	0.1	9.0	2.0	0.5	0+	0	1.0
Ginger, ground (1 teaspoon)	0.1	6.0	1.3	0.2	0.1	0	1.0
Italian Seasoning (1 teaspoon)	0+	3.0	0.6	0.1	0.1	0	1.0
Marjoram, dried (1 teaspoon)	0+	2.0	0.4	0.1	0+	0	0
Mint (1 teaspoon)	0+	3.0	0.6	0.2	0	0	2.0
Mrs. Dash (1 teaspoon)	0.1	7.0	1.7	0.2	0+	0	5.0
Mustard, dry (1 teaspoon)	0.1	12.0	0.4	0.6	0.9	0	0
Nutmeg, ground (1 teaspoon)	0.1	12.0	1.1	0.1	0.8	0	0
Onion Powder (1 teaspoon)	0.1	7.0	1.7	0.2	0+	0	1.0

	Weight (oz.)	Calories	Carbo-hydrates (g.)	Protein (g.)	Fat (g.)	Cholesterol (mg.)	Sodium (mg.)
Oregano, ground (1 teaspoon)	0.1	5.0	1.0	0.2	0.2	0	0
Paprika (1 teaspoon)	0.1	6.0	1.2	0.3	0.3	0	1.0
Parsley, dried (1 teaspoon)	0+	1.0	0.2	0.1	0+	0	1.0
Pepper, black (1 teaspoon)	0.1	5.0	1.4	0.2	0.1	0	1.0
Pepper, red or cayenne (1 teaspoon)	0.1	6.0	1.0	0.2	0.3	0	1.0
Pepper, white (1 teaspoon)	0.1	7.0	1.7	0.3	0+	0	0
Rosemary, dried (1 teaspoon)	0+	4.0	0.8	0.1	0.2	0	1.0
Sage (1 teaspoon)	0+	3.0	0.6	0.1	0.1	0	0
Salt, Morton Lite (1 teaspoon)	0.2	0	0	0	0	0	975.0
Salt, table (1 teaspoon)	0.2	0	0	0	0	0	1937.9
Tarragon, ground (1 teaspoon)	0.1	5.0	0.8	0.4	0.1	0	1.0
Thyme, ground (1 teaspoon)	0+	4.0	0.9	0.1	0.1	0	1.0
Turmeric, ground (1 teaspoon)	0.1	8.0	1.4	0.2	0.2	0	1.0
Vanilla Extract (1 teaspoon)	0.2	6.0	1.5	0	0	0	0

TOPPINGS/SALAD DRESSINGS

	Weight (oz.)	Calories	Carbo-hydrates (g.)	Protein (g.)	Fat (g.)	Cholesterol (mg.)	Sodium (mg.)
Bacon, Onion, and Chive Topping, ETW recipe (2 tablespoons)	1.0	24.9	2.1	2.4	0.7	2.1	126.0
Barbecue Chicken Topping, ETW recipe (3½ ounces)	3.5	112.6	10.3	12.0	1.7	28.1	320.1
Blue Cheese Dressing, regular, w/salt (2 tablespoons)	1.1	151.2	2.2	1.4	15.7	5.1	328.2
Bread Stuffing, from mix, w/egg, table fat, moist (3½ ounces)	3.5	206.4	19.5	4.4	12.7	65.5	500.1
Bread Stuffing Mix, dry form (3½ ounces)	3.5	368.1	71.8	12.8	3.8	4.0	1320.7
Caesar Salad Dressing, ETW recipe (3½ ounces)	3.5	52.5	3.7	7.5	0.9	3.1	347.2
Celery Seed dressing, ETS recipe (2 tablespoons)	1.0	16.6	1.4	1.9	0.4	1.4	70.1
Chicken in Wine Sauce Topping, ETW recipe (2 tablespoons)	0.8	20.3	0.8	2.9	0.5	5.3	52.5
Creamy Italian Dressing, ETW recipe (2 tablespoons)	1.2	21.9	1.6	2.8	0.5	1.7	102.2

	Weight (oz.)	Calories	Carbo-hydrates (g.)	Protein (g.)	Fat (g.)	Cholesterol (mg.)	Sodium (mg.)
Creamy Russian Dressing, ETS recipe (2 tablespoons)	1.3	24.0	2.6	2.4	0.5	1.8	70.6
French Dressing, regular, w/salt (2 tablespoons)	1.2	138.0	5.6	0.2	13.2	18.0	438.0
Garlic Dressing, ETS recipe (2 tablespoons)	1.6	31.4	1.8	4.8	0.5	2.3	174.7
Garlic French Dressing, ETS recipe (2 tablespoons)	1.3	6.0	1.9	0.1	0+	0	30.9
Green Goddess Dressing, ETW recipe (2 tablespoons)	1.3	19.7	2.0	2.3	0.3	1.3	123.9
Herb Magic Italian Dressing (2 tablespoons)	1.2	8.0	2.0	0	0	0	244.0
Horseradish Topping, ETW recipe (2 tablespoons)	1.1	20.4	1.3	2.9	0.3	1.6	97.6
Italian Dressing, regular, w/salt (2 tablespoons)	1.0	140.0	3.0	0.2	14.4	20.0	236.0
Jeff's "Cream" Dressing, ETW recipe (2 tablespoons)	1.1	18.8	1.0	3.1	0.3	1.2	101.0
Mushroom Topping, ETW recipe (2 tablespoons)	1.5	23.0	1.6	3.2	0.4	1.6	100.6
Parsley Parmesan Dressing, ETS recipe (2 tablespoons)	1.1	25.3	1.6	2.7	1.0	3.1	87.9
Roquefort Cheese Dressing, regular, w/salt (2 tablespoons)	1.0	152.0	2.2	1.4	15.6	6.0	328.0
Russian Dressing, w/salt (2 tablespoons)	1.0	148.0	3.2	0.4	15.2	6.0	260.0
Snappy Cheddar Topping, ETW recipe (2 tablespoons)	0.9	25.5	0.8	3.2	1.0	3.8	127.5
Tangy Horseradish Dressing, ETS recipe (2 tablespoons)	0.9	6.7	1.8	0.2	0.1	0	43.7
Thousand Island Dressing, ETW recipe (2 tablespoons)	1.3	33.8	5.5	2.6	0.3	0.9	137.6
Thousand Island Dressing, regular, w/salt (2 tablespoons)	1.0	114.0	4.6	0.2	10.8	8.0	210.0
Tomato Dressing, ETS recipe (2 tablespoons)	1.3	17.6	1.5	2.0	0.5	1.3	62.0
V-8 Dressing, ETS recipe (2 tablespoons)	1.1	8.6	2.0	0.2	0+	0	5.7
Yogurt Tomato Dressing, ETW recipe (2 tablespoons)	1.9	15.8	2.5	1.1	0.3	0.8	74.9

VEGETABLES

	Weight (oz.)	Calories	Carbo-hydrates (g.)	Protein (g.)	Fat (g.)	Cholesterol (mg.)	Sodium (mg.)
Alfalfa Sprouts, raw (3½ ounces)	3.5	35.4	3.5	3.5	0	0	1.8
Artichoke Hearts, frozen (3½ ounces)	3.5	25.8	6.4	2.6	0.4	0	46.6
Asparagus, raw spears, boiled w/o salt, drained (1 serving)	2.6	17.3	2.8	2.4	0.1	0	0.8

	Weight (oz.)	Calories	Carbo-hydrates (g.)	Protein (g.)	Fat (g.)	Cholesterol (mg.)	Sodium (mg.)
Bamboo Shoots, raw (1 serving)							
	2.3	18.0	3.5	1.7	0.2	0	3.3
Beans, Heinz Vegetarian (1 serving)							
	5.3	50.0	9.7	2.6	0.6	0	141.7
Beans, white, raw (3½ ounces)							
	3.5	337.4	60.8	22.1	1.6	0	18.9
Beet Greens, boiled w/o salt, drained (1 serving)							
	3.5	18.0	3.3	1.7	0.2	0	76.0
Beets, red, boiled w/o salt, drained (1 serving)							
	2.9	26.7	6.0	0.9	0.1	0	35.8
Beets, red, canned, drained solids (1 serving)							
	2.9	30.8	7.3	0.8	0.1	0	196.7
Black Beans, cooked (3½ ounces)							
	3.5	117.1	21.0	7.7	0.6	0	6.9
Black Beans, dried (3½ ounces)							
	3.5	339.0	61.2	22.3	1.5	0	25.0
Black-Eyed Peas, immature seeds, boiled w/o salt, drained (1 serving)							
	3.5	130.0	23.5	8.9	0.4	0	39.0
Black-Eyed Peas, immature seeds, raw (3½ ounces)							
	3.5	126.0	21.6	8.9	0.8	0	2.0
Black-Eyed Peas, mature seeds, dry, raw (3½ ounces)							
	3.5	340.3	61.2	22.6	1.5	0	34.7
Broccoli, frozen, chopped, boiled w/o salt, drained (1 serving)							
	3.5	26.0	4.6	2.9	0.3	0	15.0
Broccoli, raw (1 serving)							
	3.5	32.0	5.9	3.6	0.3	0	15.0
Broccoli, spears, steamed w/o salt, drained (1 large)							
	3.5	26.0	4.5	3.1	0.3	0	10.0
Brussels Sprouts, boiled w/o salt, drained (1 serving)							
	2.9	30.0	5.3	3.5	0.3	0	8.3
Butternut Squash, baked w/o salt (1 serving)							
	3.5	68.0	17.5	1.8	0.1	0	1.0
Butternut Squash, boiled, mashed w/o salt (1 serving)							
	4.4	51.2	13.0	1.4	0.1	0	1.3
Cabbage, Chinese, raw (1 serving)							
	0.8	3.1	0.7	0.3	0+	0	5.1
Cabbage, common, boiled w/o salt, large amount water (1 serving)							
	2.9	15.0	3.3	0.8	0.2	0	10.8
Cabbage, common varieties, raw (1 serving)							
	1.8	12.0	2.7	0.6	0.1	0	10.0
Cannellini, canned, rinsed (3½ ounces)							
	3.5	124.3	22.7	7.9	0.6	0	4.1
Carrots, boiled w/o salt, drained (1 serving)							
	2.6	23.3	5.3	0.7	0.1	0	24.8
Carrots, canned, drained solids (1 serving)							
	2.6	22.5	5.0	0.6	0.2	0	177.0
Carrots, raw (1 serving)							
	3.5	42.0	9.7	1.1	0.2	0	47.0

	Weight (oz.)	Calories	Carbo-hydrates (g.)	Protein (g.)	Fat (g.)	Cholesterol (mg.)	Sodium (mg.)
Cauliflower, raw (1 serving)	2.9	22.5	4.3	2.2	0.2	0	10.8
Cauliflower, steamed w/o salt, drained (1 serving)	2.0	12.6	2.3	1.3	0.1	0	5.1
Cauliflower Curry, ETW recipe (1 serving)	4.7	91.9	17.7	6.6	0.4	0	36.5
Celery, boiled w/o salt, drained (1 serving)	2.2	8.8	1.9	0.5	0.1	0	55.0
Celery, stalks, raw (3 small)	1.8	10.5	2.4	0.6	0.1	0	78.7
Chard, Swiss, boiled w/o salt, drained (1 serving)	2.9	15.0	2.7	1.5	0.2	0	71.7
"Cheddar" Stuffed Potato, ETW recipe (½ average)	5.2	145.9	26.7	6.3	1.8	6.2	128.9
Chickpeas, canned (3½ ounces)	3.5	179.0	30.3	10.2	2.4	0	260.0
Chickpeas, mature seeds, dry, raw (3½ ounces)	3.5	357.2	60.5	20.3	4.8	0	25.8
Chicory, head, raw (1 serving)	2.7	11.5	2.5	0.8	0.1	0	5.4
Chives, chopped, raw (3½ ounces)	3.5	29.8	6.0	2.0	0	0	0
Collards, leaves, boiled w/o salt, large amount water (1 serving)	3.5	31.0	4.8	3.4	0.7	0	25.0
Corn, cream style, canned, solids and liquid (1 serving)	4.4	102.5	25.0	2.6	0.7	0	295.0
Corn, cream style, low-sodium, canned, solids and liquid (1 serving)	4.4	102.5	23.1	3.2	1.4	0	2.5
Corn, whole kernel, canned, solids and liquid (1 serving)	4.4	82.5	19.6	2.4	0.7	0	295.0
Corn, whole kernel, low-sodium, canned, drained solids (1 serving)	4.4	95.0	22.5	3.1	0.9	0	2.5
Corn on the Cob, steamed (1 average)	3.5	100.0	21.0	3.3	1.0	0	1.0
Cottage Fries, ETW recipe (1 serving)	9.5	231.6	48.9	7.1	1.5	2.0	56.2
Cowpeas, immature seeds, boiled w/o salt, drained (1 serving)	2.8	86.4	14.5	6.5	0.6	0	0.8
Creamed Corn, ETS recipe (1 serving)	5.8	133.1	30.5	5.1	1.2	0.6	19.5
Cucumber, raw (½ average)	2.0	7.8	1.8	0.3	0.1	0	3.3
Dandelion Greens, boiled w/o salt, drained (1 serving)	3.5	33.0	6.4	2.0	0.6	0	44.0
Dock, boiled, drained (1 serving)	3.5	19.0	3.9	1.6	0.2	0	3.0
Eggplant, boiled w/o salt, drained (1 serving)	3.5	19.0	4.1	1.0	0.2	0	1.0

	Weight (oz.)	Calories	Carbo-hydrates (g.)	Protein (g.)	Fat (g.)	Cholesterol (mg.)	Sodium (mg.)
Eggplant, raw (2 slices)	3.5	25.0	5.8	1.2	0.2	0	2.0
Endive, leaves (10 small)	0.4	2.5	0.5	0.2	0+	0	1.8
Escarole, leaves (8 small)	0.9	4.5	0.9	0.3	0+	0	2.5
Green Beans, boiled w/o salt, drained (1 serving)	3.5	25.0	5.4	1.6	0.2	0	4.0
Green Beans, canned, drained solids (1 serving)	2.2	15.0	3.2	0.9	0.1	0	147.5
Green Beans, raw (1 serving)	2.2	21.9	4.9	1.3	0.1	0	5.0
Green Bell Pepper, raw (1 large)	1.4	9.0	1.9	0.5	0.1	0	5.0
Hash Brown Potatoes, ETS recipe (1 serving)	6.5	121.4	26.4	3.6	0.6	0	150.3
Hot German Potato Salad, ETW recipe (1 serving)	10.1	168.2	35.4	5.8	1.0	0	351.2
Hubbard Squash, baked w/o salt (1 serving)	3.5	50.0	11.7	1.8	0.4	0	1.0
Jerusalem Artichoke, raw (1 serving)	3.5	41.0	16.7	2.3	0.1	0	0
Kale, leaves, boiled w/o salt, drained (1 serving)	3.5	39.0	6.1	4.5	0.7	0	43.0
Kelp, raw (3½ ounces)	3.5	0	0	0	1.1	0	2983.6
Kidney Beans, canned, rinsed (1 serving)	3.2	112.5	20.5	7.1	0.5	0	3.8
Kohlrabi, thickened bulblike stems, boiled w/o salt (1 serving)	2.6	18.0	4.0	1.3	0.1	0	4.5
Leeks, bulb and lower leaf portion, raw (1 serving)	1.8	26.0	5.6	1.1	0.1	0	2.5
Lentils, split, raw (3½ ounces)	3.5	342.3	61.3	24.5	0.9	0	29.8
Lentils, whole, mature seeds, cooked (1 serving)	2.6	79.5	14.5	5.8	0	0	9.8
Lettuce, butterhead varieties, raw (1 serving)	2.0	7.8	1.4	0.7	0.1	0	5.0
Lettuce, cos or romaine, raw (1 serving)	2.4	12.0	2.3	0.9	0.2	0	6.0
Lettuce, loose-leaf or bunching varieties (1 serving)	2.0	10.0	1.9	0.7	0.2	0	5.0
Lima Beans, boiled w/o salt, drained (1 serving)	2.8	88.8	15.8	6.1	0.4	0	0.8
Marinated Potato Salad, ETW recipe (1 serving)	9.9	178.3	39.4	6.1	0.3	0	369.4
Marinated Vegetables, ETW recipe (1 serving)	5.2	22.7	5.2	1.5	0.2	0	6.6

	Weight (oz.)	Calories	Carbo-hydrates (g.)	Protein (g.)	Fat (g.)	Cholesterol (mg.)	Sodium (mg.)
Mashed Potatoes, ETS recipe (1 serving)	11.3	187.8	38.4	7.5	0.9	2.5	138.8
Mixed Vegetables, frozen, boiled w/o salt (1 serving)	2.9	52.3	10.9	2.6	0.2	0	43.3
Mung Bean Sprouts, raw (1 serving)	1.8	17.5	3.3	1.9	0.1	0	2.5
Mushrooms, *Agaricus campestris*, canned, solids and liquid (1 serving)	3.5	17.0	2.4	1.9	0.1	0	400.0
Mushrooms, *Agaricus campestris*, raw (5 small)	1.8	14.0	2.2	1.3	0.1	0	7.5
Mustard Greens, boiled w/o salt, drained (1 serving)	3.5	23.0	4.0	2.2	0.4	0	18.0
Mustard Spinach, boiled w/o salt, drained (1 serving)	3.5	16.0	2.8	1.7	0.2	0	18.0
Neptune's Potato, ETS recipe (1 average)	10.5	276.6	52.3	13.7	1.8	36.4	117.0
New Zealand Spinach, boiled w/o salt, drained (1 serving)	3.5	13.0	2.1	1.7	0.2	0	92.0
Okra, boiled w/o salt, drained (1 serving)	3.5	29.0	6.0	2.0	0.3	0	2.0
Onion, dehydrated, flaked	3.5	347.3	81.5	8.6	1.3	0	87.3
Onion, boiled w/o salt, drained (1 serving)	3.5	29.0	6.5	1.2	0.1	0	7.0
Onion, raw (1 average)	3.0	33.0	7.5	1.3	0.1	0	8.6
Onion Soup, canned, w/equal volume water (1 serving)	8.5	57.6	8.2	3.8	1.7	12.0	1048.8
Parsley, chopped, raw (1 serving)	0.1	1.8	0.4	0.1	0+	0	1.9
Parsnips, cooked w/o salt (1 serving)	2.8	51.6	11.6	1.2	0.4	0	6.2
Peas, green, frozen, boiled w/o salt, drained (1 serving)	3.5	63.0	11.8	5.1	0.3	0	351.0
Peas and Carrots, frozen, boiled w/o salt, drained (1 serving)	2.9	44.2	8.4	2.7	0.2	0	70.0
Pepper, jalapeño (1 serving)	0.5	13.2	2.6	0.5	0.3	0	1.3
Pepper, hot chili, green, raw pods, w/o seeds (1 serving)	0.5	5.5	1.4	0.2	0+	0	3.7
Pimientos, canned, solids and liquid (½ average)	0.6	4.2	0.9	0.1	0.1	0	3.9
Pinto Beans, dry (3½ ounces)	3.5	346.2	63.2	22.7	1.2	0	9.9
Potato, baked, w/o skin (1 average)	7.5	203.6	45.2	5.6	0.2	0	8.6
Potato, baked, w/skin (1 average)	9.0	217.1	48.9	6.0	0.3	0	8.6

	Weight (oz.)	Calories	Carbo-hydrates (g.)	Protein (g.)	Fat (g.)	Cholesterol (mg.)	Sodium (mg.)
Potato, boiled w/o skin (1 average)	9.0	157.9	35.2	4.6	0.2	0	4.9
Potato, boiled, w/skin (1 average)	10.2	217.1	48.9	6.0	0.3	0	8.6
Potato, raw, w/o skin (1 average)	8.5	157.9	35.2	4.6	0.2	0	4.9
Potato, raw, w/skin (1 average)	10.0	215.5	48.6	6.0	0.4	0	9.4
Potatoes, french fried, w/o salt (1 serving)	3.5	274.0	36.0	4.3	13.2	0	6.0
Potatoes, hash browned (1 serving)	3.5	224.0	29.0	2.0	11.5	0	299.0
Potatoes, mashed, w/milk (1 serving)	3.5	65.0	13.0	2.1	0.7	2.0	301.0
Potatoes, raw (1 average)	3.5	76.0	17.1	2.1	0.1	0	3.3
Potatoes, scalloped, w/cheese, butter (1 serving)	3.3	135.9	12.8	5.0	7.4	24.0	419.0
Potatoes Parmesan, ETS recipe (1 average)	11.5	282.4	54.2	11.9	2.6	6.8	172.5
Pumpkin, raw (1 serving)	3.5	26.0	6.5	1.0	0.1	0	1.0
Radish, common, raw (10 small)	3.5	17.0	3.6	1.0	0.1	0	18.0
Red Beans, cooked (1 serving)	3.5	118.0	21.4	7.8	0.5	0	3.0
Red Bell Pepper, raw (1 large)	1.6	10.2	2.1	0.5	0.1	0	5.7
Red Kidney Beans, canned (1 serving)	4.5	115.0	20.9	7.3	0.5	0	4.0
Rutabaga, boiled w/o salt, drained (1 serving)	3.5	35.0	8.2	0.9	0.1	0	4.0
Scallions, bulb and tops, raw (3 average)	1.8	22.5	5.2	0.5	0.1	0	2.5
Shallots, bulbs, raw (1 serving)	3.5	72.0	16.8	2.5	0.1	0	12.0
Soybean Curd (1 serving)	2.9	59.6	2.0	6.5	3.5	0	5.8
Soybeans, mature seeds, cooked (1 serving)	3.5	130.0	10.8	11.0	5.7	0	2.0
Spinach, boiled w/o salt, drained (1 serving)	3.5	23.0	3.6	3.0	0.3	0	50.0
Spinach, frozen, chopped, boiled w/o salt, drained (1 serving)	3.5	23.0	3.7	3.0	0.3	0	52.0
Spinach, raw (1 serving)	2.0	14.4	2.4	1.8	0.2	0	39.4
Squash, summer, raw (1 serving)	3.1	16.7	3.7	0.9	0.1	0	0.7

	Weight (oz.)	Calories	Carbo-hydrates (g.)	Protein (g.)	Fat (g.)	Cholesterol (mg.)	Sodium (mg.)
Squash, summer, steamed w/o salt, drained (1 serving)	3.5	14.0	3.1	0.9	0.1	0	1.0
Squash, winter, baked w/o salt (¼ average)	3.5	126.0	30.8	3.6	0.8	0	2.0
Squash, winter, steamed w/o salt, drained (1 serving)	3.5	38.0	9.2	1.1	0.3	0	1.0
Squash Amandine, ETS recipe (1 serving)	8.0	221.4	16.9	11.7	13.1	9.1	293.7
Steamed Vegetable Platter, ETW approved (1 serving)	8.2	98.8	20.4	5.2	0.9	0	35.4
Sweet Potato, baked, w/skin (1 average)	10.5	254.0	58.5	3.8	0.9	0	22.0
Sweet Potato, raw, w/skin (1 average)	11.7	382.7	88.3	5.7	1.3	0	33.6
Sweet Potatoes Discipio, ETS recipe (1 serving)	10.5	296.6	67.6	4.7	1.2	1.1	30.7
Tofu (1 serving)	2.9	59.6	2.0	6.5	3.5	0	5.8
Tomato, raw (1 average)	4.7	29.3	6.3	1.5	0.3	0	4.0
Tomato Paste, canned, w/salt (3½ ounces)	3.5	81.4	18.5	3.4	0.4	0	783.9
Tomato Puree, canned, regular pack (3½ ounces)	3.5	38.7	8.8	1.7	0.2	0	395.9
Tomato Sauce, canned (3½ ounces)	3.5	36.0	7.2	1.4	0.2	0	523.3
Tomatoes, canned, solids and liquid (1 serving)	4.4	26.2	5.4	1.2	0.2	0	162.1
Tomatoes, canned, solids only (3½ ounces)	3.5	20.8	4.3	1.0	0.2	0	129.0
Turnip Greens, boiled w/o salt, drained (1 serving)	3.5	20.0	3.6	2.2	0.2	0	50.0
Turnips, boiled w/o salt, drained (1 serving)	3.5	23.0	4.9	0.8	0.2	0	34.0
Water Chestnuts, Chinese, raw (16 average)	3.5	79.0	19.0	1.4	0.2	0	20.0
Watercress, raw (1 serving)	1.8	9.5	1.5	1.1	0.1	0	26.0
Wax Beans, boiled w/o salt, drained (1 serving)	3.5	22.0	4.6	1.4	0.2	0	3.0
White Beans, cooked (1 serving)	3.5	120.0	23.0	6.3	0.5	0	338.0
Zucchini, raw (1 average)	3.1	16.7	3.7	0.9	0.1	0	0.7
Zucchini, steamed w/o salt, drained (1 serving)	3.5	12.0	2.5	1.0	0.1	0	1.0
Zucchini and Cauliflower Italian, ETS recipe (1 serving)	6.0	47.8	8.0	3.4	0.9	1.3	175.9

APPENDIXES

Nutritional Supplements: The TwinSport Formulary

TwinSport, of Ronkonkoma, New York, manufactures some of the highest quality and most scientifically advanced nutritional supplements on the market today. Each formula contains the purest and highest quality ingredients, some of which can only be obtained in foreign countries at considerable expense. At this time, my own personal vitamin program consists solely of the TwinSport Endurance brand of nutritional supplements. While there are several other nutritional-supplement manufacturers who make excellent products, at present TwinSport products meet the high standards of purity and quality I demand in nutritional supplements. If you choose another brand of nutritional supplements, select those which conform most closely to those listed below. TwinSport based their formulation of the following products to a large extent on the nutritional recommendations in *Eat to Win* and *Eat to Succeed*. I presently consult with TwinSport to insure that they consistently manufacture those products that conform to my nutritional recommendations.

A SPECIAL NOTE ABOUT NUTRITIONAL SUPPLEMENTS

Because of the biochemical uniqueness of each of our bodies, no two people possess exactly the same daily requirements for vitamins, minerals, protein, and other vital nutrients. Special circumstances, such as stress, physical activity, age, sex, illness, diet, and genetics all play a role in determining the amounts of specific nutrients we each need every day. Some people apparently remain quite healthy and free of diet-related diseases without relying on nutritional supplements. Other people find that nutritional supplements help them to enjoy greater endurance, stamina, and maximum performance.

Nutritional supplements are, in most cases, mandatory for optimal health during calorically restricted periods of weight loss. And today, more than ever before, physicians and dietitians are recommending nutritional supplements to prevent, manage, and cure a host of diet-related health problems, from anemia to heart disease.

I recommend that *anyone who begins a nutritional supplementation program consult with his or her physician, dietitian, or nutritionist before starting such a program.* Health care organizations, such as Bio-Nutronics (see Appendix III), now scientifically formulate nutritional supplements based on individual body chemistry and life-style.

The following information on the TwinSport Endurance line of products was supplied by the manufacturer. Remember to consult your physician or qualified nutritionist before beginning any nutritional supplement program.

ENDURANCE ATHLETIC STRESS FORMULA

Strenuous exercise or physical activity increases the need for water-soluble vitamins C and B-complex. This specially developed formula replenishes these antistress vitamins to help you maintain peak performance during intense physical exertion. The formula is rich in pantothenic acid, which plays a key role in energy production. Research shows that pantothenic acid can offset the stress of heavy training and is very important to athletes who perform in extreme weather conditions, especially cold. One or two hard gelatin capsules per day provides maximum protection for athletes and people with overactive schedules. (Available in bottles of 50 or 100 capsules.)

NUTRITIONAL INFORMATION

Two hard gelatin capsules provide:		% U.S. RDA			% U.S. RDA
Vitamin C	1000 mg.	1666	Vitamin B-12		
Vitamin B-1			(cobalamin		
(thiamine)	50 mg.	3333	concentrate)	250 mcg.	4166
Vitamin B-2			Biotin	100 mcg.	33
(riboflavin)	50 mg.	2941	PABA (para-		
Vitamin B-6			aminobenzoic		
(pyridoxine)	50 mg.	2500	acid)	50 mg.	*
Niacinamide	100 mg.	500	Folic acid	400 mcg.	100
Pantothenic Acid			Choline bitartrate	100 mg.	*
(from d-calcium			Inositol	100 mg.	*
pantothenate)	250 mg.	2500			

*No U.S. RDA has been established.

Each capsule is free of coatings, binders, and colors which may cause adverse reactions in people with allergies or on special diets. Also free of corn, soy, yeast, wheat, milk, egg, and all fruit and grain products.

ENDURANCE ANABOLIC FORMULA

New free-form amino acid and vitamin mix for serious bodybuilders and endurance athletes. Contains a rich blend of l-arginine, l-ornithine, and l-carnitine, as well as branched-chain amino acids l-leucine, l-isoleucine and l-valine in a special, scientifically formulated ratio that maximizes results. Studies indicate branched-chain amino acids minimize muscle protein breakdown and maximize muscle protein synthesis. Three or more hard gelatin capsules per day provide a natural alternative to steroids.

NUTRITIONAL INFORMATION

Each hard gelatin capsule provides:

L-arginine	225 mg.
L-ornithine..	225 mg.
L-carnitine	25 mg.
Branched-chain amino acid mix (l-leucine, l-valine, l-isoleucine)....	225 mg.
Vitamin B-6...	5 mg.
Pantothenic acid	10 mg.

Branched chain amino acids are the most abundant amino acids found in muscle tissue. The branched chain amino acids l-leucine, l-isoleucine, and l-valine in this formula are in a special patent pending scientifically formulated ratio for maximum utilization. B-6 is required for the natural metabolism of l-arginine and l-ornithine. Pantothenic acid is required for the natural metabolism of l-carnitine. B-6 and l-carnitine are also required for the natural metabolism of branched chain amino acids. Each capsule is free of coatings, binders, and colors which may cause adverse reactions in people with allergies or on special diets. Also free of corn, soy, yeast, wheat, milk, egg, and all fruit and grain products.

ENDURANCE DIET AID CAPSULES

Recent studies indicate that some high-fiber foods help promote weight loss. These revolutionary capsules contain a new all-natural, bulk-producing dietary fiber blend derived from fruit, vegetables, and grain. Combined with a well-balanced diet and exercise program, they will help you lose weight by increasing your consumption of bulk fiber and reducing your caloric intake—without regular use of drugs or other unnatural foods. Taking three capsules before meals increases your feeling of fullness, which helps curb your appetite. (Available in bottles of 50 or 100 capsules.)

NUTRITIONAL INFORMATION

One hard gelatin capsule provides:

Bulk-forming fiber blend (glucomannan, guar gum, psyllium seed husk, apple pectin).......................................	800 mg.

Each capsule is free of coatings, binders, and colors which may cause adverse reactions in people with allergies or on special diets. Also free of corn, soy, yeast, wheat, milk, and egg products.

ENDURANCE MAXIMUM PERFORMANCE FORMULA

A scientifically formulated competitive edge for serious athletes. Each hard gelatin capsule provides a unique synergistic combination of nutrients that help reduce muscle fatigue. Ingredients include inosine, which increases production of ATP, an important energy donor in the body, and natural sodium phosphate, which helps athletes utilize oxygen more efficiently, reducing lactic acid levels in the blood and postponing fatigue. Also contains l-carnitine, CoQ10, pantothenic acid, lipoic acid, magnesium aspartate, and other peak performance nutrients. (Available in bottles of 50 or 100 capsules.)

NUTRITIONAL INFORMATION

Three hard gelatin capsules provide:

Soluble sodium		Vitamin B-3	
phosphate	100 mg.	(niacinamide)	50 mg.
Inosine	250 mg.	Pantothenic acid	
L-carnitine	100 mg.	(from d-calcium	
CoQ10 (coenzyme		pantothenate)	500 mg.
Q_{10})	10 mg.	Biotin............	25 mcg.
Lipoic acid	100 mcg.	Bio-formed GTF	
Vitamin B-1	25 mg.	chromium	200 mcg.
Vitamin B-2	25 mg.	Magnesium	
Vitamin B-6	25 mg.	aspartate	250 mg.

The magnesium aspartate in this formula is imported from Japan and is of the highest quality available. Each capsule is free of coatings, binders, and colors which may cause adverse reactions in people with allergies or on special diets. Also free of corn, soy, wheat, milk, and egg products.

ENDURANCE MULTIVITAMIN FITNESS PAKS

The foundation of any endurance program, whether you're trying to lose weight, gain weight, build strength, stamina, or whatever. Each pak contains seven hard gelatin capsules that, taken daily, provide an optimum balance of vitamins, minerals, trace elements, and antioxidants that athletes and active people need for peak health and fitness, like B-complex vitamins, which can increase endurance by helping convert food into energy; vitamin C for fast, healthy tissue growth and repair; and high-potency antioxidant nutrients (vitamins, A, C, E, and beta carotene, plus the mineral selenium), which may help reduce oxygen toxicity and protect the body from air pollution. Key minerals include calcium, magnesium, iodine, iron, chromium, and zinc. Each capsule is easy to swallow and assimilate. (Available in box of 30 paks, a 30-day supply.)

NUTRITIONAL INFORMATION

Each Endurance Multi Vitamin Fitness Pak contains seven hard gelatin capsules which supply the following:

VITAMIN A, BETA-CAROTENE, VITAMIN D, AND VITAMIN E (1 capsule)

One capsule contains:		%U.S. RDA
Dry vitamin A (oil-free, water dispersed, from vitamin A acetate) ..	10,000 IU	200
Dry beta-carotene (oil-free, water dispersed, pro–vitamin A activity)	15,000 IU	300
Total vitamin A activity......................................	25,000 IU	500
Dry vitamin D (oil-free, water dispersed, from natural form vitamin D-3)..	400 IU	100
Dry natural vitamin E (oil-free, water dispersed, d-alpha tocopherol succinate)	400 IU	1333

VITAMIN C (1 capsule)

One capsule contains:

Vitamin C...	1000 mg.	1666

VITAMIN B-COMPLEX (1 capsule)

One capsule contains:

Vitamin B-1..	50 mg.	3333
Vitamin B-2..	50 mg.	2941
Vitamin B-3 (niacinamide).................................	50 mg.	250
Vitamin B-6..	50 mg.	2500
Pantothenic Acid..	50 mg.	500
Vitamin B-12...	50 mcg.	833
Folic Acid...	400 mcg.	100
Biotin	50 mcg.	16
PABA	50 mg.	*
Choline bitartrate.......................................	50 mg.	*
Inositol	50 mg.	*

MULTIMINERALS (4 capsules)

Four capsules contain:

Calcium (from natural oyster shell and calcium orotate)...........	1000 mg.	100
Magnesium (from natural magnesium oxide, magnesium aspartate, and magnesium orotate)................................	500 mg.	125
Zinc (chelated as zinc gluconate and zinc orotate)...............	30 mg.	200
Manganese (chelated as manganese gluconate)..................	10 mg.	*
Iron (chelated as ferrous fumarate)	10 mg.	100
Copper (chelated as copper gluconate).......................	2 mg.	100
Iodine (from kelp)..	150 mcg.	100
Natural Form Selenium....................................	200 mcg.	*
Natural Trivalent Chromium................................	200 mcg.	*
Natural Molybdenum.....................................	500 mcg.	*

*No RDA has been established

Each capsule is free of coatings, binders, and colors which may cause adverse reactions in people with allergies or on special diets. Also free of corn, yeast, wheat, milk, and egg products.

ENDURANCE WEIGHT GAIN POWDER

Mixed with low-fat milk, Endurance Weight Gain Powder becomes a great-tasting and nutritious food supplement rich in bodybuilding elements. Because it's low in fats and oils, it contains more natural weight-gaining carbohydrates for extra energy, high-quality milk and egg proteins for proper muscle growth and development, and a unique blend of vitamins, minerals, dietary fiber, and digestive enzymes to aid absorption of nutrients. A healthy supply of crystalline fructose provides more sustained energy than glucose, which is used in many competitive products. Two servings per day combined with resistive exercise or weight training promote lean bodybuilding weight gain. (Available in 16-ounce can.)

NUTRITIONAL INFORMATION

Serving size: 1 rounded measuring scoop (42 grams)
Servings per container: 10

Each Serving Provides	1 Serving with 16 Oz. Low-Fat Milk (1% Milk Fat)
Calories	410
Protein	24 g.
Carbohydrate	52 g.
Fat..................	6 g.
Fiber................	4.2 g.

Percentage of Adult U.S. Recommended Daily Allowance (U.S. RDA)

Protein...................	50	Phosphorus	65
Vitamin A................	45	Iodine...................	35
Vitamin C (ascorbic acid)....	40	Magnesium	45
Thiamine (vitamin B-1)	40	Zinc	40
Riboflavin (vitamin B-2).....	60	Copper..................	35
Niacin...................	35	Biotin	35
Calcium	75	Pantothenic acid	45
Iron.....................	35	Manganese	1 mg.*
Vitamin D	60	Potassium................	75 mg.*
Vitamin E	35	Selenium.................	10 mcg.*
Vitamin B-6	40	Chromium................	10 mcg.*
Folic acid	30	Molybdenum.............	10 mcg.*
Vitamin B-12	50		

*No U.S. RDA established

Ingredients: Nonfat dry milk, crystalline pure fructose, whey, maltodextrin (a natural complex carbohydrate), calcium caseinate (milk protein), egg albumin (egg white protein), fiber blend (cellulose, oat bran, soy bran, psyllium seed husk, guar gum), lecithin, vanilla flavor, wheat germ, digestive enzyme mix (bromelain, papain, pancreatin 4NF), and the following vitamins and minerals: magnesium oxide, ascorbic acid, vitamin E acetate, iron, niacinamide, calcium pantothenate, zinc oxide, manganese, copper gluconate, vitamin A palmitate, vitamin D, vitamin B-12, pyridoxine, hydrochloride, thiamine, riboflavin, biotin, folic acid, potassium iodide, natural form selenium, chromium, and molybdenum.

ENDURANCE MEAL REPLACEMENT AND WEIGHT CONTROL FORMULA

A nutritionally balanced low-calorie powdered diet drink formulated to replace one or two meals per day and help you lose weight. Mixed with 8 fluid ounces of fortified skim milk, each serving is only 190 calories. Contains a rich supply of crystalline fructose to provide extra energy while you're dieting. Studies also show that crystalline fructose helps suppress appetite with less food intake, which may make dieting easier for you. Endurance formula can be used as a complete fitness and pregame meal, too. Because it's a liquid, it digests easily. It also assures an intake of fluid while contributing extra energy for competition. The best-tasting product of its kind ever developed. (Available in chocolate or vanilla flavors in 16-ounce can.)

NUTRITIONAL INFORMATION

Serving size: 1 ounce
Servings per container: 16

Each serving provides	1 Serving Plain	1 Serving with 8 Oz. Protein-Fortified Skim Milk
Calories........	90	190
Protein	5 g.	15 g.
Carbohydrate ...	18 g.	31 g.
Fat .. less than	1 g.	1 g.
Fiber..........	2 g.	2 g.

Percentage of Adult U.S. Recommended Daily Allowance (U.S. RDA)

Protein	10	35	Folic acid	20	25
Vitamin A......	25	35	Vitamin B-12 ...	20	35
Vitamin C			Phosphorus.....	15	40
(ascorbic acid).	30	35	Iodine	35	35
Thiamine			Magnesium.....	25	35
(vitamin B-1) .	30	35	Zinc..........	30	35
Riboflavin			Copper	35	35
(vitamin B-2) .	10	35	Biotin	35	35
Niacin	35	35	Pantothenic acid	25	35
Calcium	15	50	Manganese	1 mg.*	1 mg.*
Iron	35	35	Potassium	240 mg.*	680 mg.*
Vitamin D......	10	35	Chromium	10 mcg.*	10 mcg.*
Vitamin E......	35	35	Selenium	10 mcg.*	10 mcg.*
Vitamin B-6	30	35	Molybdenum ...	10 mcg.*	10 mcg.*

*No U.S. RDA established.

Ingredients: Nonfat dry milk, crystalline pure fructose, whey powder, calcium caseinate (milk protein), fiber blend (cellulose, oat bran, soy bran, psyllium seed husk, guar gum), cocoa or vanilla flavor, maltodextrin (a natural complex carbohydrate), lecithin, wheat germ, carrageenin, and the following vitamins and minerals: magnesium oxide, tricalcium phosphate, potassium citrate, iron, vitamin E acetate, ascorbic acid, niacinamide, vitamin A palmitate, zinc oxide, copper gluconate, calcium pantothenate, manganese, vitamin B-12, pyridoxine hydrochloride, vitamin D, thiamine, riboflavin, biotin, folic acid, potassium iodide, natural form selenium, chromium, and molybdenum.

ENDURANCE QUICKFIX

A delicious, all-weather powdered drink that energizes and refreshes by replacing vital body fluids lost during exercise and intense physical exertion. Low-calorie scientific formula mixes with water to replenish potassium and magnesium electrolytes and aspartates, thus helping reduce muscle fatigue and cramping. Easily digested complex carbohydrates replace spent muscle glycogen for energy. Also contains antistress vitamins C and B-complex. No added sugar or salt (sodium). (Available in 5.6-ounce jar of 20 servings.)

NUTRITIONAL INFORMATION

Serving size: 1 tablespoon (8 grams)
Servings per container: 20

Calories	23
Protein	0
Fat	0
Carbohydrate	6 g.

		% U.S. RDA			% U.S. RDA
Vitamin C	500 mg.	833	PABA	1 mg.	*
Vitamin B-1	1.5 mg.	100	Choline bitartrate	2 mg.	*
Vitamin B-2	1.7 mg.	100	Inositol	2 mg.	*
Vitamin B-3 (niacinamide)	5 mg.	25	Potassium (from potassium aspartate and potassium citrate)	100 mg.	*
Vitamin B-6	2 mg.	100			
Pantothenic acid	10 mg.	100			
Vitamin B-12	6 mcg.	100			
Folic acid	100 mcg.	25	Magnesium (from magnesium aspartate)	50 mg.	13
Biotin	100 mcg.	33			

*No RDA has been established.

The potassium and magnesium aspartate in this product are imported from Japan and are of the highest quality available. No preservatives, artificial color or flavors.

Ingredients: maltodextrin (a natural complex carbohydrate), ascorbic acid, citric acid, 100% natural orange flavor, potassium aspartate, magnesium aspartate, potassium citrate, aspartame*(Nutra-Sweet Brand),† beta-carotene, and the following vitamins: vitamin C, pantothenic acid (from d-calcium pantothenate), niacinamide, choline bitartrate, inositol, vitamin B-6, vitamin B-2, vitamin B-1, PABA (para-aminobenzoic acid), folic acid, biotin, vitamin B-12.

*Phenylketonurics: contains phenylalanine.
†Nutra-Sweet is a trademark of G. D. Searle & Co.

Liquid Meal Replacement Formulary

TWINSPORT ENDURANCE MEAL REPLACEMENT AND WEIGHT CONTROL FORMULA

Serving size: 1 ounce
Servings per container: 16

TwinSport
Twin Laboratories
2120 Smithtown Avenue
Ronkonkoma, NY 11779

Each Serving Provides	*1 serving with 8 oz. of Protein-Fortified Skim Milk*
Calories	190
Protein	15 g.
Carbohydrates	31 g.
Fat..................	1 g.
Fiber................	2 g.

Percentage of Adult U.S. Recommended Daily Allowance (U.S. RDA)

Protein	35	Iodine................	35
Vitamin A	35	Magnesium	35
Vitamin C (ascorbic acid)	35	Zinc	35
		Copper...............	35
Thiamine (vitamin B-1)..	35	Biotin	35
Riboflavin (vitamin B-2) .	35	Pantothenic acid........	35
Niacin................	35	Manganese	1 mg.*
Calcium	50	Potassium..............	680 mg.*
Iron	35	Chromium.............	10 mcg.*
Vitamin D	35	Selenium	10 mcg.*
Vitamin E	35	Molybdenum...........	10 mcg.*
Vitamin B-6...........	35	Oat bran	†
Folic acid.............	25	Soy bran	†
Vitamin B-12..........	35	Psyllium seed husk	†
Phosphorous	40	Guar gum	†

*No U.S. RDA established.
†Product contains fiber, but label does not specify amount.

297

YOUR LIFE NATURAL WEIGHT LOSS PLAN

Serving size: 1 ounce
Servings per container

Your Life Products, Inc.
Torrance, CA 90501

	1 Serving with 8 Oz. Protein-Fortified Skim Milk
Each Serving Provides	
Calories	190
Protein	13 g.
Carbohydrates	29 g.
Fat...................	3 g.
Fiber................	2 g.

Percentage of Adult U.S. Recommended Daily Allowance (U.S. RDA)

Protein...............	30	Iodine................	35
Vitamin A.............	35	Magnesium	35
Vitamin C (ascorbic acid)		Zinc	35
....	35	Copper...............	35
Thiamine (vitamin B-1)..	35	Biotin	35
Riboflavin (vitamin B-2) .	35	Pantothenic acid.......	35
Niacin................	35	Manganese	1 mg*
Calcium	45	Potassium.............	620 mg.*
Iron	35	Chromium.............	N
Vitamin D.............	35	Selenium	N
Vitamin E	35	Molybdenum...........	N
Vitamin B-6...........	35	Oat bran	N
Folic acid.............	35	Soy bran	N
Vitamin B-12..........	35	Psyllium seed husk	N
Phosphorus	40	Guar Gum.............	N

*No U.S. RDA established.
N: Product does not contain this substance.

SLIM FAST

Serving size: 1 ounce
Servings per container: 16

Thompson Medical Company, Inc.
919 Third Avenue
New York, NY 10022

	1 Serving with 8 Oz. Protein-Fortified Skim Milk
Calories...............	190 g.
Protein...............	15 g.
Carbohydrates	32 g.
Fat	1 g.
Fiber	2 g.

Percentage of Adult U.S. Recommended Daily Allowance (U.S. RDA)

Protein	35	Iodine	35
Vitamin A	35	Magnesium	35
Vitamin C (ascorbic acid)		Zinc	35
	35	Copper	35
Thiamine (vitamin B-1)	35	Biotin	35
Riboflavin (vitamin B-2)	35	Pantothenic acid	35
Niacin	35	Manganese	1 mg.*
Calcium	50	Potassium	680 mg.*
Iron	35	Chromium	N
Vitamin D	35	Selenium	N
Vitamin E	35	Molybdenum	N
Vitamin B-6	35	Oat bran	N
Folic acid	25	Soy bran	N
Vitamin B-12	35	Psyllium seed husk	N
Phosphorus	40	Guar gum	N

*No U.S. RDA established.
N: Product does not contain this substance

DIETENE

Serving Size: 1 ounce
Servings per container: 16

Creighton Product Corporation
New York, NY 10158

Each Serving Provides	*1 Serving with 8 Oz. Protein-Fortified Skim Milk*
Calories	190
Protein	16 g.
Carbohydrates	29 g.
Fat	1 g.
Fiber	N

Percentage of Adult U.S. Recommended Daily Allowance (U.S. RDA)

Protein	35	Iodine	50
Vitamin A	35	Magnesium	35
Vitamin C (ascorbic acid)		Zinc	35
	35	Copper	35
Thiamine (vitamin B-1)	35	Biotin	50
Riboflavin (vitamin B-2)	45	Pantothenic acid	35
Niacin	35	Manganese	N
Calcium	50	Potassium	650 mg.*
Iron	35	Chromium	N
Vitamin D	50	Selenium	N
Vitamin E	35	Molybdenum	N
Vitamin B-6	35	Oat bran	N
Folic acid	35	Soy bran	N
Vitamin B-12	35	Psyllium seed husk	N
Phosphorus	40	Guar gum	N

*No U.S. RDA established.
N: Product does not contain this substance.

CARNATION DO-IT-YOURSELF DIET PLAN

Serving size: 1.06 ounce
Servings per container: 12

Carnation
5045 Wilshire Boulevard
Los Angeles, CA 90036

Each Serving Provides	1 Serving with 6 Oz. Protein- Fortified Skim Milk
Calories	200
Protein	11 g.
Carbohydrates	30 g.
Fat.................	5 g.
Fiber................	1.5 g.

Percentage of Adult U.S. Recommended Daily Allowance (U.S. RDA)

Protein	25	Iodine...............	25
Vitamin A	25	Magnesium	25
Vitamin C (ascorbic acid)		Zinc	25
....	25	Copper...............	25
Thiamine (vitamin B-1)..	25	Biotin...............	25
Riboflavin (vitamin B-2) .	25	Pantothenic acid.......	25
Niacin................	25	Manganese	N
Calcium	25	Potassium.............	N
Iron	25	Chromium.............	N
Vitamin D	25	Selenium	N
Vitamin E	25	Molybdenum...........	N
Vitamin B-6...........	25	Oat bran	N
Folic acid.............	25	Soy bran	N
Vitamin B-12..........	25	Psyllium seed husk	N
Phosphorus	25	Guar gum	N

N: Product does not contain this substance.

PILLSBURY INSTANT BREAKFAST

Serving size: 1.3 ounce (1 pouch)
Servings per container: 10

Pillsbury Company
Minneapolis, MN 55402

Each Serving Provides	1 Serving with 8 Oz. Milk
Calories...............	290
Protein	14 g.
Carbohydrate	38 g.
Fat.................	9 g.
Fiber................	N

Percentage of Adult U.S. Recommended Daily Allowance (U.S. RDA)

Protein	25	Thiamine (vitamin B-1)..	25
Vitamin A	30	Riboflavin (vitamin B-2) .	25
Vitamin C (ascorbic acid)	30	Niacin................	25

Calcium	25	Biotin	N	
Iron	25	Pantothenic acid	N	
Vitamin D	25	Manganese	N	
Vitamin E	25	Potassium	620 mg.*	
Vitamin B-6	25	Chromium	N	
Folic acid	25	Selenium	N	
Vitamin B-12	25	Molybdenum	N	
Phosphorus	25	Oat bran	N	
Magnesium	25	Soy bran	N	
Iodine	25	Psyllium seed husk	N	
Zinc	N	Guar gum	N	
Copper	N			

*No U.S. RDA established.
N: Product does not contain this substance.

CARNATION INSTANT BREAKFAST

Serving size: 1.25 ounce (1 envelope)
Servings per container: 6

Carnation
5045 Wilshire Boulevard
Los Angeles, CA 90036

Each Serving Provides	1 Serving with 8 Oz. Milk
Calories	280
Protein	15 g.
Carbohydrates	34 g.
Fat	9 g.
Fiber	N

Percentage of Adult U.S. Recommended Daily Allowance (U.S. RDA)

Protein	35	Iodine	30
Vitamin A	40	Magnesium	30
Vitamin C (ascorbic acid)		Zinc	25
	50	Copper	25
Thiamine (vitamin B-1)	25	Biotin	N
Riboflavin (vitamin B-2)	30	Pantothenic acid	25
Niacin	25	Manganese	N
Calcium	40	Potassium	N
Iron	25	Chromium	N
Vitamin D	25	Selenium	N
Vitamin E	25	Molybdenum	N
Vitamin B-6	25	Oat bran	N
Folic acid	25	Soy bran	N
Vitamin B-12	25	Psyllium seed husk	N
Phosphorus	25	Guar gum	N

N: Product does not contain this substance.

SLENDER DIET MEAL FOR WEIGHT CONTROL

Serving Size: 10 fluid ounces
Servings per container: 1

Carnation
5045 Wilshire Boulevard
Los Angeles, CA 90036

Each Serving Provides

Calories...............	220
Protein...............	11 g.
Carbohydrate.........	34 g.
Fat...................	4 g.
Fiber................	N

Percentage of Adult U.S. Recommended Daily Allowance (U.S. RDA)

Protein................	25	Iodine................	25
Vitamin A.............	25	Magnesium............	25
Vitamin C (ascorbic acid)		Zinc.................	25
....	25	Copper...............	25
Thiamine (vitamin B-1)..	25	Biotin................	25
Riboflavin (vitamin B-2) .	25	Pantothenic acid........	25
Niacin................	25	Manganese	N
Calcium...............	25	Potassium.............	N
Iron	25	Chromium.............	N
Vitamin D.............	25	Selenium	N
Vitamin E.............	25	Molybdenum...........	N
Vitamin B-6...........	25	Oat bran	N
Folic acid.............	25	Soy bran	N
Vitamin B-12..........	25	Psyllium seed husk	N
Phosphorus	25	Guar gum	N

N: Product does not contain this substance.

MERITENE

Serving size: 1.14 ounce
Servings per container: 14

Sandoz Nutrition
5320 West Twenty-Third Street
P.O. Box 370
Minneapolis, MN 55440

Each Serving Provides	*1 Serving with 8 Oz. Milk*
Calories...............	275
Protein	18 g.
Carbohydrate.........	31 g.
Fat...................	9.1 g.
Fiber................	N

Percentage of Adult U.S. Recommended Daily Allowance (U.S. RDA)

Protein................	40	Thiamine (vitamin B-1)..	25
Vitamin A.............	25	Riboflavin (vitamin B-2) .	40
Vitamin C (ascorbic acid)	25	Niacin................	25

Calcium	60	Biotin	25
Iron	25	Pantothenic acid	25
Vitamin D	25	Manganese	1.0 mg.*
Vitamin E	25	Potassium	.73 mg.*
Vitamin B-6	25	Chromium	N
Folic acid	25	Selenium	N
Vitamin B-12	30	Molybdenum	N
Phosphorus	50	Oat bran	N
Iodine	25	Soy bran	N
Magnesium	25	Psyllium seed husk	N
Zinc	25	Guar gum	N
Copper	25		

*No U.S. RDA established.
N: Product does not contain this subtance.

ENSURE

Serving size: 2 ounces
Servings per container: 7

Ross Laboratories
Columbus, OH 43216

Each Serving Provides	1 Serving with 6 Oz. Milk
Calories	250
Protein	8.8 g.
Carbohydrates	34.3 g.
Fat	8.8 g.
Fiber	N

Percentage of Adult U.S. Recommended Daily Allowance (U.S. RDA)

Protein	14	Iodine	12.5
Vitamin A	12.5	Magnesium	12.5
Vitamin C (ascorbic acid)	62.5	Zinc	25
Thiamine (vitamin B-1)	25	Copper	12.5
Riboflavin (vitamin B-2)	25	Biotin	12.5
Niacin	25	Pantothenic acid	12.5
Calcium	12.5	Manganese	.5 mg.*
Iron	12.5	Potassium	1.5 g.*
Vitamin D	12.5	Chromium	N
Vitamin E	19	Selenium	N
Vitamin B-6	25	Molybdenum	N
Folic acid	12.5	Oat bran	N
Vitamin B-12	25	Soy bran	N
Phosphorus	12.5	Psyllium seed husk	N
		Guar gum	N

*No U.S. RDA established.
N: Product does not contain this substance.

APPENDIX III

The Haas-Recommended List of Nutrition Organizations

The following health organizations provide excellent nutritional counseling and health advisory services consistent with the state-of-the-art research in nutritional science. Each organization will provide program details and information upon request.

BIO-NUTRIONICS

Bio-Nutrionics is a New York City–based health care organization that uses state-of-the-art computer programs and nutritionists to evaluate, analyze, and construct diets, nutritional supplement programs, and exercise regimens for the general public. I have consulted with this organization for the last two years and have seen impressive results in weight loss, blood lipid and blood pressure reductions, and general improvement in the health and well-being of program participants. I believe that Bio-Nutrionics will become a major U.S. health care organization for people who want to lose excess body fat, gain energy, and achieve maximum performance and a high-quality life. The Bio-Nutrionics program closely follows much of the nutritional philosophy of my *Eat to Win/Eat to Succeed* programs.

BIO-NUTRIONICS
1345 AVENUE OF THE AMERICAS
NEW YORK, NY 10105
(212)586-8455

DOCTOR'S HOSPITAL

Doctor's Hospital offers a three-day intensive VIP in-patient program based on the Haas diet. The program includes complete medical/nutritional evaluation and diet and exercise education. The hospital's staff of dietitians has been specially trained in creating high–complex carbohydrate, low-fat/low-cholesterol diets.

DOCTOR'S HOSPITAL
1859 VAN BUREN STREET
HOLLYWOOD, FL 33020
(315)920-9000

304

FIT FOR THE ROAD

Fit for the Road is a health-care system for touring musicians and performers who must sustain high energy levels while on the road. Fit for the Road provides individual exercise trainers, cooks, and special diets to well-known musical groups and solo artists, as well as to actors and actresses. The organization also provides "in-town" personalized programs for its Los Angeles–based clients.

FIT FOR THE ROAD
22458 VENTURA BOULEVARD
SUITE E
WOODLAND HILLS, CA 91364

COOPER CLINIC AEROBICS CENTER

Dr. Kenneth Cooper, who founded the Aerobics Center, was one of the first health-care professionals to recognize the importance of regular aerobic exercise in a total health program of diet and exercise. The Cooper Clinic Aerobics Center provides fitness evaluations and nutritional counseling.

COOPER CLINIC AEROBICS CENTER
12202 PRESTON ROAD
RICHARDSON, TX
(214)239-7223

KUSHI INSTITUTE

The Kushi Institute is devoted to the study and teaching of the macrobiotic way of life. Macrobiotics is a dietary and philosophical program that teaches adherents how to balance their diets and other aspects of their lives through the Oriental principles of opposites (called yin and yang). The macrobiotic diet is a high-complex carbohydrate, low-fat, low-protein regime composed of ordinary and exotic foods.

KUSHI INSTITUTE
17 STATION STREET
BOSTON, MA
(617)731-0564

PRITIKIN LONGEVITY INSTITUTE

The Pritikin Longevity Institute offers a series of live-in and walk-in health programs based on the dietary philosophy of the late Nathan Pritikin. The Pritikin diet is a complex carbohydrate–based regimen.

PRITIKIN LONGEVITY INSTITUTE
1910 OCEANFRONT WALK
SANTA MONICA, CA
(213)870-2944

THE HAAS HEALTH LETTER

For those interested in staying abreast of the latest nutritional discoveries, current trends in health-related issues, newly developed Haas recipes, and Haas-recommended foods, supplements, and exercise products, I have created the *Haas Health Letter*, a quarterly publication devoted to health and nutrition. It gives you vital new health-related information, tips, and recipes long before the general public learns about them. Those interested in receiving a free copy of this newsletter and subscription information may write to me at:

P.O. BOX 69-3912
NORLAND BRANCH
MIAMI, FL 33169

Eat to Win™ Computer Software

What Is the *Eat to Win*™ Computer Program?

The *Eat to Win* computer program is a nutrition spread sheet and data base manager for foods, recipes, menus, daily food intake, and body weight. Its main functions are to:

• Monitor daily food intake and body weight for an unlimited number of people, over any length of time.

• Compare nutrition in foods, recipes, and daily menus; calorie, carbohydrate, protein, fat, sodium, and cholesterol values are recorded.

• Determine the percent of calories from carbohydrate, protein, and fat.

• Manage the nutritional information for up to 2,000 individual foods: 1,187 foods have been provided; you may add 813 more.

• Adjust recipes and menus to meet individual needs. Three hundred recipes/menus can be stored per data diskette; ninety-four recipes from the book *Eat to Win*, by Dr. Robert Haas, have been provided.

• List recipes and menus that contain a particular food.

• Select food quantities by weight, capacity, servings, slices, or whole items; grams, kilograms, ounces, pounds, milliliters, liters, teaspoons, tablespoons, fluid ounces, cups, quarts, and gallons are available.

• Convert food quantities from one unit of measure to another.

• Select food quantities by decimal numbers or common fractions (e.g., 3.5 or 3½ ounces).

• Select food quantities based on nutritional value. For example, request that a food provide 15 grams of protein and the *Eat to Win* computer program will determine the proper amount of that food.

• Print graphs, tables, and food lists. See the sample reports that follow.

What Is the *Eat to Win*—Calorie Burner™ Computer Program?

The *Eat to Win*—Calorie Burner computer program is a spread sheet and data base manager for daily activities and body weight. It will allow you to:

• Monitor the daily activity and body weight of an unlimited number of people, over any length of time.

EAT TO WIN™ SOFTWARE
(DIAGRAMMATIC OVERVIEW)

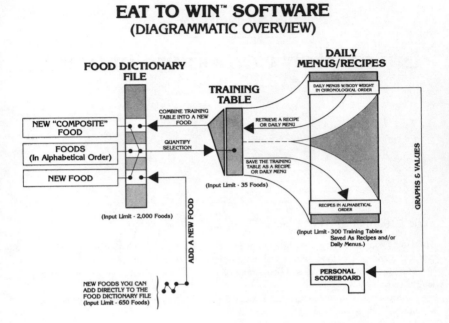

- Compare the number of calories burned by various activities.
- Adjust daily activity schedules to meet individual needs.
- Determine how much time various activities require to burn a desired number of calories. For example, you wish to know how much time you must spend walking at 3 mph to burn 300 calories; the program will determine the necessary amount of time based on your current body weight.

Eat to Win computer programs are available from:
Small Planet Systems Corporation
P.O. Box 4011
Tallahassee, FL 32315-4011
(904)224-9004

Eat to Win computer programs are available for IBM and IBM-compatible computers, CP/M computers, and Apple computers.

SAMPLE REPORTS

BODY WEIGHT

Pounds	150	155	160	165	170	175	180
01-Aug-84—Wed						*	
02-Aug-84—Thu					*		
03-Aug-84—Fri					*		
04-Aug-84—Sat					*		
05-Aug-84—Sun					*		
06-Aug-84—Mon					*		
07-Aug-84—Tue					*		
08-Aug-84—Wed					*		
09-Aug-84—Thu				*			
10-Aug-84—Fri				*			
11-Aug-84—Sat				*			
12-Aug-84—Sun				*			
13-Aug-84—Mon				*			
14-Aug-84—Tue				*			
Daily Average				*			

TOTAL CALORIES

	1000	1080	1160	1240	1320	1400	1480
01-Aug-84—Wed			*				
02-Aug-84—Thu	*						
03-Aug-84—Fri		*					
04-Aug-84—Sat	*						
05-Aug-84—Sun	*						
06-Aug-84—Mon				*			
07-Aug-84—Tue	*						
08-Aug-84—Wed			*				
09-Aug-84—Thu							*
10-Aug-84—Fri						*	
11-Aug-84—Sat						*	
12-Aug-84—Sun						*	
13-Aug-84—Mon	*						
14-Aug-84—Tue		*					
Daily Average		*					

Graphs are also available for daily intake of carbohydrate, protein, fat, cholesterol, sodium, and total weight of food and drink.

BODY WEIGHT AND CALORIC BREAKDOWN

	Weight (lb.)	Calories	Carbo.	Protein	Fat
01-Aug-84—Wed	170.0	1213	77%	14%	9%
02-Aug-84—Thu	169.0	1103	72%	18%	10%
03-Aug-84—Fri	169.5	1132	73%	17%	10%
04-Aug-84—Sat	169.0	1051	77%	16%	7%
05-Aug-84—Sun	168.0	1070	69%	21%	10%
06-Aug-84—Mon	169.0	1272	77%	14%	9%
07-Aug-84—Tue	168.0	1002	72%	20%	8%
Daily Average	168.9	1121	74%	17%	9%

BODY WEIGHT AND TOTAL NUTRITION

Weight (lb.)	Food (oz.)	Calories	Carbo. (g.)	Protein (g.)	Fat (g.)	Choles. (mg.)	Sodium (mg.)
August 01, 1984—Wednesday							
170.0	58.7	1213	250.7	44.2	13.0	25	785
August 02, 1984—Thursday							
169.0	47.6	1103	208.1	53.2	13.1	61	1466
August 03, 1984—Friday							
169.5	55.0	1132	210.4	49.0	12.1	38	1078
August 04, 1984—Saturday							
169.0	50.1	1051	214.6	44.1	8.0	6	741
August 05, 1984—Sunday							
168.0	49.0	1070	190.5	57.3	11.8	28	1829
August 06, 1984—Monday							
169.0	55.2	1272	262.8	48.6	13.1	15	1503
August 07, 1984—Tuesday							
168.0	60.9	1002	191.6	53.9	9.1	20	1199
Daily Averages							
168.9	53.8	1121	218.4	50.0	11.5	28	1240

LUNCH NUTRITION BREAKDOWN

Weight (oz.)	Calories	Carbo. (g.)	Protein (g.)	Fat (g.)	Choles. (mg.)	Sodium (mg.)
Quarter Pounder w/cheese, McDonald's (1 average)						
6.8	518	33.0	30.9	28.6	96	1206
French Fries, McDonald's (1 serving)						
2.4	211	25.0	3.1	10.6	10	112
Coca-Cola (12 fluid ounces)						
12.7	144	36.0	0	0	0	1
Totals: 21.9	873	94.0	34.0	39.2	106	1319

Lunch Calories: 43% carbohydrate, 16% protein, 41% fat

DAILY MENU FOR AUGUST 3, 1984

BREAKFAST
Oatmeal Royale (1 serving)

LUNCH
Indian Vegetable and Rice Casserole (1 serving)
Salad, w/lettuce, tomato (1 large)
Herb Magic Italian Dressing (1 tablespoon)
Apple, raw, w/skin (1 average)

DINNER
Coq au Vin Casserole (1 serving)
Salad, w/lettuce, tomato (1 large)
Green Goddess Dressing (2 tablespoons)
Banana Bread (½ slice)

SNACKS
Potato, baked in skin w/o salt (1 average)
Bacon, Onion, and Chive Topping (2 tablespoons)

Total Calories: 1132
Caloric Breakdown: 73% carbohydrate, 17% protein, 10% fat

RECIPE/MENU LIST

Component Food: Cottage Cheese, 1% fat
(All recipes listed below contain cottage cheese.)

CASSEROLES/COMBINATIONS
Brown Rice and Cottage Cheese
Chicken Casserole
Coq au Vin Casserole
Crabmeat au Gratin
Eggplant Moussaka
Potato Casserole
Spinach Noodle Casserole

PASTA
Macaroni and Cheese Lombardo
Pasta and Garlic Sauce
Tini Linguini

SAUCES/SPREADS/CREAMS
Dill Sauce Deluxe
Haas Mayonnaise Spread

SALADS/SALAD DRESSINGS
Creamy Italian Dressing
Green Goddess Dressing
Jeff's "Cream" Dressing
Thousand Island Dressing
Yogurt Tomato Dressing

TOPPINGS/STUFFINGS
Bacon, Onion, and Chive Topping
Chicken in Wine Sauce Topping
Horseradish Topping
Mushroom Topping
Snappy Cheddar Topping

VEGETABLE DISHES
"Cheddar"-Stuffed Potatoes

BIBLIOGRAPHY

Abdulla, M. 1981. "Nutrient intake and health status of vegans; chemical analyses of diets using the duplicate portion sampling technique." *Am. J. Clin. Nutr.* 34:2464.

Abernathy, R. "Lack of response to amino acid supplements of preadolescent girls." *Am. J. Clin. Nutr.* 25:980.

Abraham, S., et al. 1980. "Prevalence of severe obesity in adults in the United States." *Am. J. Clin. Nutr.* 33:364–69.

Adams, C. F. 1975. "Nutritive value of foods in common units." U.S. Dept. of Agriculture. Agriculture Handbook No. 456.

Addy, D. 1976. "Infant feeding: a current view." *Br. Med. J.* 1:1268.

Alberts, D. S., et al. 1978. "Carnitine prevention of adriamycin toxicity in mice." *Biomedicine.* 29:265–68.

Alfin-Slater, R. B., and Aftergood, L. 1980. "Lipids." In *Modern Nutrition in Health and Disease*, 6th ed., R. S. Goodhart and M. E. Shils, eds. Philadelphia: Lea & Febiger. P. 128.

Allen, L. 1979. "Protein-induced hypercalcuria: a long-term study." *Am. J. Clin. Nutr.* 32:741.

Aloia, J. 1978. "Prevention of involutional bone loss by exercise." *Ann. Intern. Med.* 89:356.

Anand, C. 1974. "Effect of protein intake on calcium balance of young men given 500 mg calcium daily." *J. Nutr.* 104:695.

Anderson, J. R., et al. 1980. "Mineral and vitamin status on high-fiber diets: long-term studies of diabetic patients." *Diab. Care.* 3:38–40.

Andersson, H. 1974. "Fat-reduced diet in the treatment of hyperoxaluria in patients with ileopathy." *Gut.* 15:360.

Angelini, C., et al. 1976. "Carnitine deficiency of skeletal muscle: report of a treated case." *Neurology.* 26:633–37.

Angelini, C., et al. 1978. "Carnitine deficiency: acute postpartum crisis." *Ann. Neurol.* 4:558–61.

Anonymous. 1980. "The regulation of fatty acid synthesis and oxidation by malonyl-CoA and carnitine." *Nutr. Rev.* 38:25–27.

Anonymous. 1981. "Research highlights: techniques for diagnosing and treating patients with systemic carnitine deficiency." *Research Resources Reporter.* 5:13–14.

Apfelbaum, M. 1976. "The effects of very restrictive high protein diets." *Clin. Endocrinol. Metab.* 5:417–30.

Arroyave, G. 1972. "Nutritive values of dietary proteins: for whom?" Proc. 9th Int. Congr. Nutr., Mexico. 1:43.

Astrand, P.-O., et al. 1977. *Textbook of Work Physiology.* 2nd ed. New York: McGraw-Hill. Pp. 483–521.

Aubia, J., et al. 1980. "Carnitine in haemodialysis patients." *Lancet.* 2:1028.

Bahna, S. 1978. "Cow's milk allergy: Pathogenesis, manifestations, diagnosis, and management." *Adv. in Pediatr.* 25:1.

———. 1980. *Allergies to Milk.* New York: Grune & Stratton.

Balke, B. 1962. "Human tolerances." FAA No. AD421156.

Barnard, R. J., et al. 1981. "Effects of an intensive, short-term exercise and nutrition program on patients with coronary heart disease." *J. Cardiac Rehab.* 1:99–105.

Barnard, R. J., et al. 1982. "Response of non-insulin-dependent diabetic patients to an intensive program of diet and exercise." *Diab. Care.* 5:370–74.

Barrows, C. H., and Kokkonen, G. 1975. "Protein synthesis, development, growth and life span." *Growth.* 39:525–33.

Bartel, L. L., et al. 1981. "Perturbation of serum carnitine levels in human adults by chronic renal disease and dialysis therapy." *Am. J. Clin. Nutr.* 34:1314–20.

Barzel, V. 1970. *Osteoporosis.* New York: Grune & Stratton. Pp. 1–37.

Bazzato, G., et al. 1979. "Myasthenia-like syndrome associated with carnitine in patients on long-term haemodialysis." *Lancet.* 1:1041–42.

Bazzato, G., et al. 1981. "Myasthenia-like syndrome after d,l- but not l-carnitine." *Lancet.* 1:1209.

Beaton, G. H., and Swiss, L. D. 1974. "Evaluation of the nutritional quality of food supplies: prediction of 'desirable' or 'safe' protein: calorie ratios." *Am. J. Clin. Nutr.* 27:485–504.

Bellinghieri, G., et al. 1983. "Correlation between increased serum and tissue L-carnitine levels and improved muscle symptoms in hemodialyzed patients." *Am. J. Clin. Nutr.* 38:523–31.

Bell, F. P. 1983. "Carnitine esters: novel inhibitors of plasma lecithin: cholesterol acyltransferase in experimental animals but not in man (homo sapiens)." *Int. J. Biochem.* 15:133–36.

Bendezu, R., et al. 1976. "Certain metabolic consequences of jejunoileal bypass." *Am J. Clin. Nutr.* 29:366–70.

Benotti, P. N., et al. 1976. "Role of branched-chain amino acids (BCAA) intake in preventing muscle proteolysis." *Surg. Forum.* 27(7)–10.

Bieber, L. L., et al. 1981. "Carnitine acyltransferases in rat liver peroxisomes." *Arch. Biochem. Biophys.* 211:599–604.

Bieber, L. L., et al. 1982. "Possible functions of short-chain and medium-chain carnitine acyltransferases." *Fed. Proc. Fed. Am. Soc. Exp. Biol.* 41:2858–62.

Bingham, S., and Cummings, J. H. 1980. "Sources and intakes of dietary fiber in man." In *Medical Aspects of Dietary Fiber,* Spiller and Kay, eds. New York: Plenum Press. Pp. 261–84.

Bistrian, B. R. 1978. "Clinical use of a protein-sparing modified fast." *JAMA,* 240:2299-302.

Bizzi, A., et al. 1978. "Accelerated recovery of post-dialysis plasma carnitine fall by oral carnitine." *Biomedicine.* 29:183–84.

Blackburn, G. L., et al. 1979. "Branched-chain amino acid administration and metabolism during starvation, injury and infection." *Surgery.* 86(2):307–15.

Blethrow, J. G., et al. 1977. "Emergency escape of handicapped air travelers." FAA No. ADA043269/OGI.

Bliznakov, E. G., et al. 1975. "Coenzyme Q deficiency in mice following infection with friend leukemia virus." *J. Vit. Nutr. Res.* 45:388–95.

Bliznakov, E. G., et al. 1978. "Partial reactivation of impaired immune competence in aged mice by synthetic thymus factors." *Biochem. Biophys. Res. Commun.* 80:631–36.

Blum, K., et al. 1971. "The pharmacology of d- and l-carnitine and d- and l-acetylcarnitine: comparison with choline and acetylcholine." *J. Pharmacol. Exp. Ther.* 178:331–38.

Boat, T. 1975. "Hyperactivity in cow's milk in young children with pulmonary hemosiderosis and cor pulmonale secondary to nasopharyngeal obstruction." *J. Pediatr.* 87:23.

Bock, William, et al. 1967. "The effects of acute dehydration upon cardiorespiratory endurance." *J. Sports Med.* 5(2):67.

Bohles, H., et al. 1982. "Decreased serum carnitine in valproate induced Reye's syndrome." *Eur. J. Pediatr.* 139:185–86.

Bohmer, T., and Molstad, P. 1980. "Carnitine transport across the plasma membrane." In *Carnitine Biosynthesis, Metabolism, and Functions,* R. A. Frenkel and J. D. McGarry, eds. New York: Academic Press. Pp. 73–89.

Bohmer, T., et al. 1977. "Carnitine uptake into human heart cells in culture." *Biochim. Biophys. Acta.* 465:627–33.

Bohmer, T., et al. 1978. "Carnitine deficiency during intermittent haemodialysis for renal failure." *Lancet* 1:126–28.

Bohmer, T., et al. "Carnitine levels in human serum in health and disease." *Clin. Chim. Acta.* 57:55–61.

Bolourich, S. 1968. "Wheat flour as a source of protein for adult subjects." *Am. J. Clin. Nutr.* 21:827.

Booze, C. F. 1978. "The morbidity experience of air traffic control personnel, 1967–1977." FAA No. ADA056053/26I.

Booze, C. F., et al. 1980. "Postmortem coronary atherosclerosis findings in general aviation accident pilot fatalities: 1975–1977." FAA No. ADA089428/7.

Booze, C. F., Jr. 1974. "Characteristics of medically disqualified airman applicants during calendar year 1971." FAA No. AD781684.

Borum, P. R. 1981. "Possible carnitine requirement of the newborn and the effect of genetic disease on the carnitine requirement." *Nutr. Rev.* 39:385–90.

———. 1983. "Carnitine." *Ann. Rev. Nutr.* 3:233–259.

Borum, P. R., and York, C. M. 1982. "Red cell carnitine binding protein." *Fed. Proc. Fed. Am. Soc. Exp. Biol.* 41:537.

Borum, P. R., et al. 1979. "Carnitine content of liquid formulas and special diets." *Am. J. Clin. Nutr.* 32:2272–76.

Borum, P. R., et al. 1983. "Epididymal carnitine binding protein." Abstract. *Fed. Proc. Fed. Am. Soc. Exp. Biol.* 42:1855.

Bougneres, P. F., et al. 1979. "Hypolipaemic effect of carnitine in uraemic patients." *Lancet.* 1:1401–2.

Bray, G. A. 1976. *The Obese Patient.* Major Problems in Internal Medicine, vol. 9. Philadelphia: W. B. Saunders.

———, ed. 1979. "Obesity in America." NIH Publication No. 79-359. Bethesda, Md.: National Institutes of Health. Available from Publications Unit, Fogarty International Center, Bldg. 16A, Rm 205, National Institutes of Health, Bethesda, MD 20205.

Bremer, J. 1977. "Carnitine and its role in fatty acid metabolism." *Trends Biochem. Sci.* 2:207–9.

Brenner, B. M., et al. 1982. "Dietary protein intake and the progressive nature of kidney disease: the role of hemodynamically mediated glomerular injury in the pathogenesis of progressive glomerular sclerosis in aging, renal ablation, and intrinsic renal disease." *N. Eng. J. Med.* 307:652–69.

Bricker, M. 1947. "The protein requirement of the adult rat in terms of the protein contained in egg, milk, and soy flour." *J. Nutr.* 34:491.

Bricker, M., et al. 1945. "The protein requirements of adult human subjects in terms of the protein contained in individual foods and food combinations." *J. Nutr.* 30:269–84.

Briggs, M. 1974. "Vitamin E supplements and fatigue." *N. Eng. J. Med.* 290:579–80.

Brodribb, A. J. M., and Humphreys, D. M. 1976. "Diverticular disease: three studies. Pt. I—relation to other disorders and fibre intake; pt. II—treatment with bran; pt. III—metabolic effect of bran in patients with diverticular disease." *Brit. Med. J.* 1:424–30.

Bronner, F. 1976. "Vitamin D deficiency and rickets." *Am. J. Clin. Nutr.* 29:1307–14.

Brooks, D. E., et al. 1974. "Carnitine and glycerylphosphorylcholine in the reproductive tract of the male rat." *J. Reprod. Fertil.* 36:141–60.

Brooks, G. A., and Fahey, T. D. 1984. *Exercise Physiology: Human Bioenergetics and Its Applications.* New York: John Wiley. 7:128–31.

Brooks, H., et al. 1977. "Carnitine-induced effects on cardiac and peripheral hemodynamics." *J. Clin. Pharmacol.* 17:561–68.

Broquist, H. P. 1982. "Carnitine biosynthesis and function: introductory remarks." *Fed. Proc.*

Fed. Am. Soc. Exp. Biol. 41:2840–42.

Broquist, H. P., and Borum, P. R. 1982. "Carnitine biosynthesis: nutritional implications." In *Advances in Nutritional Research*, H. H. Draper, ed. Vol. 4. New York: Plenum Press. Pp. 181–204.

Brown, J. M., et al. 1978. "Cardiac complications of protein-sparing modified fasting." *JAMA*. 240:120–22.

Buisseret, P. 1978. "Common manifestations of cow's milk allergy in children." *Lancet*. 1:304.

Burkitt, D. P., ed. 1975. *Refined Carbohydrate Foods and Disease: Some Implications of Dietary Fibre*. New York: Academic Press.

———, et al. 1972. "Effects of dietary fibre on stools and transit-times, and its role in the causation of disease." *Lancet*. 2:1408–12.

Burnet, F. M. 1970. "An immunological approach to aging." *Lancet*. 2:358–60.

———. 1976. *Immunology, Aging, and Cancer*. San Francisco: W. H. Freeman.

Buxe, M. G., et al. 1972. "Oxidation of branched-chain amino acids by isolated hearts and diaphragms of the rat. The effect of fatty acids, glucose, and pyruvate respiration." *J. Biol. Chem.* 24(24):8085–96.

Cade, R., et al. 1984. "Effects of phosphate loading on 2,3-diphosphoglycerate and maximal oxygen uptake." *Medicine and Science in Sports and Exercise*. 16:263–68.

Campbell, T. C. 1982. Quoted in "In the war against cancer, the latest weapons are fruits and vegetables." *People*, July 12, pp. 65–68.

Cantrell, C. R., and Borum, P. R. 1982. "Identification of a cardiac carnitine binding protein." *J. Biol. Chem.* 257:10599–604.

Carlson, S. E. 1979. "Significance of carnitine in infant diets." Prepared for the Food and Drug Administration under Contract No. 223-76-2091 by the Committee on Nutrition, American Academy of Pediatrics, Evanston, Ill.

Carroll, J. E., et al. 1980. "Carnitine 'deficiency': lack of response to carnitine therapy." *Neurology*. 30:618–26.

Carroll, K. K. 1978. "The role of dietary protein in hypercholesterolemia and atherosclerosis." *Lipids*. 13:360–65.

Cederblad, G. 1976. "Plasma carnitine and body composition." *Clin. Chim. Acta*. 67:207–12.

Cederblad, G., and Lindstedt, S. 1971. "Excretion of l-carnitine in man." *Clin. Chim. Acta*. 33:117–23.

———. 1972. "A method for the determination of carnitine in the picomole range." *Clin. Chim. Acta*. 37:235–43.

———. 1976. "Metabolism of labeled carnitine in the rat." *Arch. Biochem. Biophys.* 175:173–80.

Cederblad, G., et al. 1982. "Urinary excretion of carnitine and its derivatives in new borns." *Biochem. Med.* 27:260–65.

Cederblad, G., et al. 1983. "Urinary excretion of carnitine in multiply injured patients on different regimens of total parenteral nutrition." *Metabolism*. 32:383–89.

Cerqueira, M. T., et al. 1979. "The food and nutrient intakes of the Tarahumara Indians of Mexico." *Am. J. Clin. Nutr.* 32:905–15.

Cerra, F., et al. 1982. "Branched-chains support post-operative protein synthesis." *Surgery*. 92(2):192–99.

Chalmers, J. 1970. "Geographic variations of senile osteoporosis." *J. Bone and Joint Surgery*. 52B:667.

Chan, M. K., et al. 1980. "Carnitine in haemodialysis patients." *Lancet*. 2:1028–29.

Chan, M. K., et al. 1982. "Response patterns to dl-carnitine in patients on maintenance haemodialysis." *Nephron*. 30:240–43.

Chapoy, P. R., et al. 1980. "Systemic carnitine deficiency—a treatable inherited lipid-storage disease presenting as Reye's syndrome." *N. Eng. J. Med.* 303:1389–94.

Charney, E., et al. 1976. "Childhood antecedents of adult obesity: do chubby infants become obese adults?" *N. Eng. J. Med.* 295:6–9.

Christophersen, B. O., and Norseth, J. 1981. "Arachidonic acid synthesis studied in isolated liver cells: effects of (−)-carnitine and of (+)-decanoylcarnitine." *FEBS Lett.* 133:201–4.

Clark, H. 1973. "Nitrogen balances of adult human subjects fed combinations of wheat, beans, corn, milk, and rice." *Am. J. Clin. Nutr.* 26:702.

Cohen, H. M. 1973. "Fatigue caused by vitamin E?" *Calif. Med.* Pp. 119–72.

Committee on Nutrition of Mother and Preschool Child. 1978. "Fetal and infant nutrition and susceptibility to obesity." *Am. J. Clin. Nutr.* 31:2026–30.

Community Nutrition Institute. 1980. "Diet aids boom." *CNI Weekly Report.* 10(14):4.

Connor, W. 1964. "The interrelated effects of dietary cholesterol and fat upon human serum lipid levels." *J. Clin. Invest.* 43:1691.

Connor, W. 1982. "Reply to letter by Oster." Letter. *Am. J. Clin. Nutr.* 36:1261.

Connor, W. E., et al. 1978. "The plasma lipids, lipoproteins, and the diet of the Tarahumara Indians of Mexico." *Am. J. Clin. Nutr.* 31:1131.

Consumer Reports. 1978. "Too much sugar?" March.

Corrigan, J. J., and Marcus, F. I. 1974. "Coagulopathy associated with vitamin E ingestion." *JAMA.* 230:1300–1.

Corrigan, J. H., and Ulfers, L. L. 1981. "Effect of vitamin E on prothrombin levels in warfarin-induced vitamin K deficiency." *Am. J. Clin. Nutr.* 34:1701–5.

Coulombel, C., et al. 1981. "Transglycosylation reactions catalysed by two beta-mannanases." *Biochem. J.* 195:333–35.

Council on Foods and Nutrition, American Medical Association. 1974. "A critique of low-carbohydrate ketogenic weight reduction regimens: a review of Dr. Atkins' Diet Revolution." *JAMA.* 224:15–22.

Cox, R. A., and Hoppel, C. L. 1973. "Biosynthesis of carnitine and 4-n-trimethylaminobutyrate from 6-n-trimethyl-lysine." *Biochem. J.* 136:1083–90.

Crapo, P., and Kolterman, O. 1984. "The metabolic effects of 2-week fructose feeding in normal subjects." *Am. J. Clin. Nutr.* 39:525–34.

Crocetti, A. F., and Guthrie, H. A. 1982. *"Eating Behavior and Associated Nutrient Quality of Diets."* New York: Anarem System Res. Corp.

Cummings, J. 1979. "The effect of meat protein and dietary fiber on colonic function and metabolism, changes in bowel habit, bile acid excretion, and calcium absorption." *Am. J. Clin. Nutr.* 32:2086.

Currens, J. H., et al. 1951. "Metabolic effects of rice diet in treatment of hypertension." *N. Eng. J. Med.* 245:354–59.

Dahlberg, K. 1980. "Medical care of Cambodian refugees." *JAMA.* 243:1062.

Dark, S. J. 1976. "Characteristics of medically disqualified airman applicants in calendar years 1973 and 1974." FAA No. ADA032603/3GI.

Dark, S. J. and Davis, A. W., Jr. 1978. "Characteristics of medically disqualified airman applicants in calendar years 1975 and 1976." FAA No.ADA058158/7GI.

Daubs, J. 1980. "Flight crew exposure to ozone concentrations affecting the visual system." *Am. J. Opt. Phys. Optics.* 57:95–105.

Dayton, S., et al. 1962. "A controlled clinical trial of a diet high in unsaturated fat." *N. Eng. J. Med.* 266:1017–23.

Dayton, S., et al. 1969. "A controlled clinical trial of a diet high in unsaturated fat in preventing complications of atherosclerosis." *Circ.* 40, supple. 2:1–63.

DeBusk, B. G. 1955. "Effect of lipoic acid on the growth rate of young chicks and rats." *Arch. Biochem. Biophys.* Vol. 55.

DeHaven, J., et al. 1980. "Nitrogen and sodium balance and sympathetic-nervous-system activity in obese subjects treated with a low calorie protein or mixed diet." *N. Eng. J. Med.* 302:477–82.

Decombaz, J., et al. 1979. "Biochemical changes in a 100 KM run: free amino acids, urea and creatine." *Eur. J. Appl. Physiol.* 41:61–72.

De Grandis, D., et al. 1980. "Myasthenia due to carnitine treatment." *J. Neurol. Sci.* 46:365–71.

Demelia, L., et al. 1981. "Carnitine in hemodialysis patients." Abstract submitted for presentation in the 18th Congress of the European Dialysis and Transplant Association, Paris, July 5–8.

Dempsey, J. A., et al. 1971. "Muscular exercise, 2,3-DPG and oxy-hemoglobin affinity." *Int. Z. Physiol.* 30:34–39.

Department of Health and Social Security. 1974. "Present day infant feeding practice report." No. 9.

De Simone, C., et al. 1982. "Reversibility of l-carnitine of immunosuppression induced by an emulsion of soya bean oil, glycerol and egg lecithin." *Arzneimittelforsch.* 32:1485–88.

DeVries, H. 1974. *Physiology of Exercise for Physical Education and Athletics.* Dubuque: William C. Brown. Pp. 26–34.

DiBendetto, R. J. 1967. "Chronic hypervitaminosis A in an adult." *JAMA.* 201:700–2.

"Diet and urinary calculi." 1980. *Nutr. Rev.* 38:75–76.

Dille, J. R., and Mohler, S. R. 1968. "Drug and toxic hazards in general aviation." FAA No. AD686670.

Dill, B. D., et al. "Work tolerance: age and altitude." FAA No. AD603932.

Donald, P., et al. 1981. "Body weight and composition in laboratory rats: effects of diets with high or low protein concentrations. *Sci.* 211:185–86.

Drenick, E. J., et al. 1978. "Renal damage with intestinal bypass." *Ann. Intern. Med.* 5:594.

Du, J. I., et al. 1977. "Protein biosynthesis in aging mouse tissues." *Exp. Gerontol.* 12:181–91.

Dwyer, J. 1982. "Nutritional status of vegetarian children." *Am. J. Clin. Nutr.* 35:204.

Eastham, E. 1979. "Adverse effects of milk formula ingestion on the gastrointestinal tract—an update." *Gastroenterology.* 76:365.

Eaton, J., et al. 1969. "Role of red cell 2,3-DPG in the adaptation of man to altitude: mechanism and effect." *J. Lab. Clin. Med.* 73:603–9

Edwards, C. 1971. "Utilization of wheat by adult man: nitrogen metabolism, plasma amino acids and lipids." *Am. J. Clin. Nutr.* 24:181.

Eisenstein, R., and Zeruolis, L. 1964. "Vitamin D–induced aortic calcification." *Arch. Path.* 77:27. (Abstract of JAMA, 1964; 187:186.)

Elliott, J. 1978. "More help for the morbidly obese: gastric stapling." *JAMA.* 240:1941.

Ellis, F. 1977. "The health of vegans during pregnancy." *Proc. Nutr. Soc. Abstracts of Communication.* 36:46A.

Embden, G., et al. 1921. "Increase of working capacity through administration of phosphate." *Z. Physiol. Chem.* 113:67–107.

Engel, A. G. 1980. "Possible causes and effects of carnitine deficiency in man." In *Carnitine Biosynthesis, Metabolism and Functions*, R. A. Frenkel and J. D. McGarry, eds. New York: Academic Press. P. 271–84.

Engel, A. G., and Angelini, C. 1973. "Carnitine deficiency of human skeletal muscle with associated lipid storage myopathy: a new syndrome. *Sci.* 179:899–902.

Engel, A. G., and Rebouche, C. J. 1982. "Pathogenic mechanisms in human carnitine deficiency syndromes. In *Disorders of the Motor Unit*, D. L. Schotland, ed. New York: John Wiley. Pp. 643–56.

Englard, S. 1979. "Hydroxylation of γ-butyrobetaine to carnitine in human and monkey tissues." *FEBS Lett.* 102:297–300.

Englard, S., and Carnicero, H. H. 1978. "γ-butyrobetaine hydroxylation to carnitine in mammalian kidney." *Arch. Biochem. Biophys.* 109:361–64.

Englard S., and Midelfort, C. F. 1978. "Stereochemical course of γ-butyrobetaine hydroxylation to carnitine." Abstract. *Fed. Proc. Fed. Am. Soc. Exp. Biol.* 37:1806.

FAA Aviation Medical Library. 1964. "Aviation medical papers and reports: a bibliography." FAA No. AD613364.

Fanelli, O. 1978. "Carnitine and acetyl-carnitine, natural substances endowed with interesting pharmacological properties." *Life Sciences* 23:2563–70.

FDA Drug Bulletin. 1978. "Liquid protein and sudden cardiac deaths—an update." May-July.

Felig, P. 1971. "Amino acid metabolism in exercising man." *J. Clin. Invest.* 50:2703.

———. 1978. "Four questions about protein diets." *N. Eng. J. Med.* 298:1025–26.

Fiorica, V., et al. 1968. "Contribution of activity in the circadian rhythm in excretion of magnesium and calcium." FAA No. 674416.

Fisher, H., et al. 1969. "Reassessment of amino acid requirements of young women on low nitrogen diets. I. Lysine and tryptotophan." *Am. J. Clin. Nutr.* 22:1190–96

Fisher, H., et al. 1971. "Reassessment of amino acid requirement of young women on low nitrogen diets. II. Leucine, methionine, and valine." *Am. J. Clin. Nutr.* 24:1216–23

Flute, P. T. 1974. "Acquired disorders of blood coagulation. In *Blood and Its Disorders*, R. M. Hardisty and D. J. Weatherall, eds. Oxford: Blackwell Scientific Pub. P. 1081.

Folkers, K., and Yamamura, Y. 1977. *Biomedical and Clinical Aspects of Co-enzyme Q*. Amsterdam: Elsevier North-Holland Press.

——— 1981. *Biomedical and Clinical Aspects of Co-enzyme Q*. Vol. 3, Elsevier Publishing.

Folkers, K., et al. 1972. "Survey and new clinical studies on coenzyme Q in human muscular dystrophy." *Int. J. Vit. Nutr. Res.* 42:139–63.

Folkers, K., et al. 1977. "Biomedical and clinical research on coenzyme Q." In *Biomedical and Clinical Aspects of Co-enzyme Q*, Edited by K. Folkers and Y. Yamamura, eds. Amsterdam: Elsevier North-Holland Biomedical Press. Pp. 299–313.

Forbes, G. B. 1967. "Present knowledge of vitamin D." *Nutr. Rev.* 25:225–28.

Franklin, B. A., et al. 1980. "Losing weight through exercise." *JAMA*, 244:377.

Fraser, D., and Scriver, C. R. 1976. "Familial forms of vitamin D–resistant rickets revisited. X-linked hypophosphatemia and autosomal recessive vitamin D dependency." *Am. J. Clin. Nutr.* 29:1315–29.

Frattali, V. P. 1979. "Deaths associated with the liquid protein diet." FDA, by-lines No. 4.

Frenkel, R. A., and McGarry, J. D., eds. 1980. *Carnitine Biosynthesis, Metabolism and Functions*. New York: Academic Press.

Freund, H., et al. 1978. "The role of the branched-chain amino acids in decreasing muscle catabolism in vivo." *Surgery.* 83(6):611–18.

Freund, H., et al. 1979. "Infusion at the branched-chain amino acids in postoperative patients. Anticatabolic properties." *Ann. Surg.* 190(1):18–23.

Freund, H. R., et al. 1978. "Amino acids derangement in patients with sepsis: treatment with branched-chain amino acid rich infusions." *Ann. Surg.* 188(3):423–30.

Friedberg, W., and Neas, B. R., eds. 1980. "Cosmic radiation exposure during air travel." FAA No. ADA084801/0.

Friedberg, W., and Nelson, J. M. 1971. "Calibration of the Concorde radiation detection instrument and measurements of SST altitude." FAA No. AD732789.

Friedberg, W., et al. 1978. "Radiobiological aspects of high altitude flight: relative biological effectiveness of fast neutrons in suppressing immune capacity to an infective agent." FAA No. ADA053204/4GI.

Friedman, M., et al. 1965. "Effect of unsaturated fats upon lipemia and conjunctival circulation." *JAMA.* 193:110–14.

Fritz, I. B., and Marquis, N. R. 1965. "The role of acylcarnitine esters and carnitine palmityltransferase in the transport of fatty acyl groups across mitochondrial membrane." *Proc. Nat. Acad. Sci.* 54:1226–33.

Fritz, I. B., and Schultz, S. K. 1965. "Carnitine acetyltransferase. II. Inhibition of carnitine analogues and by sulfhydryl reagents." *J. Biol. Chem.* 240:2188–92.

Frnster, L. 1977. "Facts and ideas about the functions of coenzyme Q in mitochondria." In *Biomedical and Clinical Aspects of Coenzyme Q*, K. Folkers and Y. Yamamura, eds. Amsterdam: Elsevier North-Holland Biomedical Press. Pp. 15–21

Frohlich, J., et al. 1978. "Effect of fasting on free and esterified carnitine levels in human serum and urine: correlation with serum levels of free fatty acids and y-hydroxybutyrate." *Metab. Clin. Exp.* 27:555–61.

Frolich, W., and Lyso, A. 1983. "Bioavailability of iron from wheat bran in pigs." *Am. J. Clin. Nutr.* 37:31–36.

Fuller, R. K., and Hoppel, C. L. 1983. "Elevated plasma carnitine in hepatic cirrhosis." *Hepatology* 3:554–58.

Garn, S., et al. 1975. "Does obesity have a genetic basis in man?" *Ecol. Food Nutr.* 4:57.

Garzya, G., and Amico, R. M. 1980. "Comparative study on the activity of racemic and laevoratatory carnitine in stable angina pectoris." *Int. J. Tissue React.* 2:175–80.

Genuth, S. M. 1976. "Effect of high fat vs. high carbohydrate feeding on the development of obesity in weanling ob/ob mice." *Diabetologia.* 12:155–59.

Gerathewohl, S. J. 1977. "Psychophysiological effects of aging: developing a functional age index for pilots: I. A survey of the pertinent literature." FAA No. ADA040322/0GI.

Gerrard, J. 1967. "Milk allergy: clinical picture and familial incidence." *Can. Med. Ass. J.* 97:780.

Girandola, R. N. 1977. "Body composition changes resulting from ingestion and dehydration." *Research Quarterly.* 48(2):301.

Glasgow, A. M., et al. 1980. "Systemic carnitine deficiency simulating recurrent Reye syndrome." *J. Pediatr.* 96:889–91.

Golden, M. H. N. 1982. "Protein deficiency, energy deficiency and the oedema of malnutrition." *Lancet.* 1:1261–65.

Goldrick, R. B., et al. 1970. "An assessment of coronary heart disease and coronary risk factors in a New Guinea highland population." In *Atherosclerosis: Proceedings of the Second International Symposium*, R. J. Jones, ed. Berlin: Springer-Verlag. Pp. 366–68.

Gordon, J. 1963. "Weaning diarrhea." *Am. J. Med. Sci.* 245:129.

Grace, C. S., et al. 1970. "Blood fibrinolysis and coagulation in New Guineans and Australians." *Aust. Ann. Med.* 4:328–33.

Gravine, E., and Gravina-Sanvitale, G. 1969. "Effect of carnitine on blood acetoacetate in fasting children." *Clin. Chim. Acta.* 23:376–77.

Greenberg, I., et al. 1979. "Obesity: facts, fads, and fantasies." *Compr. Ther.* 5:68–76.

Greenberg, J. 1978. "The fat American." *Science News.* 113(12):188–89.

Griggs, R. C., et al. 1981. "Treatment of myopathic carnitine deficiency: quantitation of response to prednisone and carnitine." *Trans. Am. Neurol. Assoc.* 106:199–202.

Grinker, J. 1978. "Obesity and sweet taste." *Am. J. Clin. Nutr.* 31:1078–87.

Gross, C. J., and Henderson, L. M. 1983. "Carnitine absorption by the rat small intestine." Abstract. *Fed. Proc. Fed. Am. Soc. Exp. Biol.* 42:1320.

Guarnieri, G. F., et al. 1980. "Lipid-lowering effect of carnitine in chronically uremic patients treated with maintenance hemodialysis." *Am. J. Clin. Nutr.* 33:1489–92.

Haber, G. B., et al. 1977. "Depletion and disruption of dietary fiber: effects on satiety, plasma glucose and serum insulin." *Lancet.* 2:679–82.

Hahn, P., and Skala, J. P. 1975. "The role of carnitine in brown adipose tissue of suckling rats." *Comp. Biochem. Physiol.* 51B:507–15.

Hahn, P., et al. 1982. "Plasma carnitine levels during total parenteral nutrition of adult surgical patients." *Am. J. Clin. Nutr.* 36:569–72.

Hall, J. A., et al. 1982. "Effects of diet and exercise on peripheral vascular disease (case report)." *Phys. Sportsmed.* 10:90.

Harper, A. 1961. "Some implications of amino acid supplementation." *Am. J. Clin. Nutr.* 9:553.

———. 1972. "Adaptive changes to low nutrient intake, metabolic adaption to adequate and inadequate amino acid supply." *Proc. 9th Int. Congr. Nutr.*, Mexico. 1:1.

Hartroft, W. S. 1960. "The pathology of obesity." In *The Prevention of Obesity*, R. L. Craid, ed. Dallas: American Heart Association. Pp. 32–41.

Hartz, A., et al. 1977. "Relative importance of the effect of family environment and heredity on obesity." *Ann. Human Genet.* 41:185–93.

Hauty, G. T., and Adams, T. 1965. "Phase shifts of the human circadian system and performance deficit during the periods of transition: I. East-West flight." FAA No. AD639637.

————. 1965. "Phase shifts of the human circadian system and performance deficit during the periods of transition: II. West-East flight. FAA No. AD689811.

————. 1965. "Phase shifts of the human circadian system and performance deficit during the periods of transition: III. North-South flight. FAA No. AD689812.

————. 1965. "Pilot fatigue: intercontinental jet flight: Oklahoma City–Tokyo." FAA No. 621433.

"Hazards of overuse of vitamin D." 1974. *Nutr. Rev.* 33:61–62.

Hegsted, C. 1946. "Protein requirements of adults." *J. Lab. Clin. Med.* 31:261.

Hegsted, D. 1955. "'Lysine and methionine supplementation of all-vegetable diets for human adults." *J. Nutr.* 56:555.

Hegsted, D. M. 1968. "Minimum protein requirements of adults." *Am. J. Clin. Nutr.* 21:352–57.

Hegsted, D. M., et al. 1946. "Protein requirements of adults." *J. Lab. Clin. Med.* 31:261–84.

Hegsted, M. 1974. "Energy needs and utilization." *Nutr. Rev.* 32:33–36.

Henderson, L. M., et al. 1982. "Mammalian enzymes of trimethyllysine conversion to trimethylaminobutyrate." *Fed. Proc. Fed. Am. Soc. Exp. Biol.* 41:2843–47.

Higgins, E. A., et al. 1975. "The effects of a 12-hour shift in the wake-sleep cycle on the physiological and biochemical responses and on multiple-task performance." FAA No. ADA021518/GGI.

Higgins, E. A., et al. 1978. "The effects of altitude and two decongestant-antihistamine preparations on physiological functions and performance." FAA No. ADA054793/5GI.

Higgins, E. A., et al. 1979. "Effects of ozone on exercising and sedentary adult men and women representative of the flight attendant population." FAA No. ADA080045/8

Higgins, E. A., et al. 1981. "Physiological, biochemical, and performance responses to a 24-hour crash diet." FAA No. ADA103143/4.

Higgins, E. A., et al., 1970. "Blood alcohol concentrations as affected by combinations of alcoholic beverage dosages and altitudes." FAA No. AD709328.

Higgins, I. T. 1976. "Fatness similarities in adopted pairs." Letter. *Am. J. Clin. Nutr.* 29:1067–68.

Hill, D. 1979. "The spectrum of cow's milk allergy in childhood." *Acta Paediatr. Scand.* 68:847.

Hillman, N. M., et al. 1978. "Protein deprivation in primates. X. Test performance of juveniles born of deprived mothers." *Am. J. Clin. Nutr.* 31:388–93.

Hillman, R. W. 1958. "Tocopherol excess in man: creatinuria associated with prolonged ingestion." *Am. J. Clin. Nutr.* 5:597–600.

Hirokawa, K., and Makinodan, T. 1975. "Thymic involution: effect on T cell differentiation." *J. Immunol.* 114:1659–64.

Holman, R. T. 1978. "How essential are essential fatty acids?" *J. Am. Oil Chem Soc.* 55:774a–82a.

Holme, E., et al. 1982. "Uncoupling in the y-butyrobetaine hydroxylase reaction by d- and l-carnitine." *Biochem. Biophys. Res. Commun.* 107:518–24.

Holt, E. 1960. *Protein and Amino Acid Requirements of Early Life*. New York: University Press. P. 12.

Hoppel, C. L. 1982. "Carnitine and carnitine palmitolytransferase in fatty acid oxidation and ketosis." *Fed. Proc. Fed. Am. Soc.Exp. Biol.* 41:2853–57.

Hoppel, C. L., and Genuth, S. M. 1980. "Carnitine metabolism in normal-weight and obese human subjects during fasting." *Am. J. Physiol.* 238:E409-15.

Hornstra, G., et al. 1979. "Fish oils, prostaglandins, and arterial thrombosis." *Lancet.* 2:1080.

Hosking, G. P., et al. 1977. "Oral treatment of carnitine myopathy." *Lancet.* 1:853.

Howe, J. 1972. "Nitrogen retention of adults fed six grams of nitrogen from combinations of rice, milk, and wheat." *Am. J. Clin. Nutr.* 25:559.

Hoyt, C. S., et al. 1977. "Low-carbohydrate diet and optic neuropathy." *Med. J. Austr.* 1:65-66.

Huang, Y. S., et al. 1982. "Most biological effects of zinc deficiency corrected by gamma-linolenic acid (18: 3 omega 6) but not by linolenic acid (18: 2 omega 6)." *Atherosclerosis.* 41:193-207.

Huenemann, R. L., et al. 1980. "Cultural factors in the development, maintenance, and control of obesity." *Cardiovascular Reviews & Reports.* 1:21-26.

Hultman, E. 1976. "Adverse effects of high fat, low CHO diet on performance." American Heart Association Monograph. 15:106.

"Humans as walking legumes." 1971. *Nutr. Rev.* 29:223-26.

Hunt, S. M., and Schofield, F. A. 1969. "Magnesium balance and protein intake level in adult human females." *Am. J. Clin. Nutr.* 22:367-73.

Huth, P. J., and Shug, A. L. 1980. "Properties of carnitine transport in rat kidney cortex slices." *Biochim. Biophys. Acta.* 602:621-34.

Huth, P. J., et al. 1979. "Stereospecificity and properties of carnitine transport in rat brain and kidney cortex slices" Abstract. *Fed. Proc. Fed. Am. Soc. Exp. Biol.* 38:246.

Huth, P. J., et al. 1981. "The uptake of carnitine by slices of rat cerebral cortex." *J. Neurochem.* 36:715-723.

"Hypervitaminosis E and coagulation." 1975. *Nutr. Rev.* 33:269-70.

Iacono, J. M., et al. 1975. "Reduction in blood pressure associated with high polyunsaturated fat diets that reduce blood cholesterol in man." *Preventive Med.* 4:426-33.

Insull, W., et al. 1969. "Studies of arteriosclerosis in Japanese and American men. I. Comparison of fatty acid composition of adipose tissue." *J. Clin. Invest.* 48:1313-27.

Irwin, M. I., and Hegsted, D. M. 1971. "A conspectus of research on protein requirements of man." *J. Nutr.* 101:385-430.

Jakubczak, L. F. 1976. "Behavioral aspects of nutrition and longevity in animals." In *Nutrition, Longevity, and Aging,* M. Rockstein and M. L. Sussman eds. New York: Academic Press. Pp. 103-22.

Jayarjan, P., et al. 1980. "Effect of dietary fat on absorption of B-carotene from green leafy vegetables in children." *Indian J. Med. Res.* 71:53-56.

Jergensen, K. A., and Dyerberg, J. 1983. "Platelets and atherosclerosis." *Adv. Nutr. Res.* 5:57-75.

Johnson, D., et al. 1977. "Therapeutic fasting in morbid obesity: long-term follow-up." *Arch. Intern. Med.* 137:1381-82.

Johnson, D. D., et al. 1980. "Reactive hypoglycemia." *JAMA.* 243:1151-55.

Johnson, G. O. 1982. "Effects of a 16-week marathon training program on normal college males." *J. Sports Med.* 22(2):225.

Jowsey, J. 1976. "Osteoporosis: its nature and the role of diet." *Postgrad. Med.* 60:75-79.

————. 1976. "Prevention and treatment of osteoporosis." In *Nutrition and Aging,* M. Winick, ed. New York: John Wiley. Pp. 131-44.

Kamikawa, T., et al. 1985. "Effects of Coenzyme Q-10 on exercise tolerance in chronic stable angina pectoris." *Am. J. Cardiol.* 56:247-251.

Kannel, W., et al. 1967. "Relation of adiposity to blood pressure and development of hypertension. Framingham study." *Ann. Intern. Med.* 67:48-59.

Karam, J. H. 1979. "Obesity: fat cells—not fat people." *West J. Med.* 130(2):128-32.

Karim, B., et al. 1972. "A preliminary study of maximal control force capability of female pilots." FAA No. AD753987.

Karpati, G., et al. 1975. "The syndrome of systemic carnitine deficiency." *Neurology.* 25:16-24.

Karpovich, P., and Sinning, W. 1971. *Physiology of Muscular Activity.* Philadelphia: W. B. Saunders.

Keller, W., and Kraut, H. 1959. "Work and nutrition." *World Rev. Nutr. Diet.* 3:65–81.

Kempner, W. 1945. "Compensation of renal metabolic dysfunction; Treatment of kidney disease and hypertensive vascular disease with rice diet." *N. Carolina Med. J.* 6:61, 117.

Kempner, W. 1949. "Treatment of heart and kidney disease and of hypertensive and arteriosclerotic vascular disease with the rice diet." *Ann. Intern. Med.* 31:821–56.

Kempner, W., et al. 1975. "Treatment of massive obesity with rice/reduction diet program." *Arch. Intern. Med.* 135:1575–84.

Kennedy, D., et al. 1978. "Protein diets." *FDA Drug Bulletin.* Jan.–Feb.

Khairallah, E. A., and Wolf, G. 1967. "Carnitine decarboxylase." Abstract. *J. Biol. Chem.* 242:32.

Khan, L., and Bamji, M. S. 1979. "Tissue carnitine deficiency due to dietary lysine deficiency: triglyceride accumulation and concomitant impairment in fatty acid oxidation." *J. Nutr.* 109:24–31.

Khan-Siddiqui, L., and Bamji, M. S. 1980. "Plasma carnitine levels in adult males in India: effects of high cereal, low fat diet, fat supplementation, and nutrition status." *Am. J. Clin. Nutr.* 33:1259–63.

———. 1983. "Lysine-carnitine conversion in normal and undernourished adult men—suggestion of a nonpeptidyl pathway." *Am. J. Clin. Nutr.* 37:93–98.

Kies, C. 1965. "Determination of first limiting nitrogenous factor in corn protein for nitrogen retention in human adults." *J. Nutr.* 86:350.

Kik, M. D. 1962. "Nutritive value of chicken meat and its value in supplementing rice protein." *J. Agr. Food Chem.* 10:59–61

Kirkham, W. R. 1980. "Medical and toxicological factors in aircraft accidents." FAA No. ADA087690/4.

Knapp, J., et al. 1973. "Growth and nitrogen balance in infants fed cereal proteins." *Am. J. Clin. Nutr.* 26:586–90.

Kofranyi, E. 1970. "The minimum protein requirements of humans, tested with mixtures of whole egg plus potatoes and maize plus beans." *Z. Physiol. Chem.* 351:1485.

Kofranyi, E., and Jekat, J. 1965. "Zur Bestimmung der biologischen Wertigkeit von Nahrungsproteinen, XI. Die Wirkung von Methionin auf den Stickstoffbedarf." (The determination of the biological value of dietary protein, XI. The effect of methionine on nitrogen requirement.) *Z. Physiol. Chem.* 342:248.

Kolata, G. B. 1977. "Obesity: A growing problem." *Research News.* Dec. Pp. 905–6.

Kon, S. 1928. "The value of whole potatoes in human nutrition." *Biochemical J.* 22:258.

Korycka, M., et al. 1970. "Influence of fat level in the diet on carotene and Vitamin A utilization." *Acta Physiol. Pol.* 20:662–67.

Kruse, C. A. 1964. "Treatment of fatigue with aspartic acid salts." *Clin. Med.* Jan.

Kudo, Y., et al. 1983. "Study on the risk factors of eschemic heart disease in patients with chronic hemodialysis, with special reference to the role of plasma l-carnitine." *Nippon Jinzo Gakkai Shi.* 25:429–38.

Kuldau, J. M., et al. 1980. "Jejunoi-leal bypass: general and psychiatric outcome after one year." *Psychosomatics.* 21(7):534–39.

Kummerow, F. 1977. "The influence of egg consumption on the serum cholesterol level in human subjects." *Am. J. Clin. Nutr.* 30:664.

Kuthra, A. 1970. "The nutritional, clinical, and economic aspects of vegan diets." *Pl. Fds. Hum. Nutr.* 2:13.

Lacour, B., et al. 1980. "Carnitine improves lipid anomalies in haemodialysis patients." *Lancet.* 2:763–65.

Lala, V. R., and Reddy, V. 1970. "Absorption of B-carotene from green leafy vegetables in undernourished children." *Am. J. Clin. Nutr.* 23:110–13.

Lampman, R. M., et al. 1980. "Type IV hyperlipoproteinemia: effects of a caloric restricted type IV diet versus physical training plus isocaloric type IV diet." *Am. J. Clin. Nutr.* 33:1233–43.

Lantigua, R. A., et al. 1980. "Cardiac arrhythmias associated with a liquid protein diet for the treatment of obesity." *N. Eng. J. Med.* 303:735–38.

Lantigua, R. A., et al. 1980. "Cardiac arrhythmias associated with a liquid protein diet for the treatment of obesity." *N. Eng. J. Med.* 303: 735–38.

Lategola, M. T., et. al. 1980. "Effects of ozone on symptoms and cardiopulmonary function in a flight attendant surrogate population." *Aviat. Space Environ. Med.* 51:237–46.

Lawlor, T., et al. 1969. "Metabolic hazards of fasting." *Am. J. Clin. Nutr.* 22:1142–49.

Lee, C., et al. 1971. "Nitrogen retention of young men fed rice with or without supplementary chicken." *Am. J. Clin. Nutr.* 24:318–23.

Leeper, R. C., et al. 1973. "Study of control force limits for female pilots." FAA No. AD777839.

Leibovitz, B. E. 1984. *Carnitine: The Vitamin Bt Phenomenon.* New York: Dell.

Lemon, P. 1981. "Effects of exercise on protein and amino acid metabolism." *Med. Sci. Sports Exerc.* 13:141.

Lennon, D. L., et al. 1983. "Effects of acute moderate-intensity exercise on carnitine metabolism in men and women." *J. Appl. Physiol.* 55:489–95.

Leto, S., et al. 1976. "Dietary protein, life-span, and physiological variables in female mice." *J. Geront.* 31:149–54.

Levine, L, et al. 1983. "Fructose and glucose ingestion and muscle glycogen use during submaximal exercise." *J. Appl. Physiol.* 55(6):1767–71.

Lewis, M. F., and Ferraro, D. P. 1973. "Flying high: the aeromedical aspects of marihuana." FAA No. AD775889.

Liedtke, A. J., and Nellis, S. H. 1979. "Effects of carnitine in ischemic and fatty acid supplemented swine hearts." *J. Clin. Invest.* 64:440–47.

Liedtke, A. J., et al. 1981. "Effects of carnitine isomers on fatty acid metabolism in ischemic swine hearts." *Circ. Res.* 48:859–66.

Linkswiler, H. M., et al. 1974. "Calcium retention of young adult males as affected by level of protein and of calcium intake." *Trans. N.Y. Acad. Sci.*, ser 2. 30:333–40.

Lopez, de Romana, G. 1980. "Utilization of the protein and energy of the white potato by human infants." *J. Nutr.* 110:1849.

———. "Fasting and postprandial plasma free amino acids of infants and children consuming exclusive potato protein." *J. Nutr.* 111:1766.

Lui, N. S. T., and Roels, O. A. 1980. "The vitamins: A. Vitamin A and carotene." In *Modern Nutrition in Health and Disease*, 6th ed., R. S. Goodhart and M. E. Shils, eds. Philadelphia: Lea & Febiger. P. 156.

Luyken, R., et al. 1964. "Nutrition studies in New Guinea." *Am. J. Clin. Nutr.* 14:13–27.

Maccari, F., and Ramacci, M. T. 1981. "Antagonism of doxorubicin cardiotoxicity by carnitine is specific of the l-diasteroisomer." *Biomedicine.* 35:65–67.

Maccari, F., et al. 1982. "L-carnitine depletion from rat tissues after treatment with d-carnitine." Abstract. 21st Congresso della Societa Italiana di Farmacologia.

Maebashi, M., et al. 1976. "Urinary excretion of carnitine in man." *J. Lab. Clin. Med.* 87:760–66.

Maebashi, M., et al. 1978. "Lipid-lowering effect of carnitine in patients with type-IV hyperlipoproteinemia." *Lancet.* 2:805–7.

Mahalko, J. R., et al. 1983. "Effect of a moderate increase in dietary protein on the retention and excretion of Ca, Cu, Fe, Mg, P, and Zn by adult males." *Ann. J. Clin. Nutr.* 37:8–14.

Margen, S. 1974. "Studies in calcium metabolism, the calciuretic effect of dietary protein." *Am. J. Clin. Nutr.* 27:584.

Marquis, N. R., and Fritz, I. B. 1964. "Enzymological determination of free carnitine concentrations in rat tissues." *J. Lipid Res.* 5:184–87.

Mattson, F. 1972. "Effects of dietary cholesterol on serum cholesterol in man." *Am. J. Clin. Nutr.* 25:589.

Mayhowk, J. C. 1981. "Prediction of body density, fat, weight, and lean body mass." *J. Sports Med.* 21(4):385.

Mazess, R. 1974. "Bone mineral content of North Alaskan Eskimos." *Am. J. Clin. Nutr.* 27:916.

McGarry, J. D., and Foster, D. W. 1973. "Acute reversal of experimental diabetic ketoacidosis in the rat with (+)-decanoylcarnitine." *J. Clin. Invest.* 52:877–44.

———. 1976. "An improved and simplified radioisotopic assay for the determination of free and esterified carnitine. *J. Lipid Res.* 17:277–81.

———. 1980. "Regulation of hepatic fatty acid oxidation and ketone body production." *Ann. Rev. Biochem.* 49:395–420.

McKean, C. M. 1970. Growth of phenylketonuric children on chemically defined diets." *Lancet.* 1:148.

Mclaren, D. 1966. "A fresh look at protein-calorie malnutrition." *Lancet.* 2:485.

Med. Trib. 1979. "Somach-stapling corrects obesity and preserves digestive tissue." 20(Oct. 10).

Med. World News. 1978. "Stapling creates mini-stomach for obese patients." 19(Oct. 16):17–18.

Melton, C. E. 1980. "Effects of long-term exposure to low levels of ozone: a review." FAA No. ADA094426/4.

Melton, C. E., et al. 1973. "Physiological, biochemical, and psychological responses in air traffic control personnel: comparison of the 5-day and 2-2-1 shift rotation patterns. FAA No. AD778214.

Melton, C. E., et al. 1978. "Stress in air traffic controllers: a restudy of 32 controllers 5 to 9 years later." FAA No. ADA065767/6GA.

Melton, C. E., Jr., et al. 1974. "Comparison of Opa Locka Tower with other ATC facilities by means of a biochemical stress index." FAA No. ADA008378.

Metzner, H. L., et al. 1977. "The relationship between frequency of eating and adiposity in adult men and women in the Tecumseh Community Health Study." *Am. J. Clin. Nutr.* 30:712–715.

Michiel, R. R., et al. 1978. "Sudden death in a patient on a liquid protein diet." *N. Eng. J. Med.* 298:1005–7.

Miller, J. D. B., et al. 1977. "Effect of deep surgical sepsis on protein-sparing therapies and nitrogen balance." *Am. J. Clin. Nutr.* 30:1528–32.

Mingardi, G., et al. 1980. "Carnitine balance in hemodialyzed patients." *Clin. Nephrol.* 13:269–70.

Mitchell, M. E. 1978a. "Carnitine metabolism in human subjects. I. Normal metabolism." *Am. J. Clin. Nutr.* 31:293–306.

———. 1978b. "Carnitine metabolism in human subjects. II. Values of carnitine in biological fluids and tissues of 'normal' subjects." *Am. J. Clin. Nutr.* 31:481–91.

———. 1978c. "Carnitine metabolism in human subjects. III. Metabolism in disease." *Am. J. Clin. Nutr.* 31:645–59.

Mohler, S. R. 1965. "Fatigue in aviation activities." FAA No. AD620022.

———. 1966. "Oxygen in general aviation." FAA No. AD645497.

Mohler, S. R., et al. 1968. "Circadian rhythms and the effects of long-distance flights." FAA No. AD672898.

Molstad, P. 1980. "The efflux of l-carnitine from cells in culture (CCL 27)." *Biochim. Biophys. Acta.* 597:166–73.

Molstad, P., et al. 1977. "Specificity and characteristics of carnitine transport in human heart cells (CCL 27) in culture." *Biochim. Biophys. Acta.* 471:296–304.

Moore, C. V. 1973. "Iron." In *Modern Nutrition in Health and* Disease, R. S. Goodhart and M. E. Shills, eds. Philadelphia: Lea & Febiger. Pp. 301–4.

Moorthy, A. V., et al. 1983. "A comparison of plasma and muscle carnitine levels in patients on peritoneal or hemodialysis for chronic renal failure." *Am. J. Nephrol.* 3:205–8.

Morcos, S. R., et al. 1981. "Protein-rich food mixtures for feeding the young in Egypt." *Z. Ernährungswiss.* 20:275–82.

Morris, E. R., et al. 1980. "Trace element nutriture response of adult men consuming dephytinized wheat bran." In *Trace Substances in Environmental Health-XIV.* Columbia: Univ. of Missouri Press. Pp. 103–9.

Nagle, F. J., et al. 1963. "The mitigation of physical fatigue with Spartase." FAA No. AD429001.

Nakamura, R., et al. 1973. "A new enzymatic assay for human deficiencies of coenzyme Q-10, " *Int. J. Vit. Nutr. Res.* 43:526–36.

Nash, D. T., et al. 1979. "Progression of coronary atherosclerosis and dietary hyperlipidemia." *Circulation.* 56:363–65.

National Research Council, Committee on Diet, Nutrition, and Cancer. 1982. *Diet, Nutrition and Cancer.* Washington, D.C.: Nat. Acad. Sci. Pp. 1-5, 5-20, 5-21.

National Research Council, Food and Nutrition Board, Committee on Dietary Allowances. 1974. *Recommended Dietary Allowances,* 8th rev. ed. Washington, D.C.: Nat. Acad. Sci.

———. on 1980. *Recommended Dietary Allowances,* 9th rev. ed. Washington, D.C.: Nat. Acad. Sci.

Neely, J. R., and Morgan, H. E. 1974. "Relationship between carbohydrate and lipid metabolism and the energy balance of heart muscle." *Ann. Rev. Physiol.* 36:413–59.

Nelson, R. A. 1974. In "Are we eating too much protein?" *Med. World News.* Nov. 8, p. 106.

Novak, M., et al. 1981a. "The effects of l-carnitine supplementation of soy bean formula on plasma lipids." Abstract. *Clin. Res.* 29:877A.

———. 1981b. "Carnitine in the perinatal metabolism of lipids. I. Relationship between maternal and fetal plasma levels of carnitine and acylcarnitines." *Pediatrics* 67:95–100.

Nutr. Rev. 1974. "Current status of jejuno-ileal bypass for obesity." 32(11):33–38.

Nutr. Rev. 1975. "Obesity, jejuno-ileal bypass and death." 33(2):38–40.

Nutr. Rev. 1978. "The nature of weight loss during short term dieting." 36(3):72–74.

Nutr. Rev. 1980. "Urinary calculi and dietary protein." 38:9–10.

"Nutrition." 1976. *Metabolism* 25(11):1287–1302.

"Obesity in children: environment or genes?" 1977. *JAMA.* 238:2009.

O'Brien, B. 1980. "Human plasma lipid response to red meat, poultry, fish and eggs." *Am. J. Clin. Nutr.* 33:2573.

O'Connor, W. F., and Pendergrass, G. E. 1966. "Effects of decompression on operator performance." FAA No. AD675774.

Ohtani, Y., et al. 1982. "Carnitine deficiency and hyperammonemia associated with valproic acid therapy." *J. Pediatr.* 101:782–85.

Opie, L. H. 1979. "Role of carnitine in fatty acid metabolism of normal and ischemic myocardium." *Am. Heart J.* 97:375–88.

Osborne, T. B., and Mendel, L. B. 1914. "Amino-acids in nutrition and growth." *J. Biol. Chem.* 17:325–49.

Oski, F. A. 1969. "Red cell 2,3-DPG levels in subjects with chronic hypoxemia." *N. Eng. J. Med.* 280:1165–66.

———. 1971. "The vitro restoration of red cell 2,3-DPG levels in banked blood." *Blood.* 37:52–56.

Pande, S. V., and Parvin, R. 1976. "Characterization of carnitine acylcarnitine translocase system of heart mitochondria." *J. Biol. Chem.* 251:6683–91.

Parfitt, M. D., et al. 1978. "Metabolic bone disease after intestinal bypass for treatment of obesity." *Ann. Intern. Med.* 2:193.

Parish, W. 1960. "Hypersensitivity to milk and sudden death in infancy." *Lancet*. 2:1106.
Patel, M. S. 1977. "Age-dependent changes in the oxidative metabolism in rat brain." *J. Gerontol*. 32:643–46.
Paulson, D. L., and Shug, A. L. 1981. "Tissue specific depletion of l-carnitine in rat heart and skeletal muscle by d-carnitine." *Life Sci*. 28:2931–38.
Pease, C. N. 1962. "Focal retardation and arrestment of growth of bones due to vitamin A intoxication." *JAMA*. 182:980–85.
Pecora, L. J., and Hundley, J. M. 1951. "Nutritional improvement of white polished rice by the addition of lysine and threonine." *J. Nutr*. 44:101–12.
Pediatric Ann. 1978. "Obesity in childhood." June.
Pellett, P. 1980. "Nutritional evaluation of protein foods." *Food and Nutrition Bulletin*, supp. 4. United Nations Univ. Press. Pp. 1–6.
Penn, D., et al. 1981. "Decreased tissue carnitine concentrations in newborn infants receiving total parenteral nutrition." *J. Pediatr*. 98:976–78.
Penn, D., et al. 1982. "Possible carnitine deficiency in parenterally alimented newborn infants." *Acta Pediatr. Scand. Supp*. 296:113–14.
Pennington, J. A. T. 1976. *Dietary Nutrient Guide*. Westport, Conn.: AVI.
Pi-Sunyer, F. X. 1976. "Jejunal bypass surgery for obesity." *Am. J. Clin. Nutr*. 29:409–16.
Pipes, T. V. 1974. "Body composition characteristics of male and female track and field athletes." *Research Quarterly*. 14(2):144.
Pola, P., et al. 1980. "Carnitine in the therapy of dyslipidemic patients." *Curr. Ther. Res*. 27:208–16.
Prasad, J. S. 1980. "Effect of vitamin E supplementation on leukocyte function." *Am. J. Clin. Nutr*. 33:606–8.
Proceedings of the Nutrition Society. 1983. 42:473–87.
Rabinowitz, D. 1970. "Some endocrine and metabolic aspects of obesity." *Ann. Rev. Med*. 21:241–58.
Rebouche, C. J. 1982. "Sites and regulation of carnitine biosynthesis in mammals." *Fed. Proc. Fed. Am. Soc. Exp. Biol*. 41:2848–52.
———. 1983. "Effect of dietary carnitine isomers and y-butyrobetaine on l-carnitine biosynthesis and metabolism in the rat." *J. Nutr*. 113:1906–13.
Rebouche, C. J., and Engel, A. G. 1981. "Primary systemic carnitine deficiency. I. Carnitine biosynthesis." *Neurology* (N.Y.). 31:813–18.
———. 1983. "Carnitine metabolism and deficiency syndromes." *Mayo Clin. Proc*. 58:533–40.
Rebouche, C. J., and Mack, D. L. 1983. "Na+-gradient-stimulated transport of l-carnitine by rat renal brush border membranes." Abstract. *Fed. Proc. Fed. Am. Soc. Exp. Biol*. 42:1053.
Reddy, V. 1971. "Lysine supplementation of wheat and nitrogen retention in children." *Am. J. Clin. Nutr*. 24:1246–49.
Renaud, S., et al. 1982. "Comparative beneficial effects on platelet functions and atherosclerosis of dietary linolenic and gamma-linolenic acids in the rabbit." *Atherosclerosis*. 45:43–51.
Reynolds, H. M., and Allgood, M. A. 1975. "Functional strength of commercial-airline stewardesses." FAA. No. ADA021836/2GI.
Richardson, D. P., et al. 1979. "Quantitative effect of an isoenergetic exchange of fat for carbohydrate in dietary protein utilization in healthy young men." *Am. J. Clin. Nutr*. 32:2217–26.
Rickman, F., et al. 1974. "Changes in serum cholesterol during the Stillman diet." *JAMA*, 228:54–58.
Riopelle, A. M., and Shell, W. F. 1978. "Protein deprivation in primates. XI. Determinants of weight change during and after pregnancy." *Am. J. Clin. Nutr*. 31:394–400.
Rizek, R. L., and Jackson, E. M. 1980. *Current Food Consumption Practices and Nutrient*

Sources in the American Diet. Hyattsville, Md.: USDA.

Roberts, S. 1981. "Does egg feeding (i.e. dietary cholesterol) affect plasma cholesterol levels in humans? The results of a double-blind study." *Am. J. Clin. Nutr.* 34:2092.

Robertson, W. G., et al. 1979. "Should recurrent calcium oxalate stone formers become vegetarians?" *Br. J. Urol.* 51:427–31.

Rodgers, S. 1977. "Jaw wiring in the treatment of obesity." *Lancet.* 2:1221–22.

Rodin, J. 1978. "The puzzle of obesity." *Human Nature.* Feb. pp. 38–47.

———. 1984. "Taming the hunger hormone." *American Health.* Jan.-Feb.

Roe, C. R., and Bohan, T. P. 1982. "L-carnitine therapy in propionicacidaemia." *Lancet.* 1:1411–12.

Rose, W. 1955. "The amino acid requirements of man. XIII. The sparing effect of cystine in methionine requirement." *J. Biol. Chem.* 216:763.

———. 1955. "The amino acid requirements of man. XIV. The sparing effect of tyrosine on phenylalanine requirement." *J. Biol. Chem.* 217:95.

Rose, W. C. 1957. "The amino acid requirements of adult man." *Nutr. Abstr. Rev.* 27:631–47.

Rosenberg, H. R., et al. 1959. "Lysine and threonine supplementation of rice." *J. Nutr.* 69:217–28.

Ross, M. 1979. "Cardiovascular complications during prolonged starvation." *West. J. Med.* 130(2):170–77.

Ross, M. 1959. "Protein, calories and life expectancy." *Fed. Proc.* 18:1190–1207.

Rossi, C. S., and Siliprandi, N. 1982. "Effect of carnitine on serum HDL-cholesterol: report of two cases." *Johns Hopkins Med. J.* 150:51–54.

Rudman, D., et al. 1977. "Deficiency of carnitine in cachectic cirrhotic patients." *J. Clin. Invest.* 60:716–23.

Rudman, D., et al. 1980. "Carnitine deficiency in cirrhosis." In R. A. Frenkel and J. D. McGarry, eds. *Carnitine Biosynthesis, Metabolism and Functions*. New York: Academic Press. Pp. 307–19.

Sacca, J. 1971. "Acute ischemic colitis due to milk allergy." *Ann. Allergy.* 29:268.

Sacks, J., et al. 1937. "Carbohydrate and phosphorus changes in prolonged muscular contractions." *Am. J. Physiol.* 118:232–40.

Sanders, T. 1978. "Studies of vegans: the fatty acid composition of plasma choline phosphogylcerides, erythrocytes, adipose tissue and breast milk, and some indicators of susceptibility to ischemic heart disease in vegans and omnivore controls." *Am. J. Clin. Nutr.* 31:805.

Schaper, W., et al. 1981. "Protective action of l,carnitine compared with d,carnitine on infarct size area in mongrel dogs." Abstract. *J. Molec. Cell. Cardiol.* 13 (suppl. 1):83.

Schmidt-Sommerfeld, E., et al. 1978. "Carnitine and development of newborn adipose tissue." *Pediatr. Res.* 12:660–64.

Schmidt-Sommerfeld, E., et al. 1982. "Carnitine blood concentrations and fat utilization in parenterally alimented premature newborn infants." *J. Pediatr.* 100:260–64.

Schuette, S. A., et al. 1980. "Studies on the mechanism of protein-induced hypercalciuria in older men and women." *J. Nutr.* 110:305–15.

Schwartz, R. S., et al. 1978. "Increased adipose-tissue lipoproteinlipase activity in moderately obese men after weight reduction." *Lancet.* 1:1230–31.

Seccombe, D. W., et al. 1982. "L-carnitine for methylmalonicaciduria." *Lancet.* 2:1401.

Sedar, A. W., et al. 1978. "Fatty acids and the initial events of endothelial damage seen by scanning and transmission electron microscopy." *Atherosclerosis* 30:273–84.

Seelig, M. S. 1970. "Are American children still getting an excess of vitamin D? Hyperreactive children at risk." *Clin. Pediatr.* 9:380–83.

Seipel, J. H., and Wentz, A. E. 1964. "Unsuspected neurologic disease in aviation personnel: survival following seizures in flight." FAA No. AD453580.

Shagrin, J. W., et al. 1971. "Polyarthritis in obese patients with intestinal bypass." *Ann. Intern. Med.* 75:377–80.

Shaw, R. D., et al. 1983. "Carnitine transport in rat small intestine." *Am. J. Physiol.* 245:G376–81.

Shekelle, R. B., et al. 1981. "Dietary vitamin A and risk of cancer in the Western Electric Study." *Lancet.* 2:1186–90.

Sherr, H. P., et al. 1974. "Bile acid metabolism and hepatic disease following small bowel surgery for obesity." *Am. J. Clin. Nutr.* 27:1369–79.

Shlosberg, A., and Egyed, M. N. 1983. "Examples of poisonous plants in Israel of importance to animals and man. *Arch. Toxicol.* 6:194–96.

Shug, A. L., et al. 1982. "The distribution and role of carnitine in the mammalian brain." *Life Sci.* 31:2869–74.

Siegel, P. V., et al. 1969. "Time-zone effects on the long-distance air traveler." FAA No. AD702443.

Siliprandi, D., et al. 1973. "Restoration of some energy linked processes lost during the ageing of rat liver mitochondria." *Biochem. Biophys. Res. Commun.* 55:563–67.

Simpson, K. M., et al. 1981. "The inhibitory effect of bran on iron absorption in man." *Am. J. Clin. Nutr.* 34:1469–78.

Sinclair, H. M. 1980. "Prevention of coronary heart disease: the role of essential fatty acids." *Postgrad. Med. J.* 56:579–84.

Sinnett, P. R., and Whyte, H. M. "Epidemiological studies in a highland population of New Guinea: environment, culture, and health status." *Human Ecol.* 1:245–77.

Sirkis, J. A. 1972. "The benefits of the use of shoulder harness in general aviation aircraft." FAA No. AD739943.

Slonim, A. E., et al. 1981. "Dietary-dependent carnitine deficiency as a cause of nonketotic hypoglycemia in an infant." *J. Pediatr.* 99:551–56.

Smith, P. W. 1962. "Toxic hazards in aerial application." FAA No. AD421158.

Smith, R. 1966. "Epidemiologic studies of osteoporosis in women of Puerto Rico and south-eastern Michigan with special reference to age, race, national origin, and to other related and associated findings." *Clin. Orthop.* 45:31.

Smith, R. C. 1974. "A realistic view of the people in air traffic control." FAA No. ADA006789.

Snow, C. C., et al. 1975. "Anthropometry of airline stewardesses." FAA No. ADA012965.

Snow, C. C., et al. 1970. "Survival in emergency escape from passenger aircraft." FAA No. AD735388.

Synder, A., et al. 1983. "Maltodextrin feeding immediately before prolonged cycling at 62% VO$_2$ Max increases time to exhaustion." *Med. Sci. Sports Exercise* 15:126.

Snyder, R. G. 1963. "Human survivability of extreme impacts in free-fall." FAA No. AD425412.

Soltesz, G., et al. 1983. "The relationship between carnitine and ketone body levels in diabetic children." *Acta Paediatr. Scand.* 72(4):511–15.

Soufir, J. C., et al. 1981. "Free l-carnitine in human seminal plasma." *Int. J. Androl.* 4:388–97.

Southgate, D. A. T., et al. 1976. "A guide to calculating intakes of dietary fibre." *J. Human Nutr.* 30:303–13.

Sproles, C., et al. 1976. "Circulatory responses to submaximal exercise after dehydration and rehydration." *J. Sports Med.* 16(2):101.

Srivastava, K. C. 1980. "Effects of dietary fatty acids, prostaglandins and related compounds on the role of platelets in thrombosis." *Biochem. Exp. Biol.* 16:317–38.

Stamler, J. 1978. "Lifestyles, major risk factors, proof and public policy." *Circulation* 58:3–19.

Steiguer, de D., et al. 1978. "Aircrew and passenger protective breathing equipment studies." FAA No. ADA051002/4GI.

Stein, M. R., et al. 1976. "Ineffectiveness of human chorionic gonadotropin in weight reduction: a double blind study." *Am. J. Clin. Nutr.* 29:940–48.

Storey, R., et al. 1982. *Popular Diets: How They Rate.* Los Angeles District, California Dietetic Assn.

Stunkard, A. J. 1977. "Obesity and the social environment: current status, future prospects."

New York Academy of Science. *Food and Nutrition in Health and Disease*. 300:298–320.

Sumner, E. 1938. "The biological value of milk and egg protein in human subjects." *J. Nutr.* 16:141.

Suzuki, Y., et al. 1981. "Effects of l-carnitine on tissue levels of acyl carnitine, acyl coenzyme A and high energy phosphate in ischemic dog hearts." *Jpn. Cir. J.* 45:687–94.

Takahashi. 1966. "Effect of inosine on white blood cells of radioactivity exposed mice." Lecture at the regular meeting of plastic surgery, Tokyo Jikeikai University Medical School, June.

Tanphaichitr, V., et al. 1980. "Carnitine status in Thai adults." *Am. J. Clin. Nutr.* 33:876–80.

Taube, L. 1978. *Food Allergy and the Allergic Patient.*, 2nd ed. Springfield, Ill.: Charles C. Thomas. P. 22.

Taylor, H. L., et al. 1955. "Maximal oxygen uptake as an objective measure of cardio-respiratory perfume." *J. Appl. Physiol.* 8:73–80.

Teasdale, C., et al. 1976. "Age dependence of T lymphocytes." *Lancet.* 1:1410–11.

Thackray, R. I., and Touchstone, R. M. 1969. "Recovery of motor performance following startle." FAA No. AD704472.

Thomsen, J. H., et al. 1979. "Improved pacing tolerance of the ischemic human myocardium after administration of carnitine." *Am. J. Cardiol.* 43:300–6.

Topping, D. C., et al. 1977. "Synthesis of macromolecules by intestinal cells incubated with ammonia." *Am. J. Physiol.* 233(4):E341–47.

"Toxic reactions of vitamin A." 1964. *Nutr. Rev.* 22:109–11.

Tripp, M. D., et al. 1981. "Systemic carnitine deficiency presenting as familial endocardial fibroelastosis." *N. Eng. J. Med.* 305:385–90.

Trowell, H. 1975. "Dietary changes in modern times." In *Refined Carbohydrate Foods and Disease*, D. P. Burkitt and H. C. Trowell, eds. London: Academic Press. P. 53.

Truelove, S. 1961. "Ulcerative colitis provoked by milk." *Br. Med. J.* 1:154.

Truswell, A. 1962. "The nutritive value of maize protein for man." *Am. J. Clin. Nutr.* 10:142.

Tsai, C., et al. 1978. "Study on the effect of megavitamin E supplementation in man." *Am. J. Clin. Nutr.* 31:831–37.

Tuttle, S. 1957. "Study of the essential amino acid requirements of men over fifty." *Metabolism.* 6:564.

U.S. Dept. of Agriculture. 1980. "Nationwide Food Consumption Survey. 1977–78." Preliminary Report No. 2.

U.S. Dept. of Health, Education, and Welfare. 1977. *HEW News*. Nov. 9.

U.S. Senate, Select Committee on Nutrition and Human Needs. 1977. "Dietary goals for the United States," 2nd ed. Washington, D.C.: GPO. P. 41.

"Urinary calcium and dietary protein." 1980. *Nutr. Rev.* 38:9.

Vacha, G. M., et al. 1983. "Favorable effects of l-carnitine treatment on hypertriglyceridemia in hemodialysis patients: decisive role of low levels of high-density lipoprotein-cholesterol." *Am. J. Clin. Nutr.* 38:532–41.

Valette, G., et al. 1984. "Hypocholesterolaemic effect of fenugreek seeds in dogs." *Atherosclerosis.* 50:105–11.

Valkner, K. J., and Bieber, L. L. 1982. "Short-chain acylcarnitines of human blood and urine." *Biochem. Med.* 28:197–203.

Van Hinsbergh, V. W., et al. 1978. "Effect of l-carnitine on the oxidation of leucine and valine by rat skeletal muscle." *Biochem. Med.* 20:115.

Van Itallie, T. B. 1980. "'Morbid'" obesity; a hazardous disorder that resists conservative treatment." *Am. J. Clin. Nutr.* 33:358–63.

Van Itallie, T. B., et al. 1977. "Current concepts in nutrition." *N. Eng. J. Med.* 297:1158–61.

Van Itallie, T. B., et al. 1979. "Appraisal of excess calories as a factor in the causation of disease." *Am. J. Clin. Nutr.* 32:2648–53.

Vary, T. C. and Neely, J. R. 1981. "Characterization of carnitine transport in isolated perfused rat hearts." Abstract. *Fed. Proc. Fed. Am. Soc. Exp. Biol.* 40:1588.

Vary, T. C., et al. 1981. "Control of energy metabolism of heart muscle." *Annu. Rev. Physiol.* 43:419–430.

Van Soest, P. M., and McQueen, R. W. 1973. "The chemistry and estimation of fibre." *Proc. Nutr. Soc.* 32:123.

Walker, A. 1965. "Osteoporosis and calcium deficiency." *Am. J. Clin. Nutr.* 16:327.

Walker, A. R. P., et al. 1948. "Studies in human mineral metabolism. I. The effect of bread rich in phytate phosphorus on the metabolism of certain mineral salts with special reference to calcium." *Biochem. J.* 42:452–62.

Walker, R. 1972. "Calcium retention in the adult human male as affected by protein intake." *J. Nutr.* (102)1297.

Watkins, D. M. 1977. "Aging, nutrition and the continuum of health care." New York Academy of Science. Food and Nutrition in Health and Disease. 300:290–97.

Watt, B. K., et al. 1963. "Composition of foods: raw, processed, prepared," rev. ed. USDA Agriculture Handbook No. 8.

Weisinger, J. R., et al. 1974. "The nephrotic syndrome: a complication of massive obesity." 81:440–47.

Welling, P. G., et al. 1979. "Pharmacokinetics of l-carnitine in man following intravenous infusion of dl-carnitine." *Int. J. Clin. Pharmacol. Biopharm.* 17:56–60.

Weltman, A., et al. 1980. "Caloric restriction and/or mild exercise effects on serum lipids and body composition." *Am. J. Clin. Nutr.* 33:1002–9.

Wentz, A. E. 1964. "Studies on aging in aviation personnel." FAA No. AD456652.

West, K. M., et al. 1966. "Glucose tolerance, nutrition, and diabetes in Uruguay, Venezuela, Malaya, and East Pakistan." *Diabetes.* 15:9–18.

Whitney, E., and Hamilton, E. M. 1979. *Nutrition: Concepts and Controversies.* West Publishing.

Williams, M. H. 1976. *Nutritional Aspects of Human Physical and Athletic Performance.* Springfield, Ill.: Charles C. Thomas. Pp. 44–75.

———. 1983. *Ergogenic Aids in Sport.* Champaign, Ill.: Human Kinetics Publishers. 2:35.

Wilson, P. D. 1973. "Enzyme changes in ageing mammals." *Gerontol.* 19:79–125.

Wilson, P. D., and Franks, L. M. 1975. "The effect of age on mitochondrial ultrastructure." *Gerontol.* 21:81-94.

Winitz, M., et al. 1970. "Studies in metabolic nutrition employing chemically defined diets. I. Extended feeding of normal human adult males." *Am. J. Clin. Nutr.* 23:525–45.

Wolf, G. *Recent research on carnitine, its relation to lipid metabolism.* Cambridge, Mass.: MIT Press. P. 61.

Worthley, L. I. G., et al. 1983. "Carnitine deficiency with hyperbilirubinemia, generalized skeletal muscle weakness and reactive hypoglycemia in a patient on long-term total parenteral nutrition: treatment with intravenous l-carnitine." *J. Parent. Ent. Nutr.* 7:1765–80.

Wotecki, C. E. 1982. "Uses and limits to the use of RDA for diet planning and food selection." Speech delivered to the Food and Nutrition Board, National Research Council, Washington, D.C., December 13.

Wretlind, A. 1982. "Standards for nutritional adequacy of the diet: European and WHO/FAO viewpoints." *Am. J. Clin. Nutr.* 36:366–75.

Wright, R. 1965. "A controlled therapeutic trial of various diets in ulcerative colitis." *Br. Med. J.* 2:138.

Wynder, E. L. 1977. "Nutritional carcinogenesis." New York Academy of Science. *Food and Nutrition in Health and Disease.* 300:360–78.

Yamamura, Y., and Folkers, K. 1980. *Biomedical and Clinical Aspects of Co-enzyme Q.* Vol. 2, I to Y. Amsterdam: Elsevier North-Holland Biomedical Press.

York, C. M., et al. 1983. "Cardiac carnitine deficiency and altered carnitine transport in cardiomyopathic hamsters." *Arch. Biochem. Biophys.* 221:526–33.

Young. J. B., et al. 1977. "Suppression of sympathetic nervous system during fasting." *Science* 196:1473–75.

Zaspel, B. J., et al. 1980. "Transport and metabolism of carnitine precursors in various organs of the rat." *Biochem. Biophys. Acta* 631:192–202.

INDEX

A

Aerobic exercise, 75
Aerobics Institute, 35
Aging, 20
and coenzyme Q_{10}, 32
and dietary proteins, 22, 23, 24
Airline food, 12. *See also* Frequent Flyer's Protection Program
Airline Pilot's Association (ALPA), 82, 86
Alcohol
consumption of, 77
use of, by pilots, 96–97
All-in-One Apple Pie, 64, 220
Amantadine, 117
American Airlines
exercise program, 98–99
special diets, 92–93, 98–99
American Diabetic Association, 19–20
American Dietetic Association, 22, 101, 103–104, 105
American Hospital Association's Patient's Bill of Rights, 111
American Medical Association, 42
American Thoracic Society, 86
Amino acids, 19. *See also* Proteins
Ammonia, in blood, 35
Amphetamine, 77, 78
Anemia, 125, 128–130
Anesthesia, protecting yourself against hazards of, 8, 112–113
Angina pectoris, 29, 32–33
Antacids, 129
Antibiotics, 117
Antioxidants, 136–137
Appetite suppressants, 77–78

Appetizers
composition of, 231
recipes, 162–166
Apple and Brown Rice Cereal, 49, 156
Apple recipes, 171, 179, 212–213, 218, 220–221
Applesauce, 50, 52, 54, 212–213
Arginine, 25, 26, 109
Arthritis, 125
Asiatic flu, 118
Aspartame, 42–43, 69
Asthma, cautions for patients with, in flying, 86, 97
Atherosclerosis, 20, 28, 29
Athletic performance, and L-carnitine, 31

B

Baked Barley, 56, 194–195
Baked Cannellini, 52, 79, 195
Baked Lentils, 59, 195–196
Banana Date Muffins, 53, 215
Banana Nut Loaf Cake, 49, 56, 221
Baruck, John, 15, 16
Beans, recipes using, 166, 169, 172, 196, 201
Bean Salad, 172
Beta carotene, 136
Beverages. *See* Drinks
Bio-Nutrionics, 106, 290, 304
Black Bean and Rice Casserole, 55, 196
Black Bean Soup, 53, 166
Blood chemistry
and determination of dietary needs, 43

332